Quinine's Predecessor

The Henry E. Sigerist Series
in the History of Medicine

Sponsored by The American Association for the History of Medicine
and The Johns Hopkins University Press

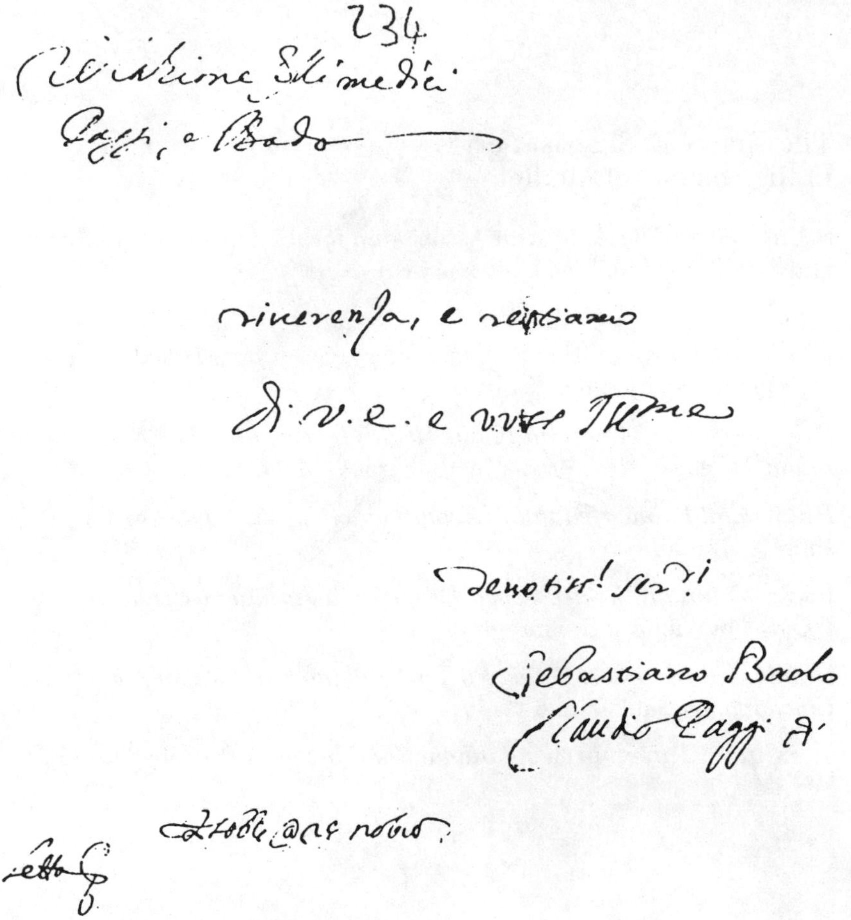
234

Relatione delli medici
Raggi, e Bado

riverenza, e restiamo
di V.E. e VV.SS. Ill.me

Devotiss.i Ser.ri
Sebastiano Bado
Claudio Raggi

Final lines of medicolegal report signed by Sebastiano Bado, Genoa, 1664. From Archivio di Stato, Genoa. Reprinted with permission.

Quinine's Predecessor

*Francesco Torti and
the Early History of Cinchona*

SAUL JARCHO, M.D.

The Johns Hopkins University Press

BALTIMORE AND LONDON

To Irma

This book has been brought to publication with the generous
assistance of the American Association for the History of Medicine

The Johns Hopkins University Press
2715 North Charles Street
Baltimore, Maryland 21218-4319
The Johns Hopkins Press Ltd., London

Library of Congress Cataloging-in-Publication Data

Jarcho, Saul.
    Quinine's predecessor : Francesco Torti and the early history of
cinchona / Saul Jarcho.
        p.   cm.—(The Henry E. Sigerist series in the history of
medicine)
    Includes bibliographical references and index.
    ISBN 0-8018-4466-5 (hc : alk. paper)
    1. Cinchona—History.   2. Malaria—Chemotherapy—History.   3.
Torti, Francesco, 1658–1741.   I. Torti, Francesco, 1658–1741.   II.
Title.   III. Series.
    [DNLM: 1. Torti, Francesco, 1658–1741.   2. Cinchona.   3.
Quinine—history.   QV 257 J365q]
RM666.C53J37   1993
616.9'362061—dc20
DNLM/DLC
for Library of Congress   92-49213
A catalog record for this book is available from the British Library.

We ought the more to give thanks to the providence of
the Almighty God, that, in so very great an obscurity, and
variety, of cases, it has favour'd us with a remedy, the
powers of which, in overcoming some dangerous fevers
at least, is prov'd by experience; though the method in
which it acts is somewhat obscure; I mean the Peruvian
bark.

Morgagni, *De Sedibus*
(Alexander's translation)

The following account . . . will, we hope, be not unacceptable to our readers. We could have made it much
larger, by adopting flying reports, and inserting unat-
tested facts; a close adherence to certainty has contracted
our narrative, and hindered it from swelling to that bulk,
at which modern histories generally arrive.

Samuel Johnson,
Life of Boerhaave

Contents

Illustrations

Preface and Acknowledgments

THE PURPOSE of this book is to relate, in ample detail, the early history of the Peruvian bark, also known as Jesuits' bark and later formally baptized cinchona. Because the term *cinchona* resulted from a famous misspelling made by Linnaeus in 1742, it will not appear often in the following pages.[1] The same is true of the word *quinine;* this drug was isolated in 1820, but its name is often used, carelessly and anachronistically, in discussions of earlier events and problems.

In 1932, Dr. C. H. La Wall, the eminent historian of pharmacy and pharmacology, wrote: "The history of quinine has never been recorded. It probably never can be completely written. . . . None of the later writers has ever taken the trouble to investigate the whole story."[2] In an extensive essay published in 1941 and oriented more toward botany than pharmacology, A. W. Haggis pointed out that the traditional history of cinchona is replete with error.

When these and other scholars were filling gaps in knowledge of cinchona, the entire field of medical historiography was being broadened, with the result that it is no longer acceptable or permissible for the medical historian to offer a mere catalog or chronicle of events. Scholars and serious readers demand that a historical presentation take into account the array of social, economic, political, religious, and other factors that can be shown to have influenced the developments that form the major theme of discussion. Ambitious programs undertaken on this principle multiply the difficulty of the research but augment the interest and value of the result. At the same time it must be admitted that even the most conscientious research coupled with endless fretful rumination may fail to reveal significant connections be-

tween individual techniques or technicalities and their economic or social bases.

The temporal limits of this history are somewhat imprecise at both
ends. It is improbable that we shall ever determine the exact date at
which the Peruvian bark first became known to a European; A.D. 1630
is a reasonable approximation. The work of Francesco Torti (1658–
1741) offers itself as an obvious terminus for the narrative, but the great
value and instructiveness of his achievement are made more accurately
appreciable if the closing date of this history is set beyond 1712, when
the first edition of Torti's *Therapeutice specialis* appeared. A yet later
date, 1738, permits us to include discussion of Torti's great contemporaries. In addition, it allows us to study in detail his second edition
(1730) and opens the gate for brief mention of the many posthumous
versions. Accordingly, the history proper ends after the death of Nic-
colò Cirillo (1734), whose *Consulti medici* did not appear until 1738. A
coda, which the reader will find in Appendix D, extends to late editions
and one translation of the *Therapeutice specialis*. These take the exposition into the nineteenth and twentieth centuries.

Since our subject exemplifies historical complexity at its fullest, the
investigation, in order not to engender a behemoth, has been limited
to the seventeenth and early eighteenth centuries. Preponderant attention is therefore given to the discovery of the Peruvian bark, its transmission to and within western Europe, the decades of contention
which ensued, and the incipient establishment of the drug as a canon-
ical part of medical practice. Special attention is often called to problems that remain to be solved and to approaches that appear promising.

Anyone who undertakes nowadays to write the history of the Peruvian bark must unfold the tale of the discovery of the drug by Europeans and its spread to Europe and then to other continents. The contributions, positive and negative, made by persons and by organizations,
both secular and clerical, must be included. The record of fevers, especially the intermittents, and the changed concepts embedded in
evolving pyretologic doctrine must be carefully examined. The medical, personal, historical, political, social, commercial, geographical,
and botanical factors that bear upon the main subject must constantly
be taken into account. This is not the work of a day or a year. Whether
the task has been performed correctly here, the reader shall judge.

The methods employed are those of standard historical investigation, applied to the diverse areas with which the subject makes contact.
Constant recourse to primary sources has been amplified and improved by discussion and correspondence with specialists in Europe,
Asia, and the Americas. I hope that my experience in clinical medicine,

pathology, and tropical medicine has adequately informed the exposition.

For readers without special knowledge of malaria, I take the liberty of explaining at this juncture a few of the concepts and technical terms used in this book.

Malaria is an infection caused by a microscopic animal known as a plasmodium, injected into man and other creatures by the bite of female mosquitoes of the genus *Anopheles* (this word means "not helpful"). Plasmodial diseases of birds are transmitted by nonanopheline mosquitoes. In the malarias of man a symptomless period of twelve to thirty days immediately after the mosquito bite is followed by attacks of chills and fever. Between attacks the patient usually feels well. In so-called tertian malaria, caused by *Plasmodium vivax*, the attacks occur on alternate days; the sickness is called tertian fever according to the ancient system, which included the first and third days of a cycle. In quartan malaria, caused by *Plasmodium malariae*, the attacks appear on the first, fourth, seventh, etc., days—every third day. The third important form of human malaria is the estivoautumnal (summer-autumn) variety, caused by *Plasmodium falciparum*, which produces pernicious malaria. It has irregular cycles and is the most deadly; it may attack any part of the body, including the brain. Much of the contribution made by Francesco Torti, eminent physician to the dukes of Modena, has to do with this form of malaria.

Since the fever in malaria is not present continuously, the disease was commonly called intermittent fever. This term, used by Torti, is now obsolete. Some authorities now consider even the newer terms—tertian, quartan, and estivoautumnal—to be obsolescent.

Malaria is not limited to the tropics. Even in recent times it has occurred in the temperate zones and has been reported from Arctic Russia. In the time of Torti much of Europe was heavily malarious. Nowadays the disease continues to be a major killer in many parts of the world.

In Algeria in 1880 Alphonse Laveran discovered malaria parasites in human blood. In 1897 Ronald Ross discovered the parasites in mosquitoes in India, and in 1898 he described the developmental cycle of malaria in birds. Similar cycles are now known to occur in human malaria.

One of the most effective drugs for the treatment of malaria is quinine, derived from the bark of cinchona, a South American tree, and first isolated in 1820. In the early seventeenth century Jesuits conveyed to Europe the earliest samples of the bark, which hence became known as Jesuits' bark and Peruvian bark. The name cinchona was invented by Linnaeus, the great Swedish botanist, in 1742.

The breadth and depth of work on this history have led to agreeable contact, usually productive, with persons, libraries, and institutions, both numerous and widely dispersed. I have therefore incurred greater debts than I can easily repay. An extensive list, regrettably and almost inevitably incomplete, appears below.

With respect to every person and each institution mentioned, I can scarcely do better than to repeat what Armand Trousseau wrote in the second edition of his *Clinique médicale de l'Hôtel-Dieu de Paris:* "Il m'en eût coûté beaucoup de ne pas leur témoigner publiquement ma vive gratitude."

In his preface to Dr. Peter Krivatsy's indispensable volume *A Catalogue of Seventeenth Century Printed Books in the National Library of Medicine* (Bethesda, 1989), the present director of that library has written, correctly, that "we hope and expect that it will serve as a contribution to the History of Medicine in particular and to 17th century scholarship in general."

About 1982–83 an unidentified bureaucrat in the office of the assistant secretary of Health Education and Welfare, perhaps in order to earn false credit for economical management, prevented the publication of Dr. Krivatsy's book, although the funds had been appropriated and disbursement had been approved. The resultant protracted delay impeded several parts of the research upon which this history is based. The guilty pathogen deserves public reproof for obstructing scholarship.

It is a pleasant obligation to thank the many persons, institutions, and agencies whose names are listed here. All have contributed information, advice, or other assistance toward the development of the research that is embodied in these pages.

My gratitude goes to the Johns Hopkins University Press, the library of the New York Academy of Medicine; the New York Public Library; the libraries of Columbia University, Yale University, Harvard University, the University of Pennsylvania, and Duke University; the Pius XII Memorial Library, St. Louis; The Boston Public Library; the library of the Wellcome Institute, London; the British Library; the National Library of Scotland; the Biblioteca Apostolica Vaticana, Vatican City; the archdiocese of Genoa; the Biblioteca Nazionale Centrale Vittorio Emanuele II, the Biblioteca della Pontificia Università Gregoriana, the Biblioteca della Università Urbaniana; the Biblioteca Comunale dell' Archiginnasio, Bologna; the Biblioteca Marciana, Venice; the Biblioteca Laurenziana, Florence; the Biblioteca Estense, Modena; the Biblioteca Civica, Genoa; the university libraries of Bologna, Milan, Genoa, and Mantua; the Public Record Office, London; the Bibliothèque Royale Albert 1er, Brussels; The Universiteits Bibliotheek KU, Louvain; the Koninklijke Bibliotheek, 's-Gravenhage; the Universiteits-Bibliotheek, Amsterdam; the Rijksuniversiteit Limburg, Maastricht; the Kongelige Bibliotek, Copenhagen; the Bibliothèque Nationale, Paris; the Austrian National Library, Vienna; the Biblioteca Nacional, Madrid; the Biblioteca de la Universidad Complutense, Madrid; the Biblioteca Nacional, Lisbon; the Biblioteca Nacional del Perú, Lima; Archivio di Stato (Bologna, Florence, Genoa, Lucca, and Modena); Stadsarchief, Antwerp; Archivio Storico degli Ospedali Civili, Genoa; Gemeentlijke Archiefdienst, Bergen op Zoom; Rijksarchief, Middelburg; Algemeen Rijksarchief te 's-Gravenhage; Servizio Affari Generale, Genoa; New York Botanical Garden; Missouri Botanical Gardens, St. Louis; Arnold Arboretum of Harvard University; Instituto de Botanica, São Paulo, Brazil; Dr. Jeanne L. Brand-Billings, North Bethesda, Maryland; Prof. J. J. McCusker, College Park, Maryland; Mrs. Dorothy Hanks, Washington; Prof. Donald R. Cooper, Columbus, Ohio; Mrs. Dorothy Claybourne, St. Louis; Mrs. Lothian Lynas, New York; Prof. Paul Potter, London, Ontario; Mr. C. Cartier, Québec; the late Dr. Leonard J. Bruce-Chwatt, London; Dr. William Bynum, London; Mr. N. H. Robinson, London; Mr. Leslie Morton, Pinner, Middlesex; Rev. Edmond Lamalle, Rome; Rev. Thomas A. Marshall, Washington; Abbé Francisque Bruel, Lyon; Rev. Paul Mech, Franchville-le-Bas; Rev. Cassiano Carpaneto da Langasco, Genoa; Rev. O. Van de Vyver, Heverlee, Belgium; Dr. J. van der Vin, Wassenaar; Prof. Dr. Ernst Braches, Amsterdam; Mr. J. J. Seegers, Amsterdam; Mr. W. I. Gnirrep, Amsterdam; Mr. G. G. A. M. Pynenborg, Nijmegen; Mr. J. Wassink, 's-Hertogenbosch; Dr. Denise Reyniers-Defourny, Antwerp; Dr. Eddy Stols, Louvain; Dr. C. Bruneel, Louvain; Prof. G. Despierres, Lyon; Mlle. J. Roubert, Lyon; Monsieur H. Hours, Lyon; Dr. Aldo Augusto, Genoa; Don Luigi Alfonso, Genoa; Dra. Laura Miani Belletti, Bologna; Dra. Isabella Zanni Rosiello, Bologna; Sra. Carmen Anton, Madrid; Dr. Angela Maria Pinho Souza Braga and Prof. Thereza Maria de Sa Carvalho, Salvador, Bahia, Brazil; Mr. Franklin Pease, Lima, Peru.

Dr. J. Worth Estes of Boston and Mrs. Jacqueline Wehmueller of Baltimore have reviewed the manuscript and made valued suggestions.

My secretary, Mrs. Françoise Duvivier Freyre, has converted multiply emended holograph into accurate typescript. My wife has been endlessly and brightly helpful and patient.

   The investigation was supported in part by the National Library of Medicine (LM-04505). This statement, required by regulations and honored by custom, is inadequate to express the full extent of my obligation to the library, its administrators, and its consultants.

Quinine's Predecessor

1 Two Rival Historical Traditions

DISCUSSIONS OF THE early history of cinchona have usually overlooked the fact that *two* traditions existed. Both are either overtly stated or less overtly traceable in the writings of the Genoese physician Sebastianus Baldus (fl. 1650–76), who, to the inconvenience of bibliographers and historians, changed his name to Sebastianus Badus.[1] Badus surmised that the two traditions might be in conflict; he says, referring to his sources, "Indeed, to be frank, I suspect that there is a certain contradiction between [the trader] Bollus and the pharmacist of the Roman College [Petrus Paulus Puccerini]."[2] It is appropriate to begin with the more romantic and famous tradition, that of the countess of Chinchon.

The Legend of the Countess

Badus states that he first heard of the Peruvian bark at Rome, from a Genoese priest named Federicus Conti, and subsequently resolved to test it in the large Genoese hospital that he headed.[3]

Badus states further that he learned the early history of the febrifugal drug from a letter written to him in Italian by Antonius Bollus,[4] a Genoese merchant who had traded with the Indians. According to Bollus, the tree that yielded the bark grew in Loxa, sixty leagues from Quito.[5] Its therapeutic properties were long known to the Indians, who kept the information secret. This opinion was destroyed with the utmost of Gallic acuity and charm by Trousseau and Pidoux, who wrote, "That an entire people should know something and that all of them should hide it for a century and a half through hatred of men whose

religion they had accepted—this is one of those ideas that are repug-
nant to common sense."[6]

Despite Indian secrecy, Bollus believed, the Spaniards ultimately
became suspicious. The drug then began to become known, but Europeans used it rarely.

Badus goes on to say that in the city of Lima, about thirty or forty
years before he wrote his book (i.e., in 1623 or 1633), the countess of
Chinchon, wife of the viceroy, fell ill of a severe tertian fever. An official
of Loxa (the *corregidor*) informed the viceroy of the virtues of the bark
and was summoned immediately to Lima. As to this part of the narrative, Hipólito Ruiz López (1754–1816),[7] a noted botanist, made the important but undocumented statement that the viceroy had the drug
tested in hospitals, presumably those of Lima. After discussion, the
bark was administered to the countess, who promptly recovered. The
happy woman thereupon procured a large amount of the wonderful
medicine, which was distributed to the fevered populace. Excellent results were again obtained. The drug became known as *pulvis comitis-
sae*, the powder of the countess.

After the lady returned to Spain, many trials of the bark made in
that country proved successful. In 1649 the drug was brought to Italy,
where it was tested under the auspices of Juan Cardinal de Lugo, a
famed Jesuit theologian.

Such is the story given by Badus. With numerous variations the tale
continued to be repeated, even as recently as 1931 and 1987. By the
late nineteenth century it had been popularized by the noted geographer, Sir Clements Markham. Somewhat earlier, Alexander von
Humboldt had expressed well-founded skepticism.[8]

The unraveling and almost complete rejection of the story are due
chiefly to the research of Joseph Rompel, S.J., Rubén Vargas Ugarte,
S.J., and Dr. A. W. Haggis and the careful supplementary studies of Dr.
Jaime Jaramillo Arango.[9] With the help of their findings we may now
consider several of the errors in the tradition.

As has been stated above, the account given by Badus is based on a
letter by Antonius Bollus. This letter is reported by no one other than
Badus; its whereabouts are unknown, and not a single supportive da-
tum has been discovered about Bollus. More significant, the story of
the countess is not mentioned by two highly regarded and well-
informed observers who lived in Peru at the time, Bernabé Cobo, S.J.
(1580–1657), and the Augustinian priest Antonio de Calancha (1584–
1654).[10]

Haggis points out that Ana de Osorio, Countess of Chinchon, died
in 1625, three years before her husband was appointed viceroy on Feb-

ruary 18, 1628.[11] Early in the month of his accession the count married Francisca Henriquez de Ribera. In January 1629 he made his entry into Lima as viceroy; his wife arrived there on April 19. An extremely detailed official diary written by a secretary, Juan Antonio Suardo, covers the period from May 15, 1629, to May 30, 1639.[12] It presents not an iota of evidence that the second countess had fever, but it records many attacks suffered by the count. The lady is reported as having had sore throat once and diarrhea on one occasion, but there is no statement that she ever had a fever.

On her return journey to Spain, the countess died of an epidemic disease and was buried in Cartagena (now part of Colombia) on January 14, 1641. The count arrived in Cadiz on June 10, 1641. Badus cites a letter by "Villerobel" [Villarroel] stating that in 1639 Dr. Michael de Barreda, a professor at Alcalà de Henares, was cured of fever by means of the bark.[13] This could not have been bark brought by the count of Chinchon, who had not yet reached Spain.

Another part of the tradition concerns Juan de Vega,[14] physician to the count of Chinchon and professor of medicine in Lima. As late as the time of Condamine (1740), it was stated that de Vega conveyed a large amount of the bark to Spain and sold it at 100 *reales* a pound.[15] Haggis has shown that de Vega never returned to Spain but remained at Lima as professor of medicine; his statement is based on a series of official documents signed by de Vega in Lima after departure of the viceroy and continuing at least as late as 1650.[16] Contradicting evidence appears in the second edition of the *Opera medica* of Petrus Michaelis de Heredia (Pedro Miguel de Heredia), which says that de Vega tested the drug in "India" [Peru] and Seville.[17] In this conflict of statements the historian is inclined to give greater weight to the series of contemporary evidences adduced by Haggis than to the evidence of Miguel de Heredia, which was at least thirty years old, yet (as will be shown) several witnesses confirm that de Vega returned to Seville. Hence this difficulty remains unresolved, unless we assume that Haggis misread the original documents or that the signatures in them were written by an amanuensis.

Another physician, Gaspar Caldera de Heredia (1591–ca. 1669), a Portuguese who practiced in Seville, refers to the drug in 1663 as the febrifugal powder of the province of Quito, western Indies, known in Rome as the powder of the most eminent Cardinal de Lugo and in Spain as that of Juan de Vega. A letter from Hieronymus Bardus, written in Rome in 1661, is included in Caldera de Heredia's book; it states that de Vega had used the bark with wonderful results (*cum admirabilibus effectibus*) in the treatment of quartans, tertians, and chronic fevers. This statement does not reveal whether de Vega had used the drug in Peru or Spain, or both, and it certainly does not support Condamine's accusation that he sold it (1740, 234).[18]

The weight of all obtainable evidence is more than enough to delete the story of the countess from the historical record. At the same time we must note a minor epiphytic tradition found in Ecuadorian writings. Dr. Hermilio Valdizan, a scholar of note, while repeating the romantic narrative, states concisely that a Jesuit priest, whose name he does not mention, conveyed the powdered bark to Lima. He adds that "in 1630 an Indian of Loja named Pedro Leyva had already made known the powders of *quina* and their febrifugal properties to the corregidor, Don Juan Lopez Cañizares, and it appears also that the qualities of the said powders were already known to Jesuit priests established in the city of Quito." [19] Most unfortunately Valdizan offers not a milligram of documentation for these important statements. This omission is in sharp contrast with the abundant documentation that he provides elsewhere in his extensive essay.

The story of Leyva or Leiva reappears in a book by Gualberto Arcos, who adds that the Jesuit was named Juan Lopez; Arcos provides no supplementary documentation. Additional repetitions, meticulously undocumented, appear in the writings of Virgilio Paredes Borja.[20]

The Iberian Tradition

Although the famous legend of the countess is recorded in Badus's *Anastasis,* evidence of a rival tradition is traceable in the selfsame book. Badus took care to include, in the introductory pages of his treatise, a section titled "Recensio eorum, qui scripsere de cortice (A review of those who have written about the bark)." His rapid summary of fifteen authors includes two Iberians whose writings are poorly represented in North American libraries and who have received adequate consideration only in an essay by Francisco Guerra, yet the historical analyst may blunder grievously if he neglects them. And, indeed, Badus did not fully recognize their value.[21]

The first of these is Gaspar Caldera de Heredia, already mentioned. His book[22] was published in Antwerp in 1663 and hence is contemporaneous with Badus's *Anastasis.* He says that in the remotest part of the province of Quito the Indians who go to the mines must cross a river. In passing from one shore to another they are immersed up to the neck and complain bitterly of cold and shivering. To alleviate the *rigor et frigor* they take the pulverized bark of a certain tree, dissolved in hot water. This brings prompt relief. Jesuit priests, observing the success of the procedure, requested samples of the bark and were given it freely.

Then, *applying an argument based on similarity*, they began to test whether the powder would also be beneficial in the cold and shivering of intermittent tertians and quartans. Performing the trial in a small series of cases, they obtained similar alleviation.[23] When a few of the priests went to Lima, they brought a large amount of the bark to a druggist named Gabriel de España, who dispensed it properly.

While the febrifugal powders, says Caldera de Heredia, were being spread through the entire province of Peru, Dr. Juan de Vega, the viceroy's physician, returned to Spain.[24] As we have seen, this statement is supported by another physician, Pedro Miguel de Heredia.[25] It is also supported, strongly, by Dr. Diego Salado Garces, a physician discussed below, and is contradicted by Haggis. De Vega brought with him a large amount of the bark, and various trials of it were made. Use of the drug began to spread in Spain, not only because the doctor recommended it but because the Jesuits returning from Peru recommended it also.

Likewise included in Badus's brief list of citations are writings by the eminent Gaspar Bravo de Sobremonte Ramirez (1603–83), who told of the new drug in his *Disputatio apologetica* and in his *Resolutionum et consultationum medicarum*. Like Caldera de Heredia, Bravo de Sobremonte used the Quechua term *quarango* for the tree later called cinchona. It was the opinion of Badus that the bark should be given in quartan fevers even in urgent circumstances, whereas Bravo de Sobremonte had declared that in such cases nothing should be done.[26]

A slightly later author, Pedro Miguel de Heredia (d. ca. 1661), mentioned above in the discussion of de Vega, was another physician of high distinction; he held the chair of medicine at Alcalá de Henares, was dean of medicine there, and was chief physician to Philip IV of Spain (Fig. 1). The posthumous second edition of his *Operum medicinalium* states that the Indians in the region of Quito use powdered "quarango"[27] bark when they have intense chills caused by exposure to cold air or to the water of a cold river crossed by swimming. By taking the powder in warm water they obtain immediate relief because heat returns to the whole body. On this observation the Jesuits made an analogy (*analogismum fecerunt*) and tested the effect of the powder in the chills of intermittent fevers. Experience confirmed what rational analogy had dictated. From this trial the matter passed on to the physicians, so that in a few years the bark was being used frequently and effectively for eradicating fevers in the entire realm of Peru. Then the news of the great remedy reached Spain through the report of "our doctor" Juan de Vega, the returned personal physician of His Excellency the count of Chinchon, viceroy of Peru, who tested the drug in many trials not only in India [Peru] but also in Seville. "Several years later," the source concludes, "while at Madrid, I saw the bark in the

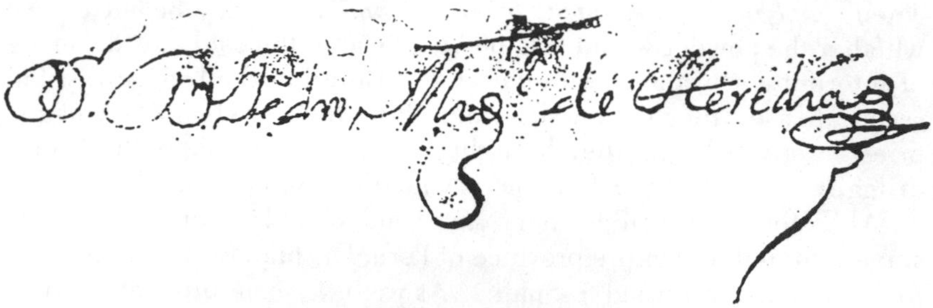

FIG. 1. Signature of Dr. D[on] Pedro Mig[uel] de Heredia [died ca. 1661],
archiater to Philip IV of Spain and a valued early commentator on
"quarango" (Peruvian bark).

home of the count of Chinchon, son of the late viceroy. It was examined
by me and by druggists skilled in botany and we found it to be simply
hot and dry in the third degree, according to Galen's teaching in several
chapters in book 4 of his *De simplicium medicamentorum* [*temperamentis et*] *facultatibus.*"[28]

I have paraphrased and quoted *in extenso* the statement of Pedro Miguel de Heredia because it contains firsthand testimony and was recorded by a learned man who had excellent opportunity to know the facts.

The treatise written by Pedro Miguel de Heredia—especially its posthumous second edition—deservedly overshadowed the writings of Pedro Miguel's forgotten unprogressive colleague Francisco Henriquez de Villacorta,[29] principal professor of medicine at Alcalà de Henares and physician to Philip II and Charles II of Spain. Henriquez's *Opera medica* (1670) includes in its prefatory material a letter from Pedro Barea y Astorga, who edited the major treatise of Miguel de Heredia and hence is more than likely to have been amply cognizant of the Peruvian bark.

The chef d'oeuvre of Henriquez de Villacorta displays the full flower of Galenic doctrine and Hispanic conservatism, not unmixed with signs of clinical judgment.[30] In discussing the pathogenesis of putrid fevers Henriquez says that fine matter is readily separated and concocted by Nature because it is less resistant than thick matter, and nothing in Galen's teaching is more familiar than attenuation and incision [of peccant humors] in the treatment of putrid fevers; hence, Henriquez says, thickening is inappropriate. This teaching has additional support because in putrid fever a thickening in fine [peccant] matter is apt to be produced by the astringents that Galen curses vigorously. No one, says Galen, uses astringent foods except because of a symptom causing faintness or because of diarrhea.

This statement may imply, indistinctly, an objection to Peruvian bark, which was considered astringent and was thought to retard expulsion of morbid matter. In the *Opera medica* of Henriquez de Villacorta I have found no mention of the bark, although either thirty or forty years had elapsed since this drug reached Spain for the first time.

The Spanish cinchonological tradition was continued by Diego Salado Garces, who is described on the title pages of his books as a native of Utrera (near Seville) and former professor of method in the University of Seville. These attributions strongly suggest that Salado Garces is likely to have been thoroughly familiar with early European occurrences in the history of the Peruvian bark. Two of his extant works, now rare, contain comment on this subject.

The earlier treatise, the *Apologetico discurso* (1678), describes, in four successive sections, the nature of powdered Peruvian bark, the objections alleged against its use, the proofs of its febrifugal property, and a refutation of the objections. Salado Garces states that Cardinal de Lugo, a native of Seville, was the first to use the drug in Europe and that Juan de Vega had used it for the rigors of tertian fever "because this very learned physician, the personal physician of the count of Chinchon . . . and primary professor and dean at the royal university, having returned to Spain, after many trials introduced its use in Seville."[31]

Among the objections Salado Garces cites,[32] from varied sources, the already familiar observations that the drug did not always prevent recurrence of the fever, that it produced no evacuation, and that it might cause a tertian to become a fever of some other kind. To these he added the allegation that the drug could only be used as a trial, but Hippocrates and Galen had declared trials to be dangerous.

The evidence in favor of the drug included successful results, cited previously, by Miguel de Heredia and Gaspar Bravo, in cases of pernicious tertian. To these Salado Garces added brief notes on four of his own cases, at least three of which gave evidence of pernicious character. Successful results were obtained in this series also.

In 1679, after the lapse of one year, Salado Garces issued a supplementary essay, his *Estaciones medicas* (1679). This work is divided into two parts, which together contain eighty-one items presented in refutation of notes sent him by an unnamed enemy of the Peruvian bark. The discussion includes brief comments on a few cases of severe intermittent fever and some remarks on the identity of Dr. Juan de Vega, who is possibly confused with a military officer of the same name.[33] The treatise also contains abundant scholastic discussion of humoral evacuation.

Such being the works and deeds of Salado Garces in Seville, it is instructive to take into account some observations made in that city *twenty-three years later*. In 1702, Giovanni Borghesi, a medical graduate of Rome(?), sojourned briefly in Seville while en route eastward. He states that the king had recently founded in that city a modern medical school, to which were attached five of the forty local physicians; the prospects seemed good. During the same visit Borghesi conversed with other practitioners. He reported that "the physicians, generally speaking, still follow the Galenic school and it would be strange news [*sarebbe la strana novella*] to speak of the circulation of the blood or fermentation of humors or other modern observations and truths of the same kind." Borghesi adds that these doctors had frequent recourse to phlebotomy, and no patient had blood drawn fewer than six or seven times.[34] Although Borghesi fails to mention the Peruvian bark, his description of superannuated opinions and methods is clear enough.

Additional comments must be intercalated at this point. First, the statement of Gaspar Caldera de Heredia and the statement in the posthumous edition of Pedro Miguel de Heredia are separated by a quarter of a century. This suggests that a separate Spanish cinchonological tradition was being formed, a tradition that deserves to be investigated in greater detail than is possible here. This tradition was not overlooked by the nineteenth-century Spanish medical historian, Antonio Hernández Morejon.[35]

Second, a discernibly separate tradition in Portuguese medicine is also beyond the scope of this history,[36] but since it cannot be ignored entirely, a few hints are offered in place of an elaborate study. At the outset one may notice a few disparaging remarks made by gifted observers. Garcia da Orta, the physician and botanist (ca. 1500–1568), wrote in his *Colloquies:* "It is true that the Portuguese are not very curious, nor are they good writers." To this we may add a comment made by a noted contemporary scholar, C. R. Boxer: "The sixteenth-century historians, João de Barros and Diogo do Couto, both complained that their countrymen were not of an inquiring turn of mind."[37] Generalizations like these are easy to ponder but difficult to weigh; total obscurity cannot be ascribed to a country or an era that produced João II, Manoel I, Vasco da Gama, and their cartographers.[38]

It is necessary to remember that Portugal is less than one-fifth as large as Spain and that the two countries were united for six decades (1580–1640). The Jesuits entered Portugal soon after their order was founded (ca. 1521) and quickly acquired great power, especially in the universities. This suggests that cinchona bark is likely to have been used in Portugal much earlier than is indicated by evidence thus far discovered. However, examination of the relatively scanty body of extant medical writing that was produced in Portugal during the first half of the seventeenth century reveals general retardation unrelieved by the presence of anyone even remotely comparable to Amatus Lusitanus, the eminent practitioner and writer, who had died before the end of the preceding century. The sole exception to this harsh dictum is Zacutus Lusitanus, who is discussed in Appendix A. He left Portugal in 1625, and most of his writing was done subsequently, in the tolerant and progressive environment of Amsterdam.

It is interesting and surprising that the treatise by Pedro Miguel de Heredia is cited almost twenty times in a manuscript volume written in Portuguese *in Pernambuco* (Brazil) around 1677.[39] Although this book discusses tertian and quartan fever, it makes no mention of the Jesuits' bark. As Guerra (1977b) has pointed out, important remarks of Miguel de Heredia, discussed above, did not appear in the first edition of his book (1665) but made their debut in the edition of 1673; hence they may have failed to reach Pernambuco by 1677, or very few copies of the book may have been available there.

A work by Andreas Antonius Castro (1636) contains routine Galenic doctrines. A slightly earlier book by Alexo de Abreu (1623) contains in its title a misleading allusion to tertian fever; the text, disappointingly, discusses the *semi*tertian. The treatise, however, is to be valued for its discussion of *mal de Loanda* (scurvy).

Third, statements of Gaspar Caldera de Heredia and Pedro Miguel de Heredia, already mentioned repeatedly, base the discovery of the drug on the use of analogy by Jesuits. In this context it should be noted that the pedagogic manual formulated and used by the Jesuits, the *Ratio atque institutio studiorum*, includes analogy among the subjects to be presented by the professor of philosophy during the teaching of logic.[40]

Much later, in 1730, Francesco Torti was to insert into the second edition of his *Therapeutice specialis* (530) a new passage in which he discussed the justification for prescribing the Peruvian bark in cases and diseases in which no trial had been made by the better practitioners but in which nevertheless a theoretical reason existed, founded either on sound hypothesis *or on several observations based on analogy.*

Miguel de Heredia clearly describes analogical reasoning tested by experimental trial. The incident merits careful attention. It is obviously an example of productive scientific method employed in the seventeenth century. In the present instance we see analogy used by obscure men who were trained in science and philosophy but whose main interests were not necessarily in these subjects.[41]

For readers who may be attracted to analogy and its history a selection of references is given in a note.[42] The selection is intended to be diverse rather than complete.

Dr. Téofilo Hernándo y Ortega, an interesting modern medical historian, has written that

at the beginning of the seventeenth century, Galileo, Harvey, and Descartes gave new orientation to scientific thought and produced discoveries of very great importance. . . . It may appear strange that we should incorporate great discoveries created by eminent men in the field of science with the finding of a drug that was popular among Peruvian aborigines, whose obstinately kept secret was revealed to the Jesuits. . . . Following the right path of the period, that of investigation and trial, they were the first to confirm the efficacy of the drug.[43]

This interpretation, impressive at first reading, loses much of its force when we remember that a large part of the discovery made by the Jesuits is attributable to their use of analogy and, further, that this process was mentioned repeatedly by Galen (see note 42). It is not unreasonable, however, to accord residues of credit to Galileo and others of the seventeenth-century pantheon if they were responsible for the investigative spirit that subsequently animated the actual trials of the medicament.

Guerra has referred to the absence of evidence that American Indians ever used cinchona in the treatment of fevers.[44] Further, he calls attention to present pharmacological opinion as to the action of quinine. Indeed, a major textbook states that "quinine increases the tension response to a single maximal stimulus delivered to the muscle directly or to the nerve, but it also increases the refractory period of muscle so that the response to tetanic stimulation is diminished. The excitability of the motor end-plate region decreases so that responses to repetitive nerve stimulation and to acetylcholine are reduced.[45] Guerra has concluded that the Indians using the bark suppressed chills caused by cold and that this result is explicable by modern pharmacological doctrine. His statement appears to be correct, although recent literature has been poor in discussion of the precise issue that is here under consideration. A paper published in 1977 by E. Satinoff on hypothermia in animals exposed to cold shows that quinine did indeed suppress shivering, a type of muscular activity that tends to counteract hypothermia.[46] From these findings we may surmise that if the Peruvian miners had ingested cinchona bark *before* crossing the river, they might have died of cold.

In his classic writings on medical thermometry Carl Wunderlich observed that in intermittent fever the use of quinine not infrequently suppresses the subjective symptoms but leaves the elevation of temperature almost equal to that of a complete paroxysm.[47] It is no quibble to

point out that Wunderlich's diagnoses of intermittent fever were made in the 1850s and 1860s; too early for corroboration or rejection by Laveranian microscopical malariology (1880). Thermometry is further discussed in Chapter 9.

2 Peru, Italy, and the Low Countries

Peru

In 1735, Joseph de Jussieu became a member of the astronomical expedition of Condamine, which he served as physician and naturalist. In 1738 he visited Loja, where he was informed that the Indians at Malacatos, about five kilometers to the south, were the earliest to discover the effectiveness of cinchona bark in intermittent fever and that an Indian *cacique* or chief had used an infusion of this material to cure an afflicted Jesuit who happened to be traveling through the district. The missionary then returned to his native land, taking with him a quantity of the bark, but he did not know from which species of tree it had been obtained. Moreover, he seems to have confounded the fever-bark tree with the Peruvian balsam tree.[1]

Jussieu's note, based on oral tradition, includes no estimate of how long the Indians had known that the bark is effective against intermittent fever. The name of the Jesuit and the date of his treatment are not stated, but the incident could hardly have occurred earlier than 1618, when missionary work in the remote region was begun.[2] The slender narrative is not incredible, nor does it necessarily conflict with the explanations given by Caldera de Heredia and Pedro de Miguel Heredia, already discussed. We cannot exclude the possibility that European knowledge of cinchona arose in more than one way during a period of ten to twenty years.

Prominent among those who have written on the early history of cinchona is Rubén Vargas Ugarte, S.J.,[3] who states that the Jesuits of Quito *must have learned* the use of cinchona from the natives of Loja. In 1618 an inhabitant of Loja, Diego de Vaca y Vega, began regional missionary work, for which Jesuits were to become famous. Contact with the Jesuits of Lima was frequent, and the discovery of the bark was imparted to them. Late in 1629 or early in 1630 the countess of Chinchon had a malignant tertian fever. When it proved resistant, Diego de Torres Vásquez, S.J., her husband's confessor, *must have advised* the use of the bark. Perhaps, Vargas Ugarte continues, her personal physician, Juan de Vega, objected, but the persuasiveness of Vasquez, who was then provincial of the order, proved decisive and successful. The Jesuits, in a meeting held not long afterward, decided to send samples of the drug to Europe; Fathers Alonso Messia (or Mexia) Venegas and Hernándo de León Garavito were designated to convey them to Spain and Rome, which they reached in 1631.[4] The countess could not have taken the cinchona to Spain because she never returned there; she died in Cartagena in 1641 (see Chapter 1).

The reader can hardly overlook the fact that Vargas Ugarte's account repeatedly fails to provide documentation—perhaps this deficiency was unavoidable—and is largely conjectural, but not incredible.

Elsewhere Vargas Ugarte states that "the slight importance which contemporaries conceded to the felicitous discovery of the bark was undoubtedly the reason for the obscurity which still surrounds the way in which it was discovered."[5] He adds that the second countess, in going from Spain to Lima, had made part of her journey from Panama to South America across malarious coastal valleys. As we have seen, she reached Lima one month before Suardo's official diary was started; hence her illness escaped mention in it.[6] In view of these facts and conjectures Vargas Ugarte was unwilling to discard entirely the story of the countess, but he recognized that she could not have brought the bark to Europe.

Vargas Ugarte drew attention to a contribution by Enrique Torres Saldamando, former conservator of the National Library at Lima, where the Jesuit documents of the region are kept. Torres Saldamando wrote a biographical note on Diego de Torres Vásquez, which includes a paragraph allegedly encountered in a letter written from Rome probably in 1631 or 1632, by Muzio Vitelleschi, general of the Jesuit order, to Nicolás Durán Mastrilli, who had succeeded to the office of provincial. The important letter expressed satisfaction at the recovery of the countess through the help of the Jesuits and acknowledged receipt of a quantity of the drug. Vargas Ugarte searched the Peruvian Jesuit archives diligently but was unable to find the original letter. Jaramillo Arango, a well-known scholar and diplomat, instituted a search in Rome, which was similarly unsuccessful.[7]

Additional comment is found in the writings of Alessandro Canezza, former director of the Biblioteca Lancisiana in Rome.[8] Canezza states that whether it was the *corregidor* of Loja or the rector of the Jesuit college who sent the bark to the countess is of secondary importance. He quotes, uncritically, a paper (replete with errors) which, entirely without documentation, makes the possibly important statement that the earliest historical notice of the drug goes back to 1620, when a Jesuit of Chuquizaca in Peru was treated with the bark by an Indian healer.[9] In a later article, unfortunately almost devoid of documentation, Canezza, unlike Vargas Ugarte, asserts that Alonso Messia Venegas, S.J. (1557–1649), procurator of the Jesuit province of Peru, went to Rome *in 1632* with cinchona in order to inform the general of the order, Muzio Vitelleschi (1563–1645), of the drug, and to present samples. In the same article Canezza states that in 1645, Bartolome Tafur, S.J., a later procurator of Peru, brought an additional quantity of the drug to Rome; this development is considered subsequently. Canezza also refers to evidence derived from the letters of contemporary physicians, "which I abstain from publishing" (*che mi riservo di pubblicare*). This evidence apparently refers to shipments of the bark or powder between 1632 and 1645.[10] At any rate, it is clear that shipment of cinchona from Peru was now beginning to become an established or at least a repeated practice.

Italy

The centralization that the Christian world inherited from the Roman Empire inevitably imprinted itself on innumerable institutions and activities; those who carefully examine the early history of cinchona find in the absorbing narrative an undeniable example of the same process. In the judgment of the historian David Ogg the seventeenth century was the period in which the religious motive was overshadowed by the economic, and the empire and the papacy were relegated to positions of little more than academic interest.[11] But the tale that we have to tell in these chapters is repeatedly characterized and diversified by the acts of royalty, nobility, and clergy. Yet no physician needs to be reminded that most malaria patients—indeed, most sick persons—could hardly have been kings or nobles or priests, and the overwhelming majority of the afflicted, having left no record, can mislead us into thinking that they were anonymous or unimportant.[12]

As we have seen, the Peruvian bark probably was brought to Rome by Jesuits in 1631 and 1632 and again in 1645, but unrecorded shipment may well have occurred between these dates. In that brief period several events occurred which are significant in this history. In 1643 Juan de Lugo, S.J., an outstanding theologian, was made a cardinal by

Urban VIII. In 1644 Innocent X became pope. Bartolome Tafur, S.J., arriving in Rome, made contact with Cardinal de Lugo, with whom he shared special interests in theology,[13] and attended the eighth general congregation of the Jesuits, which lasted from November 21, 1645, to April 14, 1646. Thus there was ample opportunity for Tafur to transmit information about the new drug to the cardinal.

According to Honoratus Fabri, a Jesuit and naturalist who wrote under the pseudonym Antimus Conygius, Cardinal de Lugo had the newly arrived Peruvian bark tested by Gabriele Fonseca, physician to Innocent X. This statement is repeated by several later authors.[14]

Fonseca (d. 1668), born in Portugal, was the son of Dr. Rodrigo Fonseca and was physician to Popes Gregory XV (1621–1623), Urban VIII (1623–1644), and Innocent X (1644–1655). He taught in Pisa and in Rome; in the latter city he held a professorship of medicine.[15]

Fonseca's known writings are few and scarce. A manuscript on dyspnea, its date unspecified, is recorded among the holdings of a library in Macerata.[16] Mandosio lists two volumes of consultations by Fonseca, dated 1622 and 1623.[17]

The only known printed work by Fonseca is a treatise on medical etiquette and deontology. This book, which appeared in 1623, approximately one or two decades before the Peruvian bark reached Rome, describes the attitude that physicians testing new drugs ought to take:

> In making a diligent search for drugs no effort should ever appear burdensome to the diligent physician. Indeed, the properties of all drugs, or at least of the main ones, should be committed to memory, as well as whatever is suitable for the expulsion of individual sicknesses. Thus the details will always be available, so that when exigency makes a demand, they will occur to us at once and those which are more proper are selected for use. . . . At the same time the physician should guard against trying out new drugs every day but should reject those which for so many centuries the most learned men have abandoned. . . . To try in the human body those drugs which have not been tested by long experience is not without danger, since the terminus of a rash experiment is the destruction of a living being.[18]

These assertions depict a careful, conscientious, and conservative physician who relied on experience and was not fanatically addicted to theories. Such was the man to whom, under the orders of Innocent X, Cardinal de Lugo entrusted the Peruvian bark for testing.

Unfortunately no detailed records of the trials and no descriptions of them are extant. Fabri, however, says: "The eminent archiater attests that he had cured many patients, declaring that they had taken this powder, whose strength and nature he diligently investigated. He found that it is a very salutary medicine and besides is safe and secure, not uncertain and doubtful, not violent and styptic, but innocent and harmless." On a later page Fabri adds that Fonseca "was informed by his own trials (*propriis experimentis edoctus*).[19]

A disappointment awaits readers of the book of Julius Caesar Benedictus, published in 1649. It contains a collection of medical epistles, several of which are dedicated to Fonseca. No part of the collection mentions the Peruvian bark.[20] A few years later, in 1657, the conservative Fonseca used the drug in treating Flavio Cardinal Chigi, nephew of Alexander VII.[21]

Juan de Lugo, S.J. (1583–1660), born in Madrid, spent his early years in Seville, which at that time was the sole Spanish entrepôt for trade with the New World. At the University of Salamanca he showed special interest in philosophy and in civil and canon law. Following the example of his elder brother Francisco (1580–1652), he entered the Jesuit order. For ten years he taught philosophy and theology in Spain. His great ability as thinker, teacher, and writer attracted the attention of Muzio Vitelleschi, general of the Jesuit order, who in 1621 transferred him to the Collegium Romanum,[22] the leading educational institution of the Jesuits. En route to his new post he traveled through southern France but apparently did not pass through Paris. Nor did he administer the bark to the dauphin (later Louis XIV), as has been alleged. He taught at the Roman College, with great distinction, from 1621 to 1643.[23]

A semipopular author has stated, without documentation, that de Lugo conducted in secrecy some experiments designed to solve certain problems in physics and mathematics and formulated a "law of inflation points," which became known as his own and which, after further experimental research by Robert Boyle, became one of the fundamental laws of modern chemistry.[24] In an extensive search of histories of physics and mathematics, and a search of writings by and about Boyle, I have found no mention of de Lugo and no evidence that he ever undertook experiments. Similarly Canezza found no trace of an interest in medicine or therapeutics in the long catalog of de Lugo's writings. An account of de Lugo's life from 1583 to 1644 by Camilo M. Abad, S.J., also yields no suggestion that he was interested in the natural sciences or mathematics.[25]

In 1643 Pope Urban VIII made de Lugo cardinal. De Lugo's acquaintance with the Peruvian bark and his interest in it began at about this time. It is considered probable that Tafur brought him the information and the drug.[26] De Lugo's high position made possible an achievement that would have been beyond the scope of an ordinary Jesuit priest or even a provincial or procurator.

A handsomely illustrated glossy volume on infection contains, in the caption of a picture, the undocumented statement that Cardinal de Lugo "conducted experiments on himself with Peruvian bark." [27] I have been able to discover no evidence that this is correct.

With his own funds de Lugo bought large amounts of the bark and distributed them at his residence. The literature of the time contains numerous contemporary reports of his generosity,[28] which led to the drug being named *pulvis cardinalis* and *pulvis de Lugo*. Sturmius, a contemporary, adds that "he gives it gratis to the fevered poor on condition that they do not sell it and that they present a physician's statement about the illness." [29]

In addition to whatever distribution de Lugo may have made at his home, there were at least two other points of distribution in Rome. One was the Ospedale di Santo Spirito. Here, according to an undocumented statement by Canezza, de Lugo, dissatisfied by hostility against the drug, took over the distribution.[30] Another site was the apothecary shop of the Collegium Romanum. In the opinion of Rompel, although cinchona bark had reached Europe in 1632, only a small amount arrived at that time, and the drug was not noticed by the then apothecary of the college.[31]

One of this functionary's successors, Pietro Paolo Puccerini[32] (1600–1661), a lay brother in the Jesuit order, became keeper of the apothecary shop at the college in 1647. In a letter to Badus in 1659 he stated that the drug had been sent to him for the first time, from Peru, in 1647. He had used it in cases of tertian and quartan fever and long intermittents, especially the protracted autumnal ones, and had given it according to the printed recipe, better known as the *Schedula Romana* (Fig. 2; see Appendix B). The drug had removed the sickness "infallibly," although a few patients had had relapses, which were readily relieved by additional doses. Puccerini had treated many thousands of patients each year; so far as he was aware, there had been no bad effects in Rome, Florence, and the papal states. Moreover, he wrote that the bark had been conveyed, by couriers and others, to Naples, Genoa, Milan, Piedmont, England, France, Flanders, and Germany; Spain, Portugal, and Austria are not mentioned.[33] Before long, Cardinal de Lugo possessed a large collection of testimonial letters.

The expulsion of the Jesuits from Venice by Pope Paul V in 1606 obviously occurred too early to affect the distribution of the Peruvian bark. Their readmission by Pope Alexander VII (Chigi) in 1656 could hardly have been other than favorable for the drug.

In 1656, Sebastianus Badus (then named Baldus) issued, under que typis Romæ Schedion, quod ex Italico sic Latinum feci:

Adfertur cortex iste ex Peruuiano Regno, vocaturque China febris; exhibetur contra febrem tertianam & quartanam, quæ cum frigore ægros prehendunt, & quæ per multos dies sunt confirmatæ. Præparatur autem in hunc modum:

ORBIS AMERICANI.   5

dum: Corticis drachmæ duæ tunduntur subtiliter, ac per setaceum traijciuntur. Tribus horis ante paroxismum puluis maceratur in vini albi potentis cyatho; dumque frigus febrile incipit, vel sentitur aliquod leue accessionis principium, sumitur tota dosis præparata, ægerque se componit in lecto. Constat experientiâ omnes ferè, qui eo puluere sunt vsi, à febre liberatos fuiße, purgato benè priùs corpore, & quaternis à sumptione diebus abstinendo ab omni alio medicamento. Sed non est assumendus nisi præuio Medici consilio, qui iudicet de modo & tempore quod sumptioni sit opportunum. Hactenus Schedion, quod à Romanis pharmacopolis corticem pretio parantibus dari solet.

FIG. 2. Chiflet's Latin translation (1653, 4–5) of the *Schedula Romana*, the earliest statement of the dosage and administration of the bark. Courtesy Wellcome Institute Library, London. The original Italian text is no longer extant. Text and discussion in Appendix B.

anonymous editorship, a collection of old and new essays by various authors. Most of the items deal with plague, but a long introductory letter in this rare and obscure volume states, "and so we see that *China Chinae,* a unique prodigy in medicine, overthrows and tramples to the ground not only quartan fevers, based on cold humor, but also tertian fevers, which are based on hot, dry, and bilious humor, and we see also that the *China* is inherently hot and dry." A later page adds, "*China*

Chinae, whose results against tertian and quartan fevers are very famous, although other men have blabbed against it . . ." Further, "My book on *China Chinae* is ready for the press." The last of these excerpts confirms the authorship of the introductory letter and supports the Badian editorship of the volume.[34]

Later in 1656—seven years before his famous *Anastasis* appeared—Badus issued his *Cortex Pervviae redivivus*. In translation the full title is: "The Peruvian bark revived; the destroyer of fevers defended against the attacks of Melippus Protimus [pseudonym of Vopiscus Fortunatus Plempius], a Belgian physician." This treatise is part of a Flemish controversy, which is discussed in Chapter 3. Badus's later and more important book on cinchona, the *Anastasis corticis Peruviae* (1663), has already been mentioned as an extensive work in which the tradition of the countess of Chinchon is transmitted but in which several traces of a different tradition can also be detected.

According to evidence accumulated by Rompel, Badus, a man of great learning, had studied medicine under Sinibaldi in Pisa and had practiced medicine in Rome during 1651–52. He was in contact with Pietro Paolo Puccerini, apothecary of the Collegium Romanum, and corresponded with him after 1652. In addition, he was acquainted with de Lugo before the latter became a cardinal. In 1652 Badus returned to Genoa, where he served as physician at the Pammatone Hospital, already mentioned, and at the Ospedale degli Incurabili. He also acted as adviser to the government.[35]

His *Anastasis* (1663) narrates the early history of the bark, argues vigorously against Jean-Jacques Chiflet, who is discussed in Chapter 3, and provides a brief review of the literature. It also describes the perplexities of the humoralist and logician who attempts to understand the action of the drug:

I admit that this problem is quite difficult if we consider it according to the Hippocratic rule and the method of contraries. For how could you counteract bile, a hot and dry humor, with the bark, which is just as hot and dry and [hence] has unsuitable qualities? How can you control fever by means of hot substances? A quartan, indeed, could be halted by hot things since it is cold, at least in its cause although not in its form. But a tertian, a continued fever, and the like, are hot, both formally and materially. These bring it about (since experience shows that these fevers are driven away just as quartans usually are) . . . that the bark must be judged to operate by hidden qualities rather than by manifest qualities, as happens also in syphilis . . . for guaiac works by hidden qualities. (138–39)

Other chapters of the *Anastasis* cope with objections that were to appear repeatedly in the literature of the next hundred years, namely, that the bark thickens the humors and hence causes such dangerous effects as constriction, constipation, and obstruction.

Badus quotes the entire text of the *Schedula Romana* from Chiflet's Latin version of the Italian original, and he subjoins a gloss exactly in the style of medieval commentators such as Gentile de Foligno, who as it happens is mentioned incidentally along with other writers. For textual comparison and medical certainty Badus also obtained a copy of the *Schedula* directly from its source, his friend the apothecary of the Collegium Romanum.[36] The fact that Badus compared two copies of the text and prepared a gloss shows that he was conscientious; this fact is to be weighed against charges of inaccuracy made by Condamine, Haggis, and others.[37]

Badus devotes the third book of the *Anastasis* to "trials of the bark and testimonials of physicians and other illustrious persons." Having given the reader a complete, verified, and glossed text of the *Schedula*, which contains details of dosage, Badus most unfortunately did not trouble to describe individual cases. While it is easy to assume that the trials conducted in the Pammatone and other Genoese hospitals were based merely on the *post hoc ergo propter hoc* principle, we cannot exclude the possibility that some form of controlled test may have been employed.

A century earlier, Nicolas Monardes, writing of the occidental bezoar as used in Germany during an outbreak of plague, made the following statement: "There being in the hospital four persons who were stricken by this sickness, it was given to two of them and not to the other two. Those who received it recovered, the other two died."[38]

It would be rash to assert that this is the earliest record of controlled experimentation. Something of the kind was proposed—not performed—by the theological writer Arnobius of Sicca (fl. A.D. 300) in his *Disputationes adversus gentes*;[39] and still earlier sources, such as Tertullian, have been suggested.[40]

It should be noted in addition that Badus prefaced his report of clinical results by proclaiming that experience, especially the evidence of sight and touch, is far more reliable than literature. He supported his contention by reference to the Gospel of Luke, to Thomas Aquinas, and to Cardinal Bellarmine.[41]

In addition to the disappointingly few case reports that are intercalated in his text (e.g., at pp. 113–18 of the *Anastasis*), usually in support of special contentions, and instead of the statistical analyses that a critical modern-day editor would demand, Badus supplied a collection of testimonial letters. A physician named Antonius Gibbonus, writing in 1658 from a large hospital in Genoa (probably the Pammatone, in whose records his name repeatedly appears) states that over a period of several years he had treated about three hundred persons suffering from quartan and tertian fever, old and recent, with complete success; a few had had relapses that yielded to additional treatment. Similar experiences are reported from the same hospital in 1660 by Dr. Antonius Vialis. Badus himself had seen more than six hundred fever patients in that hospital. He was accompanied by two younger physicians, both of whom died of plague (whereas no report in the series tells of physicians dying from intermittent fever).[42]

Badus adds that nowadays convalescents from fever, that is, tertian and quartan, are too numerous to be mentioned; the region, and the era, were obviously overwhelmed by the intermittent fevers. In a supplementary letter Dr. Cosmus Suarez, director of the Pammatone, confirms that Badus had introduced the drug there.[43] In addition the book contains laudatory letters from high-ranking nonmedical persons, especially cardinals. Although many parish priests must have struggled with the troubles of fever patients, the humble rarely receive individual mention.

An extremely important inclusion in the *Anastasis* is a letter written from Modena in November 1656 by Antonio Frassoni (1607?–1680), who stated that he had first prescribed the Jesuits' bark about ten years previously—*scito me Corticem hunc decem plus minus ab hinc annis primo propinasse*—approximately in 1646.[44] Frassoni, a central or paracentral figure in this history, requires extended consideration, which is accorded in Chapter 8.

Another important inclusion in the *Anastasis* is a letter Cardinal de Lugo wrote to Badus under date of October 4, 1659, in reference to Badus's earlier book. His letter states that daily experience confirmed the value of the drug; it was being used at Rome in quartan and tertian intermittents and even in continued fevers, with marvelous results.[45] With such extensive use, it was becoming scarce and there was a risk of falsification and adulteration, as usually happens with rare and foreign drugs.[46] Since acumen sharpened by learning is believed to be a professional trait among cardinals, it would not be astonishing if de Lugo had read discussions of adulteration in Pliny and Dioscorides.[47] It is well to observe also that while much adulteration or substitution in those times was often merely the replacement of one inert substance by another, in the case of cinchona a conspicuously and promptly effective drug was at stake.

Another high-ranking ecclesiastic mentioned in Badus's *Anastasis* is Gianstefano Donghi (d. 1669),[48] who was made cardinal by Urban VIII in 1643, at the same time as two other prelates mentioned in this history, namely Juan de Lugo and Cesare Facchinetti.[49] Cardinal Donghi suffered from *febris notha tertiana*, the so-called false (really a mixed humoral) tertian fever in Piacenza from August to October 1661. His physicians refused to prescribe the bark. In this decision three Milanese consultants concurred, and left written records of their opinions.[50] Badus disagreed, whereupon the Placentines canceled their opposition, the drug was administered, and the cardinal regained his health. The consultation reports and discussions, too elaborate to summarize here, describe the great resistance that cinchona sometimes encountered, offer ample insight into prevailing clinical opinion, and in addition provide a picture of seventeenth-century consultations and customs.[51] One of the Milanese, Dr. Christoforo Paravicino, estimated that he had treated a thousand sufferers from quartan fever during the preceding twelve years,[52] yet he objected to using the bark in tertians. The opinions produced by him and his colleagues proved influential— in part because the patient at hand was a high-ranking churchman— but they also were harmful and ultimately were recognized as obsolete.[53]

Badus quotes a statement signed by Dr. Paravicino and several colleagues and dated October 22, 1658, to the effect that the Peruvian bark had reached Milan "many years" previously (*multis abhinc annis*) and was first tried by Jesuits at the Collegium Braydense.[54] This bit of information justifies and fortifies the opinion that the spread of the drug, unlike that of other drugs, was no hit-or-miss affair but was largely (not exclusively) dependent on Jesuit organization. Paravicino's statement is compatible with the remarks of Puccerini, quoted above.

Extensive and successful experience with cinchona did not affect Badus's opinions as to pathogenesis, but it gradually altered his procedure. He accepted, with minor modification, Fernel's statement that the main site of intermittent fever is the *primae viae* and that the peccant humor lingers in "the precordial region, the stomach, diaphragm, hepatic concavity, spleen, pancreas, and omentum or mesentery."[55]

With regard to therapeutics of the intermittent fevers, medical opinion had required and emphasized pretreatment of the humors. This habit was respected by Chiflet and no less by the *Schedula Romana*. Indeed, the physician was advised to wait until the fever had been established for many days, especially if he was to use a febrifuge that was believed to be hot.

Badus, after describing these dominant opinions, says

Yet I do not know whether it was accidentally or purposely, but I began to reduce the procedure, so that not only in tertian fevers, in which the humor is more tractable, but also in quartans, in which it is usually more obstinate, I gave the bark as soon as I could, and as successfully as if the body had been purified in every way. I believe this was done not without reason and defensible arguments and, what is more important, not without experience, which is the master. (108)

In this comment it is easy to see the old doctrines yielding, albeit slowly, to new knowledge.

The importance of the Jesuits in the history of cinchona was abundantly evident in events that occurred in Peru, in Spain, and in Italy. The involvement of other clergy is recorded in Badus's *Anastasis* and is symbolized by his ample reports concerning Cardinal Donghi. Two additional aspects described by Rompel must not be allowed to escape unnoticed.[56] One is the relation between cinchona and the general meetings (known as congregations) of the Jesuit order. The other is the effect of malaria on the conclaves that were held for the election of popes.

During 1645 to 1652, while de Lugo, a Jesuit, was cardinal, the eighth, ninth, and tenth general congregations were held. Rompel felt that the eighth (1645) was the most important in the history of the Peruvian bark, although its role is likely to have been indirect. De Lugo had no official role in any of the congregations, but it is highly probable that he was influential in them. He certainly was acquainted with many of the participants and can be assumed to have exchanged information with them.

Padberg points out that about 1646 the Jesuits in Italy suffered financial stringency.[57] This fact makes even more creditable their generosity in the distribution of cinchona to the poor. Of interest also is evidence related to the papal conclaves. In August 1623, when Urban VIII was elected, de Lugo and seven cardinals were malarious. Immediately afterward a cardinalatial "hecatomb" (Celli's characterization, 1933) occurred.

Rompel believed that Cardinal de Lugo did not know of the Peruvian bark in 1644, when Innocent X was selected, but probably learned of the drug from Tafur in 1645. Malaria hastened the proceedings of the conclave and apparently prevented the French from impeding the election. By 1650, when a jubilee was held, the bark was famous in Rome and its fame was spreading elsewhere. Brunacci, an author who was well known in high social and religious circles, states clearly that the bark was first brought to Rome in 1650, by Jesuits, on the occasion of the jubilee, and was received by Cardinal de Lugo.[58] In the conclave of 1655, at which Alexander VII was elected, de Lugo was at the height of his influence, the drug was available, and malaria played no part.

The known importance of the Jesuits in the introduction of the bark raises the possibility that they played a role in introducing other drugs. The size and distribution of the order were favorable to activities of that kind. That an unidentified priest in Brazil (not necessarily a Jesuit, however) was associated with the introduction of ipecacuanha is mentioned in Chapter 13.

In the *Anastasis* Badus quotes Bollus the merchant as having written that he had received—almost certainly while he was in Peru—from Seville traders (*a mercatoribus Hispaliensibus*) a chest containing the bark and *other foreign drugs* for transmission in Rome to Cardinal de Lugo (24); the statement implies that the discovery of the bark was merely the successful part of a wider search. Investigations of this kind were part of Spanish official policy from an early period and are exemplified by the questionnaire which the Consejo de Indias issued about 1577 under the title *Instrucción y memoria de las relaciones que se han de hacer para la descripción de las Indias* (Instruction and memorandum on the reports that must be made for the description of the Indies).[59] The sixth of the fifty questions in this document specifies the transmission of information about "the herbs or aromatic plants with which the Indians treat themselves, and the medicinal or poisonous properties thereof." Whether the establishment of the famous Jesuit relations (reports) by the followers of Ignatius (Iñigo) Loyola could have inspired, or could have been inspired by, the Spanish questionnaires, is an interesting question that is beyond the scope of this history.

With respect to the activities and contributions of the Jesuits, completeness would require mention of the polypractic Athanasius Kircher (1602–80). It is repeatedly stated in the secondary literature that Kircher in his voluminous correspondence encouraged the use of the Jesuits' powder.[60] I have, however, lacked opportunity to examine these writings, most of which are preserved in Rome in the Pontificia Università Gregoriana.[61]

What has been said in the present chapter concerning the distribution of the Peruvian bark in Italy is necessarily limited to a few important cities, such as Rome and Genoa. Evidence concerning arrival of the drug in other cities is either absent or undiscovered or defective. An example is Venice. Bernardino Zendrini (1679–1747) wrote of a Camaldolese monk in that city who had a quartan fever that was refractory to orthodox medication. The patient wrote to Cardinal de Lugo, who had been his teacher of theology, and requested the febrifugal powder. A cure was obtained after the third or fourth dose. This result aroused skepticism in the attending physician, who then tested the drug in another case of quartan fever and again obtained a successful result. Unfortunately this report contains no personal names and no

dates.[62] It appears more than probable that the copious Italian literature contains detailed information concerning the earliest arrival of the
Peruvian bark in Venice and in many other places in Italy.

Belgium and the Netherlands

It is not known when the Peruvian bark first entered Belgium and the Netherlands. According to an imprecise statement by
Chiflet, after the *Schedula Romana* was issued the Jesuits brought the
bark into Belgium from Rome, where they had met in order to elect a
general of their order.[63] This could only have happened after the eighth
general congregation, which lasted from November 21, 1645, to April
14, 1646.[64] The seventh congregation had ended in 1615, too early to
be considered in this context.

Chiflet makes the additional vague statement that one Michael
Belga, "named after an old millhouse" (*a veteri molendino cognomi-
natus*) brought the bark to Brussels from Peru. This man had worked
in Lima for several years in the household of the marquis of Mancera,
who was immediate successor to the count of Chinchon as viceroy of
Peru.[65] Rompel surmised that Michael Belga's *cognomen* might translate as van Oudenmolen or something similar. Moreover, he reasoned
that Michael began to serve in Peru in 1640 and must have conveyed
the bark to Europe at some time between 1645 and 1652; hence he
could not have been the first to transmit it. Rompel pointed out in addition that Tafur reached Rome before Michael could have arrived in
Brussels.[66]

After consultation with a Dutch friend and fellow-historian, and the
help of Dutch archivists, I inferred that the probable modern equivalent
of Michael Belga's cognomen *a veteri molendino* was likely to be derived from a hamlet called Oudenmolen (51°32′N, 4°17′E) in the parish of Heeze, in the province of Noord-Brabant. Photocopies of the
baptismal register show that numerous children in the parish (1654–
99) were given the name Michael, but the register did not begin until
1649. Correspondence with the archivists of Bergen op Zoom, with the
Streekarchief Nassau-Brabant, and with official Belgian sources,
yielded no additional information on this point. Further inquiry directed to the cooperative archivists of Nassau-Brabant by a Dutch
scholar early in 1988 also yielded a negative result, attributable to the
fact that it was impossible to find clues requisite for a successful archival search.

The most promising source that remains for further exploration is
the record of Spanish travelers to the Americas. The data are in Seville,

and the catalog is in course of publication.[67] The documents are now being computerized; a search very kindly conducted by the archivists at my request did not discover the name or nicknames of Michael Belga.

Additional records are probably to be found in Lima and perhaps in Loja, Ecuador.

3 Continental Developments, 1653–1675

THE YEAR 1641 witnessed the death of Ferdinand (Hapsburg), viceroy of the Netherlands and brother of the Spanish king, Philip IV. His demise, attributed to tertian fever, occasioned an intricate controversy that at its outset was not directly related to the history of cinchona. The opening gun or arquebus in the skirmish was a four-page doctoral thesis or program issued in November 1641, two weeks after the viceroy's death, by Martinus Soers, under the direction of his teacher Vopiscus Fortunatus Plempius, professor of medicine at the University of Louvain. The text is devoted to such topics as Spanish phlebotomy methods.[1]

Soon afterward, in 1642, Soers issued another statement, the nastiness of which is suggested by its title, "Strictures against a certain . . . confused East Belgian chatterer. Controversies stirred up between Doctors Petrus Barba and V. F. Plempius on the treatment of the tertian."[2] The abusive pamphlet attacks an unnamed and allegedly unworthy person who received an academic (doctoral?) degree at Louvain in 1633. This culprit had objected to Soers's statement that the treatment of a tertian should start with the administration of a mild evacuant. Further hostilities concerned the proper use of phlebotomy. In addition, the East Belgian had dared to attack Plempius. Nowhere in the text is the Peruvian bark mentioned, but the controversy had only begun.

At an unknown date, 1642 or thereabouts, Pedro Barba (ca. 1590–1650), professor of medicine at Valladolid and physician to Philip IV, replied to Soers's thesis of 1641 in a pamphlet titled *Vera praxis de curatione tertianae*. . . . Again and again this work was later cited

incorrectly as a treatise on *cinchona*.[3] The error survived into the
fourth edition of Fielding Garrison's history of medicine and beyond.[4]

Barba's essay, like the two writings of Soers, deals mainly with phlebotomy and regimen in tertian fever. The discussion, presented in the
form of syllogisms and bolstered by citation of authors ranging from
Hippocrates to Valles Covarrubias, is a typical seventeenth-century
medical polemic. However, it repeatedly appeals to experience as well
as to reason or dogma, and it is in addition an interesting medical example of nationalistic hostility between Spanish overlords and their
northern subjects.[5] At the very end of the book Barba recounts the case
history of Viceroy Ferdinand, which had led to the controversy.

In 1642, Plempius launched a diatribe against Barba's *Vera praxis*.[6]
Barba had attacked parts of a thesis that had been issued under Plempian auspices, such as a passage that had discussed the use of a mild
laxative at the start of treatment of tertian fever and contradicted a passage on the use of phlebotomy in tertian fevers unaccompanied by plethora. In addition Plempius's tract contains much adverse comment on
Iberian therapeutic methods. Throughout the venomous text I found
no mention of Peruvian bark.[7]

While the exact chronology of the writings of Soers, Barba, and
Plempius is not clear, it is evident that Plempius and his disciple Soers
were ranged against Barba and at least one other opponent and that
the controversy dealt with the treatment of intermittent fever, especially
by means of laxatives, purges, phlebotomy, and various drugs. The series of incidents in the conflict is significant because it displays the attitudes that prevailed and were taught, and some of the practices that
existed, when the Peruvian bark first reached Belgium. Moreover, it
introduced a long-lived error into the literature about that medicament.

What has been characterized as the earliest known printed reference
to the Peruvian bark appears in a work titled *Discours et advis sur les
flus de ventre douloureux* (1643), written by Herman van der Heyden
(1572–1650?), a practitioner and public-health official in Ghent. In
discussing tertian fever, van der Heyden says, "If the patient prefers
powders alone, a drachm or less of the aforementioned diacarthamum
[saffron] powder may be beneficial, and even more, the powder that
hereabouts is called *pulvis indicus*."[8] This statement, found in van der
Heyden's discussion of tertian fever, is his sole and total reference to
what *may have been* the Peruvian bark. His chapter on quartan fever
does not mention the substance (but is interesting because it contains
some remarks about splenic "scirrhosity"[9] and dropsy as complications).

Rompel has pointed out that van der Heyden's recommendation of the bark, dated 1643, could not have been based on importations made by Tafur but must have resulted from an earlier shipment. Jaramillo Arango concluded that van der Heyden's *pulvis indicus* is not cinchona. His principal reason is that the *Antidotarium Gandavense* of 1663, the official pharmacopoeia of Ghent, mentions a *pulvis indicus*, which contains scammony and antimony but not Peruvian bark.[10] It is difficult to maintain that in the evaluation of seventeenth-century evidence a pharmacopoeia published twenty years after the event under discussion weighs heavily in the balance. In other words, the entry in the Gandavian antidotary does not tell us anything certain about the drug van der Heyden used. We must limit ourselves to the conclusion that the nature of his "Indian powder" remains unknown.

The Controverted Illness of Archduke Leopold

The illness that befell Leopold William, archduke of Austria, Belgium, and Burgundy, in the autumn of 1652, like the illness of Viceroy Ferdinand, which had occurred eleven years earlier, gave rise to vigorous controversy. Jean-Jacques Chiflet (1588–1660), one of the physicians in attendance—Pedro Barba was another—judged that the archduke was suffering from a false (i.e., impure) tertian, which turned into a double quartan.[11] The responsible physician was not eager to try out a new and poorly known drug on an illustrious patient. Reluctantly yielding to pressure from bystanders, some of whom were laymen and most of whom are likely to have been influential, he administered two drachms of powdered Peruvian bark in white wine. The fever disappeared. It returned thirty-three days later, whereupon the patient refused to take the bark again, in part because his brother, the Holy Roman Emperor Ferdinand III, had sent him a letter disapproving its use. The archduke died.

In his account of the illness Chiflet pointed out that in Brussels all quartans treated with the bark were marked by relapse. The Peruvian bark, he said, merely lengthens the intervals but does not cure the disease; the drug is not needed in Europe, where many other febrifuges are available. Chiflet himself had been cured of a double tertian in 1615 by means of gentian. In addition, he said, the bark is dangerous. By its astringency it may condense yellow bile in the gallbladder, black bile in the spleen, and impure phlegm in the stomach and intestines, making these humors immobile. They might then putrefy, liquefy, and spill over into adjacent organs, producing "prolonged and fatal diseases, mentioned by famous men."[12]

Chiflet supported these contentions with quotations from a series of ancient, medieval, and early modern (hence precinchonal) medical authors. In addition he referred to recent letters and comments—briefly quoted or merely cited—from Rome, Madrid, Naples, Florence, Vienna, and Paris; all were almost totally unfavorable to the use of the bark and were almost uniformly vague.[13]

Neither van der Heyden's indistinct brief allusion nor the *Schedula Romana*, already discussed, invalidates the assertion Rompel made in 1907 that Chiflet's work is the earliest separate book on the Peruvian bark.[14] Prepared at the request of the archduke, his statement was designed to explain and justify his own actions. Accordingly it presents his version of the case history, and it marshals such writings and such clinical experiences as would support his opinions.

Chiflet's book is useful to the historian as a description of anticinchonal attitudes. In addition it contains two paragraphs of historical information, as well as the earliest extant version of the *Schedula Romana*.[15]

Almost totally devoid of procinchonal facts or arguments, the book is by no means a balanced presentation. For example, it contains no letters reporting favorable experiences with the Peruvian febrifuge, nor does it give due weight to the concise statement in the *Schedula* that almost all who had been given the drug were relieved of their fever. The involvement of exalted personages in the *affaire Chiflet* exemplifies a trait that we have previously encountered in this history and shall meet again. It is endemic to the history of fevers.

In 1653, as we have seen, Chiflet published his book, which defended his treatment of the archduke and at the same time attacked the use of the Peruvian bark. A short while afterward, in 1655, a reply was issued by Honoré Fabri (1606–88), a Jesuit priest and nonphysician who used the pseudonym Antimus Conygius and who wrote at the request or instigation of a person pseudonymously designated as Germanus Poleconius.[16] The work had the approval of de Lugo and Fonseca, who had urged its publication.

Readers are likely to admire the cleverness of Fabri's attack against Chiflet. For example, Fabri starts with the interesting and historically significant principle that all causes are decided, and all judgments are given, on the basis of reason, authority, and experience. He then shows that Chiflet's citation of authorities is irrelevant, his interpretation of experience is false because it asserts that the powder has helped no one, and his reasoning is nil. Further, Dr. Fonseca, the papal physician, had investigated the powder at the request of de Lugo and found it harmless and very useful.[17]

As to the letters that Chiflet had received from Madrid and other cities, the question at issue involves not merely the feelings of a few but the experience of many. In a sparkling passage Fabri attacks Chiflet for belittling the value of the "increased interval" (in modern terms, the afebrile period before a relapse) that the drug produced. With equal cleverness he demolishes Chiflet's contention that the drug is unnecessary in Europe; if the bark is not needed, there is also no need of the many other febrifuges, such as theriac, myrrh, and gentian, which Chiflet mentioned without disapproval.[18]

Much as these passages may attract the admiration of logicians and lawyers, the historian reads with equal or greater interest Fabri's seventh chapter, on "the marvelous effects of this powder."[19] Here he writes that in Rome during the recently ended year, 1653, several thousand people were sick with diseases of several kinds. Many died of malignant fever. A much greater number had simple or double quartans; almost all took the powder, which *had first become known at that time*, and the results were good. If he wished, Fabri could mention by name more than a hundred persons who were benefited, including several cardinals, princes, high government officials, and persons of religion.[20]

During these events, Fabri continued, the charity of de Lugo shone forth: he bought the bark at his own expense and distributed it freely to the poor, but only on the advice of physicians, whose prescriptions he requested to see before he would dispense the drug. In Fabri's opinion de Lugo had acted in this way on the advice of leading medical doctors.

To illustrate additionally the beneficial properties of the Peruvian bark, Fabri described his own illness, which he believed to be a simple quartan that had turned into a double quartan and later a triple quartan. The fever was accompanied by chills and by very severe attacks of colicky pain. These symptoms remitted and recurred several times over a period of twenty-two weeks. On at least two occasions the fever ceased soon after the powdered bark had been administered.[21] Fabri was certain that his case demonstrated the treatment for intermittent fever, but the prominence of concomitant colicky pains—their location is not specified—suggests that he may have been suffering from an infection in the biliary or urinary tract.

In his final chapter Fabri presents an original "physical" (iatrophysical) theory of fever, based on the Harveian circulation. On this foundation he erects a pharmacodynamics of the Peruvian febrifuge. He believed that the powder contains particles that *cause* relapses. Such particles could be removed, and relapses avoided, if the bark was subjected to forty or fifty hours of maceration followed by filtration. This new method Fabri suggests to the apothecary of the Collegium Romanum. The discussion ends with an original paraphrase of the *Sched-ula Romana;* this version, surprisingly, fails to embody Fabri's proposed improvement. The book contains as a postcript Chiflet's treatise of 1653, newly reprinted.[22]

Fabri's book shows its author to have had an original mind, both analytical and inventive. The text is a typical piece of pseudonymous seventeenth-century pamphleteering. Whereas Chiflet, as we have seen, defended himself, Fabri defended the Peruvian bark and, by im-plication, the Jesuit order and its achievements. The description of his illness is typical of the times in that the recital is limited to symptoms and omits physical signs. The excursus on fevers shows humoralism giving way to iatrophysical and iatrochemical speculation untested by reference to direct observation. The Latin prose offers delightful hints of Horace, Sallust, and others.

Before the year 1655, as Rompel pointed out,[23] Plempius had writ-ten nothing against the Peruvian bark. In that year, using the pseudo-nym Melippus Protimus, he issued a pamphlet titled (in translation) *Antimus Conygius, Defender of the Peruvian Powder, Repulsed. . . .* In this essay Plempius pseudonymously reviews, chapter by chapter, Fa-bri's pseudonymous pamphlet. A pugnacious tone is heard likewise in the writing of Plempius's pupil Soers; it appears also in many of Plem-pius's publications on other medical subjects.[24]

Plempius points out that Fabri agreed with the admonition in the *Schedula Romana* that the powder should be taken only on the advice of a physician, yet though he admitted he was not a physician, he rec-ommended the drug and dared to write about it.[25]

Plempius reports that all the fever patients in Brussels who were given the bark suffered relapse. Many became cachectic and several died. He cites unfavorable results reported in letters from Paris—where the eminent Dr. René Moreau had declared that the drug was no longer used (*est morte en cette ville*)—also from Ratisbon and several Italian cities, and even from parts of Rome. The statement that Fonseca and others in Rome had had several thousand therapeutic successes is dismissed as "hyperbole." His contentions include occasional vague references to numbers of patients, but nothing is presented that later centuries would accept as genuinely quantitative evidence.[26]

Another conflict involves the interpretation of authority. Fabri had denied the value of citations from ancient and early modern authors, since these men had had no experience with the bark, but Plempius asserts that their testimony and opinions are extremely valuable be-cause they had discussed febrifuges that act in the same manner as the bark and they condemned empirical drugs that leave pyrogenic mate-rial in the body. As to contemporary physicians, the authority of the papal archiater Fonseca is counterbalanced by that of the imperial archiater Johannes Glantz and a royal archiater named Gutterius.[27] Glantz wrote from Ratisbon on May 5, 1653, that all who had taken the American febrifuge suffered relapses; another of Glantz's comments will be discussed when we consider Wolfgang Hoefer.

As we have seen, Chiflet had declared that the bark was not needed in Europe; it merely lengthens the intervals but does not remove the disease. Plempius repeats this opinion and adds that the drug is inherently pernicious.[28]

In the National Library of Medicine the polemical printed tracts by Chiflet and Fabri and a manuscript transcript of Plempius's tract have been bound together in a single volume, which also contains a fourth component. This is an undated manuscript of seventeen eighteen-line pages titled (in English translation): *Reply to the book, The Fever-Powder Discussed, by John Jacob Chiflet, Medical Doctor of the Archduke.*

This manuscript is a reply to Chiflet's attack of 1653. Probably it was composed by a Jesuit whose name was abbreviated Io[hann]es Biss: or was merely transmitted by him.[29] The author states that Chiflet had had insufficient experience with the drug, was in error as to its color and taste, and falsely accused it of astringency, which would sequestrate the peccant humors and lead ultimately to recurrence. In the current year all tertians and quartans, *however they were treated,* relapsed.[30]

This rejoinder evidently was written in 1653 (*hoc anno*). Like Chiflet's pamphlet, it was based on the case of the archduke. The author asks why the powder was not given a second time. The patient was afebrile for thirty-three days after the first dose. The second fever was not a relapse but a new illness.[31]

Two additional matters connected with the manuscript must not escape observation. First, the author had received several doses of the powder from a friend—presumably a Jesuit—who had returned from Italy. If the presumption is correct, it suggests continued functioning of the Jesuit system of distribution, which centered in Rome. Second, it had been asserted that because Europeans possess febrifuges that are safer and better known than Peruvian bark, the bark was unnecessary in Europe. The Jesuit replies: if physicians of the preceding era had argued in this way when guaiac, sassafras, and sarsaparilla were brought to us from the selfsame America—and all these are in very frequent use among us—would you not accuse them of insanity? But the Spaniards were wiser; they brought these things to us, and also gold and silver.[32]

Moreover, the author continues, the other therapeutic measures recommended by Chiflet are impracticable; and his drugs, such as theriac, myrrh, and gentian, are ineffective. The Jesuit author had cured many fever patients with a single dose of the bark, without relapse; other patients responded to a second or third dose. He had even cured some who had been sick for as long as a year and a half.[33]

At this juncture a controversy over religion obtrudes itself. In view of the political, intellectual, social, and ecclesiastical disturbances that were involved in the career of Jansenism—a movement of Belgian origin—during the times of Urban VIII (1623–44) and Innocent X (1644–55), it might be expected that, especially during the latter reign, acceptance of the Jesuits' bark would have been affected. The most that can be said is that notable early opposition to the bark was due to Plempius, who, like Cornelius Jansen, held a professorship at the University of Louvain, and that this university was important in the spread of Jansenist doctrine. However, investigation of primary and secondary sources and correspondence with Belgian scholars have revealed no clear evidence of a relation, either favorable or unfavorable, between the new belief and the still newer drug. A North American historian has written: "When in 1652 the Archduke Leopold of Austria failed to receive a cure [after having taken Jesuits' bark] and rose up in wrath against the drug, one of his chief supporters in a campaign of spite was the renowned professor of medicine at the University of Louvain, Vopiscus Plempius. Louvain was a center of Jansenism, and the tirade against quinine became lost in the larger Jansenist-Jesuit quarrel over predestination versus free will."[34] Unfortunately this statement is undocumented.

A French Jesuit historian states that at this time (the late seventeenth century) the Jesuit pharmacies, with their perfumes, hyacinth, and *quinquina*, played a picturesque role in Jansenist polemics and produced an income that was not negligible.[35]

Denmark, Italy, France, and Germany

The decade extending from 1653 to 1663 can be regarded as the period that ends the early history of the Peruvian bark. From the domain of the Hapsburgs, the site of the polemics that have just been described, the spotlight moves or diffuses to Denmark, Italy, France, and Germany. While empires expanded and contracted, the realm of the bark slowly grew.

The essay by Plempius, issued under the pseudonym Melippus Protimus, reproduces a letter dated Ratisbon (now Regensburg), May 5, 1653. It was addressed to Chiflet by Johannes Gregorius Glantz, physician to the Holy Roman emperor. This letter commends Chiflet's essay and at the same time reports that all of the patients Glantz had treated with the bark had suffered relapses. No information about place, time, season, or numbers is provided.[36]

On June 25, 1654, Heinrich von Moinichen, a Schleswig surgeon, informed his ex-teacher Thomas Bartholinus that one Joel Langelottus of Gottorp, physician to the Duke of Holstein, had sent Moinichen information about the Peruvian bark. The brief letter mentions the opinions of Chiflet and the danger that the drug (here called "gannaperide") might cause compaction of the ferment responsible for quartan fever.[37] The reader will observe that this comment transfers the alleged risk of compaction from humors to ferments.

Also in 1654, Thomas Bartholinus described an outbreak of what he called epidemic tertian fever. The sickness had occurred in and near Copenhagen in the summer of 1652. Among the features were delirium, hemorrhagic spots, and buboes. The horn of the Greenland unicorn (narwhal) was used in treatment. There is no mention of the Peruvian bark.[38]

Seven years later, in 1661, Bartholinus published a brief essay, "The Febrifugal Peruvian Powder." The text begins with the well-tempered statement that in recent years the bark of a Peruvian tree had reached Europe. Its powder is proclaimed to be very effective against tertian and quartan fevers.[39] Bartholinus included with his comment a Latin translation of the *Schedula Romana* (see Appendix B) and a picture of the Peruvian tree, obtained from Hieronymus Bardus through the mediation of Bartholinus's ex-pupil, Heinrich von Moinichen.[40] Bartholinus also excerpted the books by Chiflet and Fabri and added that he had tested the drug in a case of quartan fever, without successful result. The report shows the late arrival of the bark in Copenhagen.[41] It illustrates Bartholinus's diligence in the collection and dissemination of new knowledge and demonstrates his progressiveness, defeated in this instance by what we can now recognize as the procedural inadequacy of basing a clinical opinion on a single observation.

In 1654, the year of von Moinichen's communication with Thomas Bartholinus, Pietro Castelli (ca. 1570–1661), professor of botany in Rome, published *Chemical Response on Effervescence and Change of Colors*, which has been considered a treatise on the Peruvian bark and hence the earliest to appear under Italian authorship.[42] Not having seen this book, I am obliged to rely on commentators, both of whom were well qualified. Rompel pronounced the work a *Pseudo-China-schrift*, or false chinological text; he found no evidence that Castelli had ever had in his hand a piece of the bark or a dose of the powder. To this

condemnation Haggis added evidence that Castelli had possessed
seeds of Peruvian balsam about 1623 and later confused them with cinchona.[43]

Castelli's book being disqualified, the Italian crown must go to Fabri's (Conygius's) *Pulvis febrifugus vindicatus* of 1655. I have discussed
this contribution and also the prompt riposte of Plempius, disguised
under the pseudonym Melippus Protimus.

Attention now shifts to Genoa.[44] From this city, in the year 1656,
Sebastianus Baldus—who later changed his surname to Badus, which
I will use henceforth—issued his *Cortex Peruviae redivivus*. This publication is a direct sequel to the controversy of Chiflet, Fabri, and Plemp.
In fact, it is a transalpine extension of hostilities. To change the
metaphor, Badus's book puts the problem back in the historical main-
stream.

Badus was born at an unknown date subsequent to 1600 and was
alive and gouty in 1676.[45] He studied medicine in Pisa under Sinibaldi
and Stephanus Castrensis (Esteban Rodrigo de Castro),[46] a physician
praised by Zacutus Lusitanus. In 1651–52 he practiced medicine in the
highly malarious city of Rome. With Pietro Paolo Puccerini, apothecary of the Collegium Romanum, he established a contact that was to
last at least a decade, and he knew Juan de Lugo even before 1643,
when the latter became a cardinal. In the opinion of Rompel it is not
certain that Badus ever served as de Lugo's physician. According to his
own statement Badus first learned of the Peruvian bark while he was in
Rome, that is, in 1651 or 1652, his informant being the Reverend Federicus Conti, a Genoese priest.[47]

In 1652 Badus returned to Genoa, where he became physician to the
Pammatone Hospital and one other large hospital and, in addition, had
municipal administrative responsibilities. Convinced of the value of
the bark, he introduced it on a large scale, with great success.

He now intended, as he tells us, to write an extensive book against
Chiflet, antagonist of the Peruvian drug, but he suspended this plan in
order to write a book against the more recent work issued by a supporter of Chiflet (i.e., Plempius, masquerading as Melippus Protimus).
Badus intended the title of his new little book, *The Peruvian Bark Revived*, to counteract the Plempian sneer that the obsequies of the bark
were being celebrated.[48]

Two of the ten chapters of texts are especially valuable to the historian. Chapter 5 refers to the experiences of Dr. Gabriele Fonseca, papal
archiater, and Cardinal de Lugo; the latter had communicated the facts
about the bark directly to Badus in Rome (*primus ipse met Romae vul-
gatus*). Chapter 6 says:

In the public hospital where I practice medicine I saw it [the sickness] yield happily in all who took the bark, those who had been seized by quartans as well as those who had tertians or mixed fevers. I saw this more than a hundred times; and I saw more, the destiny and power of this wonderful medicine never changed. I know that these things happened within one and a half or two years at the most. Day after day new experiences and events, always happy, are always being observed. I saw this in the overcrowded public hospital, as did three colleagues who, with me, take care of treatment at the same place. All the attendants who were with us saw it . . . all were astonished that those fevers, against which all medicine put together is usually unavailing, could stop so quickly—virtually in a moment. I saw six or seven patients at most who had relapses. Usually they were restored by diet alone. In one or two the bark was repeated and health was regained completely. The drug constantly dispersed the remains of the fever. In that same hospital I now have in my hands a dropsical man with quartan fever and huge visceral obstruction. The bark was given to him and—a wonderful thing!—it immediately destroyed the fever. The dropsy, usually fatal, did not impede the strength and power of the bark.[49]

To this thrilling recital Badus subjoined an alphabetical list of Genoese physicians who had witnessed the power of the new drug. His narrative is obviously correct. It recounts events that were proceeding at the time the record was written. The experiences described are not the earliest trial of the new drug; as Badus tells us, the trials conducted by Fonseca—never recorded directly, but mentioned by Badus, Fabri, and Plempius,[50]—came earlier. Until further documentary discoveries are made, the account given by Badus is the earliest large trial recorded by the principal participant and bolstered by anything approaching quantitative information.

The cinchonal affairs narrated by Badus are centered in Rome and Genoa. Another Italian city for which data are extant is Milan. Again, Badus serves as a source of information.[51] In the *Anastasis* he reproduced a letter dated October 22, 1658, written by six Milanese physicians, one of whom was Christophoro Paravicino, *physicus* of the College of Physicians of Milan. This document states that the Peruvian bark had been brought to Milan "many years before" (*multis ab hinc annis*); the first to try it were some Jesuits in the College of Brera[52] who suffered from quartan fever. The authors of the letter then used the drug for ten years, with good results. The Brera pharmacy still exists, and its early records are extant.[53] It is obvious that the early history of the febrifugal bark in Milan, like its history in Rome and Genoa, shows the effect of Jesuit organization and influence.

Approximately contemporaneous with the first developments in Milan and more exactly contemporaneous with the *Cortex . . . redivivus* (1656) is a thesis presented in Paris by Franciscus Bovonier under the aegis of Daniel Arbinet. Rompel has characterized this work as devoid of relevance and substance.[54]

Probably earlier than the thesis of Bovonier is another work that bears the same publication date, 1656, but contains licenses dated 1652 and 1653. This is the *Noctes geniales, annus primus* of Johannes Nardi (ca. 1580–ca. 1655).[55] According to Haller the author was a learned Florentine.[56] Included among his conversations, which are reminiscent of Aulus Gellius, is a discussion of "the recent Chinese [*sic*] febrifuge." It yields, despite Nardi's unenthusiastic tone, the important implication that as early as 1652–53 the success of the new drug in at least occasional cases was great enough to lead to discussion about the progress of medicine, present and future.

In 1657, Wolfgang Hoefer (1614–81), a Bavarian physician who rose to the rank of Viennese *Hofrath*, published his valuable encyclopedia, titled *Hercules medicus*. This work contains a discussion of quartan fever which embodies a statement derived from Joannes Glantz, an Austrian imperial medical councillor and archiater,[57] whose letter of 1653 was mentioned earlier in this chapter. Rompel considered Glantz's statement in *Hercules medicus* (1657) to be the earliest Austrian mention of the bark.[58]

There is at least one obstacle to Rompel's interpretation. The statement by Glantz that is included in the book by Plempius and is discussed above is not relevant to Austrian priority, since it was written from Ratisbon in Bavaria, and the statement in Hoefer's book is a list of alleged febrifuges recommended by Glantz and reads as follows: *centaur. min. theriaca, arcanum duplicatum Minsichtij, Rad. China Chinae,*[59] *a ʒss. ad ʒii in vino (quae nihil aliud esse videtur, quam gentiana Indica frutex)*. Taken literally, this statement refers not to cinchona but to chinaroot, that is, Smilax. It is possible, but quite improbable, that the imperial medical councillor confounded a root with a bark. Yet the same statement quite evidently refers to a plant that was new and unfamiliar to Glantz, and chinaroot is more than likely to have been known to him. We must therefore reject Rompel's verdict and limit ourselves instead to a suspension of judgment on this minutia.

About 1654 the Spanish ambassador to the Hague received from Archduke Leopold a gift of Peruvian bark. Rolandus Sturmius, a native of Louvain and a medical alumnus of Bologna, was requested to give an opinion on this controversial drug.[60] His initial reluctance was caused by unfamiliarity with its properties, but he soon found his motivation augmented and his inexperience overcome by a large outbreak of quartan fever in 1657–58 in Delft, where he practiced medicine.

His book, published in 1659, is soundly based on his experiences and a memorable defense of the bark. It mentions Chiflet, Melippus

Protimus (Plempius), and other opponents and combatants and does not suppress their contentions.

While it does not bypass controversy, its tone is mainly not polemical, nor are its expressions vituperative. It supplies incidental historical information such as the fact, of which I find no record elsewhere, that Father François de Cleyn of Mechlin during four years as rector—no date is given—treated successfully, by means of the powder, at least fifty persons who suffered from tertian and quartan fever.[61] The significance of this fragmentary remark, completely credible although unconfirmed, lies in the fact that since the sixteenth century Mechlin (remembered by our allies as Malines) has been the ecclesiastical capital of Belgium and the seat of its primary archbishopric. Hence the drug, if it was being conveyed by a priest, would have followed the route of religion rather than that of commerce. Also mentioned by Sturmius, but without much useful detail, are favorable statements from a Dr. Julius Doniatus and from Jacob Savernel; the latter had treated several quartans successfully with the bark in Louvain.[62] Hence at this early time the drug had reached several of the major cities of Belgium.

Sturmius records the interesting fact that in Brussels in March 1658, twenty doses of the bark were priced at 60 florins, but the supply had been exhausted. He mentions also the difficulty of determining from which plant the drug was obtained.[63] To this he adds his opinion, based on abundant observation, that the bark has a peculiar febrifugal property not found in other febrifuges, especially with respect to tertians and quartans, and that the power of the drug is not attributable to its temperament alone.[64] This conclusion obviously signifies a weakening of traditions dominant for many centuries.

Transcending these considerations in importance is the fact that an entire section of Sturmius's book (*pars prior, sectio quinta*), running to thirty-two pages, is devoted to a series of thirteen case reports.[65] These histories do not omit to mention relapses and other difficulties. They show Sturmius groping toward establishment of an optimal dosage and at the same time attempting to follow the *Schedula Romana* as strictly as possible.[66] Except in one trying and confused case, two drachms of the powdered bark usually sufficed, but relapses were frequent, though usually tractable. Sturmius dispensed the drug gratis.

Sturmius's book reproduces the *Schedula Romana*, both in the original Italian and in Latin translation. Of this important document he says that the authorities in Rome are so strict that they would not have allowed it to be printed unless proper investigation had been made.[67]

The second part of Sturmius's book, slightly smaller than the first, deals with the way in which the bark acts.[68] Believing that it dissolves the febrile humor, he speculated as to the mechanism of solution, according to particulate hypotheses; he reflected also about the possible source of the activity involved. At the same time he found himself in agreement with statements made by Antimus Conygius (Fabri) in the contest with Melippus Protimus (Plempius).

Sturmius's treatise has the great merit of presenting a series of cases, which it discusses individually and in something like adequate detail. Therefore, although his experience was notably smaller than that described by Badus in 1656, his contribution is at least as interesting and instructive.

His book, a major achievement bearing the date 1659, must not cause us to overlook a small but significant item also composed in that year. This is a letter written in Rome on October 4, 1659, by Cardinal de Lugo to Sebastianus Badus. It appears as the first item after the laudatory prolegomena in Badus's *Anastasis*, which did not emerge in print until 1663. This letter was discussed in Chapter 1 and receives additional attention subsequently.

The cardinal's letter, which runs to twenty-two lines in the Latin version, acknowledges the receipt of Badus's [Baldus's] earlier volume seven years previously (it bears the publication date 1656) and states that physicians were using the bark indiscriminately for quartan and tertian intermittents, and even in continued fevers, and were seeing marvelous results. In consequence of frequent demand the bark was becoming scarce in Rome. "As for that which is on sale, I do not know if it can be protected from the danger of being adulterated, as usually happens with other expensive and foreign drugs." This cardinalatial sentence summarizes and explains much of the early history of cinchona and is specially applicable to a proportion of the failures. We may note also that while the value of the bark was being contested in Belgium, the supply in that country had been exhausted, while the supply in Rome was being threatened with both exhaustion and adulteration.

In 1659, the year in which the book by Sturmius was published and in which de Lugo sent his letter to Badus, significant developments were occurring in England. These are considered in Chapter 4, although strict chronology would require their inclusion at this point.

In 1661 Gaudentius Brunacius (1631–69) issued *On China china or the fever powder, a physiologic treatise.*[69] This work was published in Venice. The author directed the Hospital of the Holy Spirit in Rome and tested the drug there. At an unspecified time ("many years ago"),[70] he had been cured, by means of the same drug, of a double tertian intermittent that had dragged on for thirty days. Brunacius's book provides a few incidental historical details, such as the statement, cited above, that the bark had been brought to Rome in 1650 by Jesuits attending a jubilee, had been tested by de Lugo in a great many trials, and had gained a large reputation and price.[71] The treatise exemplifies well the botanical confusion and taxonomic perplexity prevalent with respect to the Peruvian tree from which the bark was obtained.[72] Brunacius's great experience was based on a large and famous hospital.[73] The reader is not told whether the patients were ambulatory or confined; the simultaneous distributions of the drug at the Collegio Romano and those conducted by Cardinal de Lugo are likely to have been for ambulatory patients and for persons treated at home.

Brunacius held the drug in high esteem. Regarding its efficacy as a well-established fact, he made no attempt to prove *that* it worked; he was interested in *why* it worked. He was concerned chiefly to determine its temperament, properties, and actions, interpreted in accordance with Galenic criteria.

He accepted the dictum that the bark is hot and dry. Prepared in strict accord with the method of the *Schedula*, it must not be given until the patient has been purged repeatedly: as was evident from the writings of Galen and Hippocrates, coction must be achieved first, then the peccant humors could be removed through any channel; many kinds of fever could be cured in this way.[74]

Unlike Sturmius, Brunacius did not present a series of case histories, although many were at his disposal. Instead, he regressed to scholastic argumentation, of which he offers a plethora. But this culminates in empiricist opinions quoted from Valeriola, Hippocrates, Stobaeus, and others, and he mentions with special approval some pragmatic comments of Caesar, Cicero, and Fernel.[75] The Belgian polemics of Chiflet and Plemp are not even mentioned. The contrast between new clinical facts and old doctrines employed for their interpretation did not elude the vigilant Rompel.[76]

During 1656–63 the Peruvian bark, contrary to the lugubrious prophecy of Plempius, failed to die. Indeed, as we have observed, it was the subject of books, letters, and notes, large or small, written *inter alios* by Nardi, de Lugo, and Brunacius in Italy, by Hoefer and Glantz in Austria, by Sturmius in Holland, by Rothmann in Germany, and by von Moenichen, Langelottus, and Thomas Bartholinus in Schleswig and Denmark.

The description in Chapter 1 of this history of the legend of the countess of Chinchon as it appears in the *Anastasis* of Sebastianus Badus (1663) hinted at perplexities associated with that narrative, even in its earliest recorded version. After a long but necessary interruption devoted to other considerations and to many countries, it was necessary, in preceding pages of the present chapter, to return to Badus, to tell of his earliest years, and to report his earliest achievements, including his *Cortex Peruviae redivivus* (1656).

As the reader may remember, Badus returned from Rome to his native Genoa in 1652 and planned to write immediately a large book against Chiflet, an influential enemy of the Peruvian bark. But the distractions of plague, private misery, and public office caused him to swerve, and he found himself publishing instead a shorter work against the violent Plempius (Melippus Protimus). This is the *Cortex Peruviae redivivus* of 1656.

By 1663, the febrifugal bark of Peru had gained acceptance widely but incompletely. The Chifletio-Plempian disturbance was still producing aftershocks that could not be ignored. So much is evident even in the title and subtitle of Badus's new book, published in 1663, the *Anastasis*, which can be rendered as "Resurrection of Peruvian Bark, or, the Defense of China-china, by Sebastianus Badus of Genoa . . . against the Diatribes of John Jacob Chiflet and the Bellowing of Vopiscus Fortunatus Plemp, Eminent Physicians." The book and some of its implications are discussed in Chapters 1 and 2.

In 1667, four years after Badus published his important *Anastasis*, a febrile disease broke out among the inhabitants of Leyden. Franciscus de le Boë Sylvius (1614–1672), the noted clinician and devoted iatrochemist, described the sickness as an intermittent fever that had changed from single to double, the paroxysms occurring on alternate days.[77] Despite the progress that the Peruvian bark had made in many parts of Europe, this drug is not mentioned by the tenacious iatrochemist. It had not displaced its predecessors, and such was to be the state of affairs for many decades. In his remarks on the treatment of tertian fever Sylvius wrote that to achieve a quick, safe, and pleasant cure the physician should use *vitrum* of antimony, or the crocus of metals [mixed oxides], or *mercurius vitae*.[78] The Jesuits' bark is not mentioned, Sylvius being far from the last to cast the old aside.

At approximately the same time, Frederick Dekkers (1648–1720), another Batavian, reported a case of quartan fever in which cure was obtained by venesection alone and another case in which Peruvian bark had been used unsuccessfully ("*frustraneo eventu*").[79] Events of this kind are not surprising to the physician or the historian; they warn us to expect no happy record of uninterrupted triumph.

In addition to publishing his own observations, Dekkers edited those of Barbette, who listed as "medicines against Feavors" approximately thirty items, which included the bark of China along with the roots of masterwort, plantain, and dandelion.[80] This compilation shows that cinchona competed not only with iatrochemical products but also with galenicals and miscellaneous botanical preparations.

As to the debut of the Peruvian bark in Dutch and Belgian pharmacopoeias, a small quantity of positive and negative information is available. The drug is not mentioned in pharmacopoeias of 1636, 1656, 1659, or 1660.[81] Mr. W. K. Gnirrep, of the library of the Dutch Society for the Promotion of Medicine, has written that the *cortex kinae kinae* is not listed in an undated edition of the *Pharmacopoea Amstelredamensis* (ca. 1701) but mention has been added in manuscript. Mr. Gnirrep adds: "As it [cortex chinae chinae] is mentioned in the Dutch translation of the Pharmacopoea, published in 1683, I suppose that the Latin edition of 1682, still unknown, should be the first to contain the substance."[82] The drug is included in the Haarlem pharmacopoeia of 1693.[83]

In a later chapter it is shown that quotations of Peruvian bark did not begin to appear in the monthly (and sometimes weekly) business reports from Amsterdam until 1777, almost a century after the earliest entry in the Amsterdam pharmacopoeia.

In 1696 the widely traveled physician, chemist, and historian, Johann Conrad Barkhausen (designated in his Dutch publications as Barckhausen), issued in Utrecht the second edition of his pharmaceutical treatise, the *Pharmacopeus synopticus.* It includes the recipe for an antipyretic powder (which is presented as a curiosity, *curiositatis gratia*): antimony, the salt of hartshorn (presumably ammoniacal), and *China chinae.*[84]

4 England after 1650

In 1651 the sixteenth edition of Robert Burton's *Anatomy of Melancholy* appeared; it was a posthumous version of an immortal work. In discussing cures for countless major and minor symptoms the author mentioned a diapason of drugs, including even "the decoction of guiacum [*sic*], china [almost certainly chinaroot, i.e., Smilax or sarsaparilla], salsaperilla, sassafras"; nor did he overlook "our new London Pharmacopoeia."[1] Burton said nothing whatever about the Peruvian bark. His book can therefore be taken as a *terminus a quo* or a chronologic remote control.

On December 30, 1670, Dr. Robert Brady wrote to Thomas Sydenham that "for twenty years (more or less) I have myself used the bark."[2] This gives us the approximate date of 1650, close to the time of Burton's sixteenth editon.

In 1785, Sir George Baker, famed for his research on lead poisoning, added to his laurels by publishing his "Observations on the Late Intermittent Fevers; to which is added a Short History of the Peruvian Bark." In this extensive and valuable essay, Baker wrote, "We may collect from Sydenham that it [the Peruvian bark] began to be in vogue" in England about the year 1655, but that after a short time the more prudent physicians were deterred from its use, in part because of occasional fatalities.[3] One of the relatively conspicuous victims was an alderman, who died in 1658. In a later passage of his essay, Baker reported "no reason to suppose that it [the bark] was, about this time, declining in its reputation, or sinking into disuse."[4]

In addition, Baker pointed out that in 1658 a London newspaper, the *Mercurius Politicus*, advertised that a quantity of powdered Jesuits' bark was for sale. More extensive review, involving also the *Publick In-*

telligencer, has revealed six advertisements, all of which appeared in 1658 and 1659.[5] A typical example, taken from *Mercurius Politicus* no. 422, June 24 to July 1, 1658, reads as follows:

These are to give notice, that the excellent powder known by the name of the Jesuits Powder, which cureth all manner of Agues, Quotidian, Tertian or Quartan, brought over by James Tompson[6] Merchant of Antwerp, is to be had at the Black-Spred-Eagle over against Black and white Court in the Old Baily, or at the shop of Mr. John Crook, at the sign of the ship in St. Pauls Churchyard, a Bookseller, with directions for using of the same.

The notices in *Mercurius Politicus* no. 545 (December 9–16, 1658) and no. 553 (February 3–10, 1659) include this statement: "Which Bark or Powder is attested to be perfectly true by Doctor [Francis] Prujean, and other eminent Doctors and Physitians who have made experience of it." No. 553 subjoins: "This is done to prevent future mistakes." It is not known whether persistence of the announcements during a period of almost eight months indicates large demand or small sales, a single shipment from Antwerp or repeated shipments.

Concerning James Tompson Merchant of Antwerp, Mme. Denise Reyniers-Defourny of the Stadsarchief of Antwerp has kindly informed me that the Cathedral of Antwerp (Onze Lieve Vrouw Zuid) records successively the baptism of a daughter and two sons of Jacobus Thompson and Maria Anna Robijns. The oldest of the three entries (November 26, 1652) adds that one of the *susceptores* at the baptism was "Guillielmus Willems nomine D. Edward Somerset Marchionis de Woester."[7] This is significant because Edward Somerset, sixth earl and second marquis of Worcester (1601–67), was a leading Roman Catholic layman and suffered persecution for his religion. Indeed, he was a prisoner in the Tower of London from July 28, 1652, to October 5, 1654.[8] Obviously, therefore, he could not have appeared in person on November 26, 1652, at the baptism of James Tompson's oldest child.

These minutiae show that the best-known early transmittal of Jesuits' bark to England was achieved by Roman Catholics via Belgium.[9] That Tompson's was not the only or the earliest shipment during this period is suggested by a letter that P. P. Puccerini, apothecary of the Collegium Romanum, wrote to Sebastianus Badus on April 5, 1659, stating that couriers and others had taken the drug from Rome to many places, such as Piedmont, England, Flanders, and Germany.[10] The routes of shipment implied in the statements of Sydenham, discussed below, have not been discovered but might perhaps be revealed by search in the records of apothecaries and in commercial records such as the London Port Books.[11] My correspondence in 1985 with appropriate authorities does not suggest that the archives of the English

Province of the Society of Jesus are a promising source of additional information, but an energetic and conscientious investigator might be rewarded by interesting discoveries.

The eminence of Sir Francis Prujean (1593–1666), president and treasurer of the Royal College of Physicians, is incontestable. There are no grounds for assuming that he either approved or disapproved the use of his name in Tompson's newspaper advertisement. I have found no mention of Prujean's opinions with respect to the Peruvian bark, and no reason to suppose that he was connected with either the Roman Catholic Church or the Jesuit order. The bookdealer John Crooke, who sold the bark in his bookshop, made a minor entry in the history of medicine: he published two editions of Sydenham's *Methodus curandi febres* (1666 and 1668).[12] William Crooke, believed to be his nephew, printed a book on "Jesuites powder."[13] These bits of antiquarianism might well inspire an investigation into possible relations between the English trade in books and that in drugs and other items.

As we have seen, the best-known transmittal of the Jesuits' bark to England was achieved by Roman Catholics via Belgium. This incident or series of incidents fits exactly the statements made by a Belgian historian, Adrien de Meeüs.[14] In his judgment the Society of Jesus was so important in Belgium that the country became a sort of Jesuit empire and was the actual center of the society for northern Europe. He notes that about the middle of the seventeenth century there were 1,574 Jesuits in Belgium, compared with only 2,000 in the whole of France and 2,283 in all of Germany.

When James Tompson was advertising the availability of Jesuits' bark, the English nation observed, with pain or joy, the death of Oliver Cromwell (1599–1658). The history was reviewed, recently and instructively, by the late Dr. L. J. Bruce-Chwatt, the eminent malariologist.[15] Cromwell had spent many years in the malarious cretaceous lowlands of Huntingdon, Cambridgeshire. Bruce-Chwatt concluded that although Cromwell had had malaria and other febrile diseases, his death was due to stone and infection in the urinary tract. The same scholarly scientist has rejected as unconfirmed the statement that Cromwell had been given Peruvian bark and the rival statement that he had refused the drug as a "Popish remedy."[16]

Appendix A devotes attention to Thomas Willis's concepts of fever. We must consider here what Willis wrote about the Jesuits' bark. This drug does not appear in his casebook of 1650–52.[17] In the first edition of Willis's "De febribus" (1659) the chapter on tertian fever contains no mention of the bark, but the chapter on quartan fever reports in its final sentence the use of a powder made from a bark obtained in the Indies: "It is said [*perhibetur*] to cure this disease most certainly; its property or action consists only in this, that it suppresses the attacking febrile paroxysms without any kind of evacuation." The placement and brevity of this sentence suggest that it was an afterthought, which is approximately compatible with the interpretation of Baker that in the "De febribus" of 1659 Willis "seems to acknowledge that at that time he had no experience of it [the Jesuits' bark]."[18]

The "De febribus" of 1660 tells a somewhat different story. Here, in the fourth chapter, on tertian fever, a final paragraph has been inserted for discussion of obstinate cases.[19] In its last sentence Willis states that febrifugal applications may be made at the wrists and soles, and a powder of Peruvian bark or a substitute, or even the bark of the ash, or tamarisk, or gentian, admixed with salt, may be given in white wine.

A much larger change appears in the sixth chapter, which discusses quartan fever. Here the last sentence of the earlier text (which ends with the words *paroxysmos febriles ingruentes inhibeat*) is followed by an important new inclusion. Willis now states that the powder of a bark recently brought from the Indies has gained approval. It cures very certainly not only quartans but also other intermittents; however, its power or action is unaccompanied by evacuation and consists only in suppression of oncoming paroxysms. Recently it has come into daily use. Willis explains the dosage and administration of the drug and mentions occasional relapses, which occur especially when reduced dosage has been employed. While he remarks that hardly one patient in a hundred has taken the drug in vain, he also gives the discordant impression that the bark, however helpful, is really a suppressant of symptoms and not a fundamental cure.[20]

Admitting inability to explain its action, Willis offers some "theses" or propositions based on carefully assembled observations (*a phaenomenis diligenter collatis*) in the hope that they will at least be a step forward. The bark acts in the blood, not the viscera. Its persistence in the blood depends on dosage. The particles of drug combine with the blood and circulate with it. Part of the ingested dose is retained in the body, where it remains active for a long time. The drug acts differently from other febrifuges.

The explanation, unsurprisingly, is based on the actions of particles and at the same time invokes concepts of fermentation. Willis says that when particles of ingested drug are mixed with blood, they force the blood into a certain new fermentation, which continuously agitates it and prevents it from accumulating dregs or feverish swellings. When the particles of drug have gone away entirely, the previous bad tendency of the blood reappears. The power of the drug is related to its bitterness, a property found also in other "antidotes," such as gentian.

As has been stated, these addenda in the fourth and sixth chapters

of the *Diatribae* are found in the second edition (1660). They are reproduced, almost verbatim, in the third edition of 1662. Since they do not
appear in the first edition (1659), there are no grounds for believing
that Willis used the bark to any great extent at an earlier time.

In his edition of Willis's casebook of 1650–52, cited above, Dewhurst traced, in an interesting and convincing manner, Willis's slow
transition from Galenism to iatrochemistry. In the same work he asserted that "by the mid-1650's Willis had considerable experience of
the 'powder of Peruvian bark' and when discussing the treatment of
quartan fevers he gives details of its preparation and use. . . . When
writing in 1657 he had obviously had considerable experience . . . as
he mentioned that 'scarce one of a hundred had tryed this Medicine'
in vain." According to Dewhurst's footnotes, the passages just quoted
are based on Pordage's translation, *The Remaining Works of . . . Dr.
Thomas Willis*, which appeared in 1681.[21] Pordage presents in English
a version of the "De febribus" identical with the one that appeared in
Latin in 1660 and 1662 and that, as I have shown above, contains material added *since* 1659. If, as Dewhurst says, Willis had great experience of powdered Peruvian bark by the mid-1650s, it is difficult to explain why the "De febribus" of 1659 omits all mention of the drug in
the chapter on tertian fever and offers no more than part of a sentence
about it in the discussion of quartans.

It should be noted that the text of the "De febribus" in the editions
of 1660 and 1662, which contains material added after the edition of
1659, reappears unaltered, except for typographical peccadilloes, in
the *Opera omnia* of 1681 and hence presumably embodies Willis's latest recorded opinions about the bark.

Willis's *Pharmaceutice rationalis* appeared in 1674 and 1675.[22] This
work opens with the incontestable judgment or platitude that the actions of drugs, and the localization of these actions, are not understood.
The third chapter of section 5 reminds us that our life is in constant
flux, hence new things must be added and old things taken away. The
reader thus admonished is dismayed to discover that the innumerable
recipes that adorn the book contain no mention of the Jesuits' bark. A
possible explanation is that the treatise contains no section on fever,
although it discusses sweating and diaphoretics.

The preface to the "De febribus" shows that Willis's incredulity toward humoralist doctrine was related to Harvey's discovery of the circulation. In the same preface there is, again, no mention of the Peruvian bark. These facts suggest—but, of course, do not prove—that *in
the weakening of belief in humoralism—a major change that was occurring at about this time—the role of the new drug was the less powerful,
just as it was also the later, of the two historical influences.*

Whatever their exact chronology, Willis's opinions about intermittent fevers and about the Peruvian bark are at once a prototype and a parallel to the generality of informed thought in his time. Especially striking are the gradual transition from Galenism to newer systems, and, in the case of the bark, the transition from apathy, caution, or skepticism to guarded acceptance.

We have now arrived at the year 1663, noteworthy because of Badus's *Anastasis*, already discussed, and also because it is the year selected by Richard Morton as marking the time when the Jesuits' bark was established.[23] On this point we can certainly accept the opinion of Morton, since he had been in very active medical practice. At the same time it must be recognized that commercial records such as the port books of London and other cities probably contain much valuable information about the quantities of bark that entered England and may reveal when importation reached large dimensions.

The career and contributions of Sir Robert Talbor (or Tabor, 1642?–1681) are important in the history of Peruvian bark and afford much insight into the medical manners and standards of the time. In part because of his unconventional behavior, self-promotional flamboyance, and great financial and social success, he was denounced as a quack. As Sir William Osler is reputed to have said, "The trouble with quacks is that they cure people."[24]

It is now known, partly through the researches of Sir George Baker,[25] that Talbor was apprenticed to an apothecary in Cambridge, from whom he obtained some pharmaceutical experience with the behavior of the Peruvian bark, and that he studied at St. John's College, Cambridge, beginning in 1663. In 1671 he removed to Essex, which was highly malarious, and apparently tested various preparations of the new drug. There are, most unfortunately, no records of this preliminary work. Talbor then set up practice in London, where he soon had a large clientele. He treated King Charles II for ague,[26] and he also treated members of the French and Spanish royal families. Louis XIV, having bought his secret remedy for a large sum of money, ordered the pharmaceutical method published.

Robert G. Latham states, apparently on the authority of Baker, that Talbor used the drug with success and confidence as early as 1666.[27] A book on agues, intended for laymen, appeared under Talbor's name in 1672. Together with some elementary explanations of the different kinds of fever, it contains the statement that the ague is a lump of vomited matter![28]

In February 1680 the *London Gazette* advertised that "the infallible Medicine of Sir *Robert Talbor,* for cure of Agues and Feavours, being in his absence rightly prepared by his Brother . . . is to be had when he is

out of Town, at Mr. Lords a Barber in St. Swithings-lane. . . . The price
a Guinea two doses."[29] It should not be assumed that this advertisement was an impropriety by seventeenth-century standards. In his
Chronicles of Pharmacy A. C. Wooton mentions a handbill dated con-
jecturally at 1675 in which Dr. Charles Goodall offered "for the public
good a very superior sort of Jesuit's Bark, ready powdered, and papered
into doses" at 4 shillings per ounce.[30] Goodall, who will reappear in
this history, was a censor, a defender, and subsequently a president, of
the College of Physicians, and obviously a man of very high repute.

Talbor's most important writing, which appeared posthumously and
was titled *The English Remedy*, tells of "quinquina . . . which we have
had knowledg of for about thirty years." This book cites important
predecessors and important differences of opinion. The comments on
Willis are judicious and unimpeachably logical. Talbor goes on to say
that "it is an error in Physick to make a hodge-podge of many ingredients . . . to satisfie one and the same indication; and therefore as Quinquina . . . is without contradiction the surest of all simple Febrifuges,
so is it the only basis of the English Remedy." Thus the veil of secrecy
was lifted.[31]

As we have seen, early in his career Talbor carried out what today
would be called field trials of the Peruvian bark. We do not know
whether he included in his procedure anything resembling a control,
nor are we warranted in supposing that he kept statistics. Later he en-
gaged in random observation under urban conditions in England and
France. We do not know from which sources he obtained the bark, but
his supplies must have been genuine and potent. He combined medical
knowledge with greater pharmaceutical expertness than ordinary physicians are likely to have possessed, and his successes helped to support
the reputation of the drug at a time when, according to some but not
all observers, it was flagging. His experiences illustrate, for not the first
or the second time, the role of eminent personages in the history of the
bark.

There are many written evidences that Talbor's intelligent adventures influenced the use of the drug. Of these we may select, and the
reader may wish to examine, the comments of Carlo Ricani and those
of Jacobo de Castro Sarmento and the judicious verdict of Sir George
Baker.[32] The commendation of Talbor by the naturalist John Ray is
considered later.

In the opinion of Dr. Donald Bates, Thomas Sydenham began to
practice medicine in Westminster about 1656.[33] In 1659 or thereabouts
Robert Brady (1627?–1700), Sydenham's colleague and correspondent, began to use Jesuits' bark.[34] Also in 1659, Willis issued the first
edition of his "De febribus," which, as we have seen, limits its comment

on the bark to a few lines. A greatly amplified comment appears in the edition of 1660. It will be remembered also that Richard Morton would later judge that by 1663 the drug had become established[35] and that, in the same year, Talbor was admitted as a sizar to St. John's College in Cambridge and Badus issued the important *Anastasis.*

In 1666, three years after these events, Sydenham published the first edition of his *Methodus curandi febres propriis observationibus superstructa* (Method of Treating Fevers, Based on Original Observations). The pyretologic doctrines in this book are discussed in Appendix A. Of drugs to be used for the cure of intermittent fever Sydenham says, "Meanwhile I consider the problem to be quite difficult and I have no doubt that it is dangerous. The powder (which they call Jesuits') furnishes a clear example. Although by using it we may be able to suppress the fermentation temporarily, the leftovers which should be dispelled in fermentation soon regain their strength and start a new war against nature." After citing some deaths attributed to administration of the powder immediately before a paroxysm, he adds, "Yet I do not want to deny that medicines of this kind, given wisely and carefully during the decline of such fevers, have sometimes been beneficial and have removed the paroxysms entirely, if they were used in a less epidemic season.[36] In view of the rather lukewarm attitude which Sydenham at this time displayed with respect to the bark, it is not surprising that the review in the *Philosophical Transactions*, written probably by Robert Hooke, fails to mention the drug.[37]

Sydenham's famous *Observationes medicae*[38] of 1676 is regarded as the third edition of his *Methodus curandi.* In this treatise he advised that spring agues "should always be left to themselves, and that they should not be meddled with. No one that I know has ever died of one." Patients suffering from autumnal tertians should be covered with blankets and sweated with a posset before the fit. Then they should be given pills containing aloes and alhandal dissolved in a mixture that contains aqua vitae and treacle.[39] With this, says Sydenham, he had obtained better results than with the usual decoction of gentian and centaury. He does not include the bark among the drugs used in tertian fever.

In the treatment of quartan fevers, Sydenham continues, the only valid drug is the Peruvian bark, and "even this checks rather than conquers them" since its effect is only transitory. Hence the powder should be repeated at short intervals. If the drug is given before the sickness has to some extent worn itself out by its own action, the life of the patient may be endangered.[40] Sydenham's significant comment on the bark as a specific is discussed in Appendix A.

Sydenham states incidentally that autumnal agues in children cannot be dispelled until the abdomen has begun to swell and harden, especially in the neighborhood of the spleen.[41] This comment deserves the attention of immunologists.

Up to this point we have been considering Sydenham's opinions as they are set forth in his *Methodus curandi* (1666) and his *Observationes medicae* (1676). In the epistle to Brady of 1679, Sydenham writes, "The Peruvian bark became my sheet-anchor." This commendation is in sharp contrast with his earlier resistance; further approval is obviously implied in the three recipes for Peruvian bark that appear in the *Processus Integri*. A valuable addendum, summarizing years of observation, occurs unexpectedly in the treatise on gout and dropsy (1683).[42] Here Sydenham writes that dogmatists had "hallucinated" with respect to the essences and cures of diseases. "Of this we have a sufficiently clear instance in the discovery of that great specific for intermittent fevers— the Peruvian bark." He refers also to "the success which attended the use of the bark itself," and adds that "such is the power of the remedy, that . . . the recovery will, generally, take place."

In Sydenham's attitude toward the Jesuits' bark, early cautious reluctance gave way slowly to judicious acceptance. The bias of medicohistorical writing tends to undervalue the undramatic virtue of caution, a trait important in the habitual attitude of the medical practitioner, who probably saves more lives by prudence than by audacity. Yet, if values are to be injected into a historical narrative, we must respect Sydenham's earlier attitudes as well as the opinions that later supplanted them. We must note also, and with interest, that his life's work bore witness to the role of the bark in assisting the decline of humoralism and to the weakening of dogma in general.

Dewhurst has stated that "in England, Willis's *Rational Therapeutics* was the more favoured medical textbook until long after Sydenham's death, when it was superseded by the latter's *Observationes medicae*."[43] The reader who wishes to estimate the extent of Sydenham's influence can easily do so by referring to the *Index-Catalogue*,[44] in which volume 14 of the first series lists forty editions of Sydenham's *Opera Omnia*, plus a plethora of editions of individual writings.

It is not surprising that in his opinions about the Jesuits' bark, however slowly they evolved, Sydenham was in advance of many contemporaries. The drug still had opponents and continued to need defenders.

In 1667, Sir Thomas Browne requested his son, a naval lieutenant, to buy in Cales [Calais?] "a box of the Jesuits powder at easie rate and bring it in the bark, not in powder."[45] The bark is not mentioned in the *Pharmacopoeia Londinensis Collegarum* of 1668. It is listed in the London pharmacopoeia of 1677 and in Salmon's translated and edited pharmacopoeia of 1678. Here Salmon says of *Peruanus*, "If the Colledge mean the Peruvian bark, of which the Jesuites powder is made, it is an Excellent thing against all sorts of Agues. . . . My own experience confirms it, for the Cure of the Rickets: Some suppose it the bark of the Sassafras tree."[46]

At this time, in the year 1678, occurred the death of Andrew Marvell, the poet, satirist, and scholar who bore the high honor of commendation by John Milton. According to Richard Morton, Marvell had intermittent fever and was killed by opium administered by an ignorant and supercilious old doctor who was opposed to the use of the bark.[47] Marvell's case made a common occurrence memorable.

Richard Morton was later to recall that after 1678 the supplies of the drug were adulterated.[48] In 1680, Charles Goodall—mentioned briefly earlier in this chapter—replied to some questions and objections raised by a correspondent.[49] In the concept of fever, Goodall's opinion did not differ radically from that of Sydenham: a *seminium febrile* from the atmosphere perverted part of the body's nutritive juice. In addition Goodall felt that the bark suppressed fermentation but also acted as a diaphoretic and purge; these effects were evidence of its desirability.[50] Recurrence of the fever was not a major objection since even a brief period of apyrexia is beneficial to the patient. Finally, the occurrence of annoying sequelae could not justifiably be attributed to the bark, and "the complaints of a few will bear no ballance with the comendations of many." Moreover, wrote Goodall, "some of the most ingenious of our modern physitians have not only called the Ancients theory into question as highly dissatisfactory to inquisitive men, but their very practice as being unhappily founded upon an erroneous opinion."

Dewhurst has called attention to the fact that Sydenham, in dedicating the *Schedula monitoria* to Goodall, included in the dedicatory letter, dated September 29, 1686, a plea that Goodall undertake extensive clinical observations in order to perfect or correct those that Sydenham had made. In Dewhurst's interpretation it was in response to this Sydenhamian stimulus that Goodall started to assemble information for a book on the Peruvian bark. In this project he was to be helped by John Locke and by Sydenham's young former pupil Hans Sloane.[51] A letter dated July 19–20, 1687, from Goodall to Locke contains questionnaires that were to be used.[52] The undertaking, like many other enterprises of great pith and moment, was abandoned.

Walter Harris (1647–1732), physician to Charles II and to William and Mary and an admirer of Sydenham, was the author of *Pharmacologia anti-empirica* (1683), noteworthy because it exemplifies the conflicts and confusion of opinion that prevailed in the final decades of the seventeenth century. Harris says that many agues can be cured with more safety and no less certainty by means other than the cortex [bark], yet

> that man must be very ignorant in modern practice, or very sowre in his natural temper, or must wish but little to the good of people, who will still deny the cortex to be a very extraordinary remedy, or would be willing to derogate from its real excellency. . . . We are all of us still in the dark, more or less, as to a great many particulars about it. . . . In quartans, and autumnal tertians, it is a remedy of greater certainty, and specifick propriety, than perhaps physick was ever furnished with before.

Harris adds that on several occasions he had cured both tertians and quartans with diaphoretic antimony. In quartans the bark is "the most absolute and certain specifick that ever has yet been known" but in some other intermittents it is one of the worst. Other febrifuges should not be forgotten, such as mithridate or theriac of Andromachus. Two drachms of the bark formerly produced a longer effect than an ounce nowadays; a possible reason is adulteration.[53]

The treatise written in 1683 by Harris's contemporary John Jones (1645–1709) exemplifies the fact, noticed again and again in this history, that even after the Peruvian bark had begun to be accepted, it did not immediately cause rival febrifuges to be discarded. Jones's opinions are discussed in detail in Appendix A.

In his classic *Historia plantarum* (1686–1704) John Ray (1627–1705) included a chapter on the febrifugal Peruvian tree called *china chinae*. Although not a physician, Ray was a close friend or colleague of major medical men; in addition, he had read widely, had traveled widely, was a careful observer, and had lived through many of the vicissitudes outlined in this chapter. He says that powdered Peruvian bark, given in proper dosage, is a safe, certain, and trustworthy remedy against all intermittent fevers, according to his own experience (*debita dosi exhibitus adversus febres omnes intermittentes tutum, certum et minime fallax est remedium, etiam experientia nostra*).[54] He adds that the eminent Thomas Sydenham calls it a very great specific, which first came to England thirty years before the time of writing. Ray recalls (*memini*) that the drug was then held in high esteem and was used often. Perhaps because it was given in excessively small doses, there were relapses and failures. It became suspect and fell into desuetude until "a few years ago" Robert Talbor boldly increased the dose and resuscitated the drug. He did not stop with scruples[55] but went on to drachms and ounces, and gained great fame for himself and for the powder.

An opponent of the Peruvian bark—a physician more vociferous and abusive than important—was Gideon Harvey (1640?–1700?). If we can trust the autobiographical statements included in one of his minor diatribes, Harvey studied medicine in Leyden and Paris and practiced in London. Late in life he became physician to Charles II, who was not automatically averse to atypical practitioners.[56]

Harvey's best-remembered writing is *The Conclave of Physicians* (1683), a bipartite work that combines an invective against the College of Physicians with an attack on Jesuits' bark. In discussing the properties of this drug he wrote that "since *per se* it neither operates by Vomit, Stool, Urin, or Sweat . . . we may safely conclude its chief Energy consists only in stopping of Ague fits . . . and the vitious Humours [are] retained and mured up, whereby either the Fits upon some short interval do return, or . . . worse Diseases are engendered." He observed that several pieces of bark in the best of the parcels differed from one another in color, taste, and grain. In another chapter he adds that "not only Steel, but the Jesuits Powder, and Laudanum, are to become the three Quack-Medicines of this Age."[57] He accuses Thomas Willis of composing "Physical Romances, and Romantick Notions" and says cleverly that Willis's caprices were always formed before experimental observation, hence Willis was obliged to strain the latter into agreement with the former.[58]

In another outburst, his *Art of Curing Diseases by Expectation*, Harvey says that in great diseases more patients owe their deaths to physicians than are saved by them. He characterizes as farrier-doctors those who prescribe iron or steel; ass-doctors are those who prescribe asses' milk, and Jesuitical doctors are those who prescribe the Jesuits' powder, "fourbs from the top to the bottom." It is not surprising that he quotes Molière's satires on physicians.[59]

While Harvey's witty thrusts contain much truth, their value is weakened by the fact that the thruster aimed at many different targets. Hence much of his attack against the bark is likely to have been motivated by endogenous hostility rather than objective fact. In this he reminds us of Plempius and foreshadows Patin, who is discussed in Chapter 5. In addition, Haggis has shown that Harvey, having denied that the bark was a new discovery, "was ascribing to Cinchona a historical fact which rightly belonged to the febrifuge bark of the Peruvian Balsam tree (*Myroxylon*)."[60]

In his *Pyretologia* (1692, 1694) Richard Morton says that the Peruvian bark is a "Herculean antidote" to the poison of intermittent fevers and, when given in proper dosage, usually returns the patient to health immediately. He says also that the poisonous ferment of this fever, whatever it may be, is rather mild compared to that of other fevers. The name Jesuits' powder, he adds, continues to cause terror among members of the public (even those who do not belong to the lowest classes), as if the drug were not a natural remedy but a poisonous diabolic artifice prepared by Jesuitic craft. The name china-china or some other synonym should be used instead. Morton's strong disapproval of Talbor ("a vagabond") contrasts with Ray's opinion, mentioned above.[61]

A few nefarious physicians, says Morton, had attempted to suppress the drug lest it cut short the fevers. Others, decent men, had misgivings about the bark because, blinded (*obcaecati*) by their belief in humoralism, they were doubtful about cures accomplished without perceptible evacuation. There had been innumerable futile controversies among highly erudite men until Sturmius in 1659 and Badus in 1663 defended the bark so learnedly and eloquently that very few physicians now dare to attack it: "As far as I know, nobody nowadays remains in doubt as to the powers of this febrifugal drug, but sometimes, because of the vehemence of the symptoms . . . these fevers not rarely simulate many other diseases, even the most acute, yet they yield to the powers of the bark, and if the bark is not given they quite often end fatally." However, he adds, because the drug nowadays is adulterated, the dosage prescribed in the *Schedula Romana* has had to be increased from two drachms to two or even three ounces.[62]

Haggis has shown that Morton's description of the Peruvian *tree* apparently was taken from the literature and applies to the Peruvian balsam tree *Myroxylon*, not to cinchona, whereas Morton's remarks about the appearance of the *bark* are correct, indicating that he had had genuine specimens of cinchona at hand.[63]

Morton presents a collection of thirty reports that describe "very recent cases" of intermittent fever.[64] These were not ordinary cases but were selected to illustrate what he calls the protean character of the disease; almost all were complicated or diagnostically difficult. The series includes subseries of cases in which diarrhea, or muscle spasms, or convulsions occurred. In these trying situations Morton tended to base the diagnosis on periodicity of symptoms and on the lateritious or rubicund appearance of the urine.[65]

In addition, he used the therapeutic result as a means of diagnosis. He says, by way of illustration, that in some cases of periodically recurring hemicrania such treatments as jugular venesection and a large number of other methods had been unsuccessful or even harmful. He had finally learned through experience that by the abundant use of Peruvian bark he could overcome the febrile poison that had caused the pain. The same reasoning was successful in cases in which intermittent fever simulated apoplexy or numerous other diseases.[66]

Like most physicians of his time, Morton observed the external appearance and the pulse but did not undertake what we today would call a complete physical examination. Even in his cases of severe abdominal pain the appearance of the abdomen is not mentioned, nor do his reports tell anything about the spleen.[67]

Morton usually tried to allay the complicating or conspicuous symptoms first. This effort involved a wide variety of drugs and such therapeutic measures as enemas and phlebotomy. After the obvious acute threat had been averted, he would treat the intermittent fever, counteracting its causative poison by means of the bark. Further treatment with additional doses of the bark was sometimes required; in several instances this was neglected and relapses occurred. He sometimes used the bark in cases of continued fever[68] and also in pulmonary hemorrhage.[69]

Although Morton included among his clinical reports a few cases in which modern physicians would question the diagnosis of intermittent fever, his *Pyretologia* gives a convincing picture of the disease. His book, a major contribution, demonstrates that the Peruvian bark is effective against many forms and many complications of the intermittent fevers, and it describes a feasible method of administration. It shows that the bark had gained full acceptance.

Preoccupation with the history of the intermittent fevers and with their treatment should not becloud the fact that the Peruvian bark was used at this time and subsequently for a range of other diseases. This much was recorded by almost all of the authors who have been discussed in this chapter and can be confirmed easily by reference to the treatises of Sydenham and Morton, and also by examination of John Locke's journals.[70] A complete catalog of the diseases and symptoms is beyond the scope of this history. Some of the most important or conspicuous are: continued fevers, phthisis, and hemoptysis; recurrent or periodic pains, including those of neuralgia and hemicrania; convulsions, hysteria, and hypochondriasis; arthralgia, rheumatism, and gout; and abdominal and intestinal disorders, including dysentery.

The amplitude of this list shows that the proper realm of the bark had yet to be defined. As late as 1764 a German writer compiled an inventory of more than twenty diseases in which the drug was alleged to be helpful. Despite the well-known dictum of Sydenham, gout is not included.[71]

Martin Lister (1638?–1712), a medical practitioner and eminent biologist, was a vigorous defender of tradition. His explanation of the conservative attitude in medicine is not without instructiveness for the modern reader.[72] Although he was strongly inclined toward observation, in his *Octo exercitationes medicinales* he repeatedly attacked both the contratheoretic Sydenham and the speculative Willis, showing in his comments a degree of acridity which was palatable in the seven-

teenth century but is not tolerated nowadays. He described Willis's remarks on smallpox as ludicrous and trifling. He (not altogether un-
justly) ridiculed as "dreams" the notion of Sydenham that epidemic
diseases are caused by subterraneous vapors, and he characterized a
statement in Sydenham's famous essay on gout as being a beautiful
and elegant fiction (*bellam atque lepidam fictionem*). But he was an
investigator as much as a scoffer, as is suggested by his attempt to ana-
lyze ascitic fluid and is demonstrated by his writings on natural history.[73]

Conservatism did not restrain Lister from admitting that those who
are taken with intermittent fevers are cured rapidly and safely by the
famous drug made from Peruvian bark; moreover, the patients do not
become dropsical. In a special addendum or *mantissa* he evidenced approval of the bark, cited many years of experience with it, and advocated an improved system of dosage. He remarked astutely that whatever money the bark had taken away from the medical profession had
been restored abundantly by untimely and protracted repetition of
dosage.[74]

Lister's experienced opinions show the Peruvian bark as victor over
grudging conservatism. His thorny writings exhibit also the polemical
tendencies of seventeenth-century medicine; hence they are strongly
reminiscent of the pamphleteering that is also conspicuous in the political and religious literature of the era.

That the vicissitudes and the reputation of the Peruvian bark continued to be complicated by difficulties in clinical diagnosis and by ob-
scurities in clinical reasoning is shown in the handsomely worded essay
of Martin Warren, who described an outbreak of fever which occurred
ca. 1727–28; he appended seven case reports.[75] The difficulties were
long to outlast the eighteenth century.

In 1727 an economic historian included in his compilations some
scattered and inconspicuous notes that explicitly or implicitly comment
on the reputation of cinchona in England in the final decades of the
seventeenth century.[76] He wrote that during 1682–83 342 pounds of
Jesuits' bark were imported into London. Under 1694–95 he noted
that 3,205 pounds of gentian root, which some considered equal to
Jesuits' bark in the cure of agues, were imported from Holland. Clearly,
the victory of bark over bitters was yet to be completed.

5 France, Germany, and Switzerland

France

France in the seventeenth century enjoyed or suffered the domination of the Bourbons, their great and centralizing power—which twice overcame the resistance of the Fronde—and their burdensome extravagance disguised as glory. This mise-en-scène had in its foreground widespread poverty, misery, and disease; fatuous wars; equally dismal religious conflicts; colonial expansion; and brilliance in philosophy, natural science, literature, and the arts. Recent research has disclosed also that disobedience, disorder, and dissent were not rare.[1] Most of these developments or occurrences were reflected in some manner in French medicine, and many of them in some manner affected the history of cinchona.

Since the vicissitudes of cinchona in seventeenth-century France and those of antimony, its principal rival, were entangled in the struggle between Catholicism and Protestantism, it is well to observe that important parts of what may be called the French Protestant domain were malarious. From the details assembled by Hirsch and more recently by Bruce-Chwatt and Zulueta, it can be seen that, apart from many isolated spots, malaria occurred especially in the western and southern parts of the country, including the coasts of Languedoc and Provence and the cities of La Rochelle, Montpellier, and Nîmes.[2] The last-named authors point out also that in 1599 Henry IV announced that "all swampy areas should be drained, but neither he nor his successor Louis XIII completed the enormous task although they sought the advice of Dutch engineers who were masters of the craft."

In the realm of French medicine and medical pedagogy, the domi-

nant force was conservatism. The opposition to new ideas and methods
was very strong, especially in Paris, and has been characterized by a
recent French author as *misonéisme*.[3] An eminent scholar had previously remarked that "Paris, which contributed little to the common enterprise, became the pitiless opponent of all innovation."[4]

In the year 1618, Théophraste Renaudot (1586–1653),[5] a Protestant
physician who had studied at Montpellier and had been designated, at
least nominally, as physician-in-ordinary to Louis XIII, devised an antimonial panacea to which he gave the Galenic name of *polychreston*.[6]
This medicament Renaudot advertised in his pioneer newspaper, the
Gazette, as beneficial in cases of paralysis, apoplexy, stone, uterine suffocation, contagious diseases, and fevers.[7] The preparation was in part
a derivative of Paracelsian iatrochemistry. It was therefore disapproved
by the Paris Faculty[8] and was denounced by Guy Patin, a leading rep-
resentative of Parisian medical and Catholic orthodoxy. In a letter written to André Falconet on October 11, 1667, Patin alleged that antimonialists, monks, and empirics supported *inter alia* the use of
quinquina.[9]

Renaudot, a social activist on behalf of the poor, ultimately became
a Roman Catholic and a supporter of Richelieu and Louis XIII.[10] With
their deaths, in 1642 and 1643 respectively, his influence faded. An
authoritative eighteenth-century chronicler has preserved the significant fact that Renaudot had been attacked in several memoirs composed by René Moreau and Jean Riolan the younger (see below), but
these diatribes were suppressed through the influence of Richelieu.[11] A
later historian has reported the additional information (which unhappily he has failed to document) that the medical faculty of Montpellier,
Renaudot's school, in extending its therapeutic range, "was soon to
adopt" the use of *quinquina* and ipecac.[12] According to an undocumented and undated statement by Dousset, Renaudot favored the Peruvian bark.[13] On chronological grounds this is possible. Renaudot's
life and work illustrate the iatrochemical inclinations of Montpellier
and French Protestants, the concomitant opposition of the Catholic
medical faculty of Paris, and the social meliorism of a poor man's physician who ultimately became incorporated, more or less, into the dominant component of French society.

In comment on René Descartes (Appendix A) attention is called to
the particles that the great philosopher and his followers mentioned in
writings composed mainly between 1629(?) and 1646. In April 1645,
or thereabouts, William Cavendish, Marquis of Newcastle, sent Descartes four questions on animal heat, fever, and spirits. In his reply
Descartes remarked that in [intermittent] fevers the fever can be cured
by an infinite number of remedies, but all are uncertain.[14] His state-

ment contrasts sharply with the early and conspicuous successes scored by the bark in the early Italian trials, such as those of Fonseca, de Lugo, and Badus. These Cartesian writings—especially the letters—suggest, but do not prove, that if the Jesuits' bark had entered France and the Netherlands by 1646, it had made no great impression, especially inasmuch as Descartes was in epistolary or personal contact with many learned and well-informed persons during this period.

A contemporary of Descartes was René Moreau (1587–1656), characterized long after his death as *un des plus Sçavans de son siècle*.[15] He was professor of medicine and surgery in Paris and served as dean of the Faculty. In addition, he was physician to Louis XIII in 1638 and to the young dauphin in 1639. His scanty clinical or clinicopedagogical writings make no mention of the Jesuits' bark.[16] By French scholars he is esteemed especially for his extensive comments on the *Schola salernitana* (1625); this contribution, however, long antedated the European advent of the drug.

When the Peruvian bark first entered France is unknown, but the problem might be solved by recourse to the records of the Jesuits.[17] That some kind of establishment existed, either as a pharmacy or as the drugstore of an infirmary, in Lyon in 1643, is reported in the letters of Guy Patin.[18] Georges Guitton, a Jesuit historian, in discussing financial difficulties the order experienced in 1698, mentions pharmacies at the four Jesuit colleges of Lyon, Avignon, Dôle, and Chambéry, and the suggestion—soon rejected—that their profits might be used to alleviate financial problems.[19]

In 1644 Patin mentioned a lawsuit in which the Jesuits of Lyon were pitted against the apothecaries.[20] Patin, characteristically, hated both.

Rompel has shown that Bartolomé Tafur, S.J., was made procurator of Peru in 1642 and traveled to Rome in order to attend the eighth congregation of the Jesuit order, at which he was present, constantly or intermittently, from August 1645 until April 1646. It is therefore possible that he gave the bark in 1643 to the five-year-old dauphin, who later became became King Louis XIV.[21]

That the Jesuits' bark is unlikely to have been in wide use in France at this time and for a decade afterward can be inferred, uncertainly, from the writings of Lazarus Riverius (1589–1655) of Montpellier, a noted protagonist of iatrochemistry. His *Observationum centuria quarta* includes ten case reports of tertian and double tertian fever, which are dated from 1646 to 1655 and which make no mention of the bark, nor is any mention of it to be found in his ample *Opera medica universa*. Indeed, Riverius remarked that "up to now quartan fever has been regarded as incurable in its onset, its rise, and its steady state. . . . The more prudent physicians advise long patience for sufferers from

the quartan and put them off until the spring." Riverius prescribed antimony, salt, and mercury. His *pulvis diaphoreticus* contained antimony
and bezoar, and at times he treated intermittent fever with sulfur and
absinthe.[22]

The combative Jean Riolan the younger (1580–1657), professor of
anatomy and botany in Paris and physician to Henry IV and Louis XIII,
was unquestionably a successful teacher and writer and a major figure
in his day. It is therefore disappointing that his medical writings (1649,
1651), which accept most Galenic traditions as well as the Harveian
circulation and reject iatrochemistry, say nothing at all about the Jesuits' bark. This deficiency is observable also in an amplified edition issued in 1661, four years after Riolan's death.

One of Riolan's writings, published in 1651, describes the therapeutic methods used by the regular physicians of Paris at that time: re-
freshing *cardiaques* (cordials), acids, and diaphoretics to purify and re-
fresh the blood; venesection; and moderate purgation. Metallic emetics
(i.e., antimonials) were disapproved, as were pearls, bezoars, and the
horn of the unicorn.[23]

Guy Patin (1601–72), a medical *apparatchik* not distinguished for
ability in medicine or science, immortalized his bile in epistolary
form.[24] Much of his gall was divided into four parts, one directed
against the Jesuits, the second against the Jesuits' bark, the third
against apothecaries, the fourth against iatrochemists and their favorite
drug, antimony. The inevitable connection between the first and the
second was influential in England, where the hatred of Catholics and
especially Jesuits was strong among Protestants, but in France the
odium and the fear, although also involved with religion, took a different course. Between the bark and the antimonial drugs the common
element, novelty, was anathematized by conservatives, and antimony
easily gained admission to their *Index expurgatorius*. The complicated
record of this drug is summarized at the end of this section on France.

The letters of Patin provide both negative and positive evidence
about the introduction of the Jesuits' bark into France. In a letter dated
July 20, 1649, Patin wrote that in Paris there were numerous cases of
continued fever. On August 12, 1649, he wrote that there were many
continued fevers, double tertians, and dysenteries. Neither of these letters mentions the Jesuits' bark or any other drug. On June 27, 1651, he
wrote that the duke of Beaufort had a continued double tertian; no
drugs are mentioned. On July 5, 1652, he stated that [François] Vautier,
who had been first physician to the king "but was last in ability," died
of a malignant continued fever; the only drug cited in this report is
antimony.[25]

On April 8, 1653, Patin informed Charles Spon that

three months ago some Jesuits of Lyon, as well as others who came from Italy, brought here a certain powder that had come from the Indies and had wonderful power against quartan fevers. This drug was immediately accredited, as all new things usually are. But soon afterward the result proved defective (*l'expérience manqua*) and those who were unwilling to use it were commended. I have spoken harshly against this innovation in many places where these very tricky priests[26] were promising miracles and where it did no good at all.[27]

This letter is Patin's earliest known reference to the drug. It fixes the arrival of the bark in Paris at January 1653.

In a letter dated December 30, 1653, and addressed to Charles Spon, Patin mentioned Chiflet's new book, the anticinchonal *Pulvis febrifugus*, discussed in Chapter 3.[28] He remarked that the *quinquina* had no repute in Paris and that a single dose cost forty francs. "See how the world goes; it is merely a fool and wants to be deceived. This powder is very hot and does not purge in any way." Soon afterward, on January 30, 1654, Patin sent word to Spon that he had never seen any good effect from the bark. On February 13, 1654, he wrote to the same correspondent that almost the only advocates of the bark are Jesuits. Another unfavorable comment appears in a letter to Spon dated March 10, 1654.[29]

Plempius quotes a letter written by Moreau to an unnamed physician on July 9, 1655: "The reputation of the Peruvian powder is so dead in this city [Paris] that it is no longer spoken of and we no longer prescribe it."[30]

If reliance were to be placed on these letters of Patin and Moreau, we would conclude that the Peruvian bark began to be used in Paris in January 1653 and disappeared from favor before July 1655. However, we cannot exclude the possibility of surreptitious use by Jesuits, nonconformists, travelers, and others.[31]

On November 19, 1656, Patin wrote that the *kinkina* of the Jesuits of Rome has cured no one in Paris and that it is not mentioned anywhere.[32] In a valuable historical treatise Maurice Raynaud (1834–81), whose eponym is well known to clinicians, mentioned a Paris thesis of 1658 by B. Dieuxyvoie and titled, in translation, *Is the Peruvian bark appropriate in quartan fever?*, the question being answered in the affirmative.[33] According to a corrective statement published by Delaunay in 1906, the thesis was the work of one Louis Gallais and was presented under the supervision of instigation of his teacher, Bertin Dieuxyvoie (1620–1710). The thesis, which favored the treatment of quartan fever by its specific, Peruvian bark, had a riotous reception, partly hostile.[34]

At a time that is difficult to determine exactly but that probably must be placed in the last third of the seventeenth century, the bark was scarce. This is evident from a statement made in 1719: "The late Monsieur Fagon [1638–1718] said on several occasions to Monsieur Boulduc, junior, that at the time when *quinquina* was still rare in France he often used *chacril*[35] successfully in intermittent fevers. . . . This febrifuge has the advantage over *quinquina* that it is active in a smaller dose and does not have to be continued as long." [36]

In 1661 Patin wrote to Falconet that the bark "performs no miracles here." On August 13, 1662, he informed Thomas Bartholinus that the febrifugal powder had deceived many people; we cannot believe the false statements issued by scoundrels, such as ointment vendors, druggists, chemists, Loyolites, and other greedy persons. On December 8, 1664, he wrote that the queen had a tertian fever; apparently the bark was not used.[37]

In April 1667 Patin described his treatment of tertians and of continued fevers: bleeding and purgation, the latter being accomplished by means of cassia, senna, and syrup of roses. He found this method to be highly successful. On October 11 of the same year he wrote that quartan fever cannot be cured by *quinquina*, which is a powder overvalued by monks and empirics—he often used the latter term as a synonym for antimonialists—"but the world wants to be deceived." [38]

From November 1675 to April 1679 John Locke was in France. According to the researches of Dewhurst, none of the many French physicians whom Locke met in his travels used the Jesuits' bark.[39] We note later that evidently Locke committed an error in the sampling of his informants. Meanwhile Sydenham, overcoming an early aversion to the drug, had resumed its use. Indeed, in 1677, when Locke had ague, Sydenham sent him advice on the dosage and administration of the bark. In the next year, 1678, Louis XIV busied his royal self with extensive construction at Versailles and Marly, two malarious places.[40] On October 12, 1678, the vigilant Mme de Sévigné wrote of the "prodigious mortality among the laborers; every night carts filled with their bodies are carried away. This sad journey is concealed, in order not to scare the laborers." [41]

Leaving the Grand Monarch at malarious Versailles, we must now return to Robert Talbor, discussed in Chapter 4. In 1672 Talbor had been presented to Charles II, whom he soon afterward treated successfully for ague. He was appointed physician to the king and subsequently was knighted. In 1678 he was in France, where he treated courtiers and was made first physician to Maria Luisa (1662–89), the young queen of Spain.[42] In 1679 he successfully treated Louis XIV for an obstinate intermittent fever. Talbor was also successful in treating the dauphin,[43] as well as Colbert and Condé. The king bought the secret formula from Talbor, gave it to his physician Antoine d'Aquin, and had it published by Blegny. The resultant writings necessarily exceed in value Talbor's book for laymen issued in 1672.[44]

Among Talbor's contributions was the introduction of useful dosage forms such as the tincture; he probably preceded Sydenham in this innovation. In addition, he sometimes combined the bark with opium, especially its tincture. As for Blegny, a man despised by all commentators,[45] we must applaud his observation that those who, in attempting to understand the action of Jesuits' bark, proposed to replace a humoral cause by an iatrochemical one, namely, alkalinity, merely explained an obscure matter by something that was still more obscure.[46]

The influence of Talbor's therapeutic success is evident in the letters of the well-placed Mme de Sévigné. On October 6, 1679, she wrote that "the Englishman is divine." On November 1 she reported that "the Englishman's remedy, which will soon be public, makes the physicians highly despicable, with their bloodlettings and medicines." On November 24 she wrote: "The physicians are strongly condemned and despised. . . . I do not think that the First Physician [d'Aquin] has the true secret."[47] On September 29, 1680, she wrote that the remedy had done marvels this year, and on October 2 that Talbor had cured everyone who had come to him. On November 8 she remarked acutely: "It is a pity that Molière is dead. He would have written a marvelous scene about d'Aquin, who is enraged at not having the good medicine, and about all the other physicians, who are overpowered by the experiences, the successes, and the virtually divine predictions of this little man." That Louis XIV had ague that was repeatedly and successfully treated with the bark at least as late as 1686 is recorded in her informative letters.[48]

Mme de Sévigné's statements report the opinions of patients at the highest levels of French society. She noticed the discomfiture that fell upon recognized and respected physicians, and indeed on all of the regular medical profession, in consequence of ancient doctrines and methods becoming abruptly discredited by new empirical observations. Necessarily she did not take account of more fundamental problems, which are discussed later in this chapter. It must be noted also that, even before the arrival of Talbor on the French medical scene, she had been skeptical and hostile toward the medical profession.[49]

As Mme de Sévigné had noted, d'Aquin at first was unacquainted with the content of Talbor's successful febrifuge. Yet the formula that the king later used is recorded as *vin de quinquina, pour le roi (d'Aquin)*: it consisted of pulverized bark of *quinquina* in Burgundy wine.[50] Further, d'Aquin's preparation was later used in Italy, under his name. For example, a letter written, probably by Ippolito Francesco Albertini about 1710, states: "I would recommend *China* [Jesuits' bark] which Dr. d'Aquin used on his king and the nobility of Paris."[51] D'Aquin therefore had become the heir of what he had not had the good luck to discover or the wit to contrive.

Somewhat later, in 1730, Francesco Torti was to write, without documentation: "We know that under this designation [prevention] the bark has been given to healthy persons also and that it was given annually to the late Louis XIV, unconquered king of France."[52] Moreover, as this chapter later asserts, the strong personal influence of Louis XIV is justly credited with having favored the acceptance of the Peruvian bark in France. It is therefore surprising that there is almost no evidence of a similarly favorable effect in the field of prophylaxis. Here is a theme worthy of further study.

To this statement there is a single small exception. The diary tells us that the king was given the bark therapeutically for the first time in 1686, and again in 1687. In March 1688, say the physicians, "having noticed that all the fevers that had been cured last autumn, especially by the use of the bark, were renewing themselves strongly, we wanted to save His Majesty from a relapse of this kind. For this reason he took his purgative bouillon on March 22 . . . and on the same day he took two doses of *quinquina*. He took four on the 23d, three on the 24th, 25th, 26th, 27th, and 28th and thereafter he seemed perfectly well."[53] The next month he had a double tertian. No prophylactic doses are recorded thereafter. Unquestionably, the doses given on March 22–28 were administered with prophylactic intent.

The truly royal success of Talbor and his Jesuits' bark could not fail to be reflected in both the medical and the nonmedical literature. Conspicuous in the panorama is a work by François Monginot, the younger.[54] Monginot had studied at Montpellier, had worked in Lyon, and had been imprisoned for the crime of Protestantism.[55] His book, the *Traité de la guérison des fièvres par le quinquina*, appeared in Lyon in 1679 and went through other editions (1680–86) there and in Paris.[56]

Monginot says that *quinquina* is unquestionably the surest and best remedy thus far discovered. The drug, known in Europe for about thirty years, had been virtually abandoned, but it has been given for a long time by a London physician [Morton]. The sole effective ingredient is *quinquina;* substances added for disguise may impair its effectiveness. The action of the drug is really not understood. Preliminary phlebotomy is usually requisite but must be employed carefully, and preliminary purgation is essential when the abdomen contains abundant "impurities." Often, he adds, the *quinquina* produces no evacuation, because there is nothing to be evacuated. To those who object that the residual material of the fever will become active if there is no evacuation, Monginot replies that when the treatment is given properly, reactivation does not occur. The bark has been found to be effective also against obstructions of the spleen [i.e., splenomegaly, often malarial] and other structures.[57]

Monginot describes the composition, dosages, and use of several preparations of *quinquina*, solid and liquid. He uses such expressions as "experience has often shown," and "reason and experience make one see." He adds, "These are the preparations that I have used very successfully," and "you can be assured that I shall propose nothing that has not been based on a very large number of experiences."[58] These remarks, published in 1680, show that John Locke had committed an oversight in 1675–79 when he found no French physician who had used the bark.[59]

Monginot remarks incidentally that the "vapors" were cured by the bark.[60] This malady is regarded nowadays as being probably equivalent to what was also called hypochondriasis or hysteria. Scoffers should remember that the symptom complex included migratory muscle spasms and abdominal cramps, and that the latter in many cases are due to intestinal infection, bacterial, viral, and protozoal. It is now recognized that the spasms may be alleviated by quinine. This applies also to some of the infections, especially those that are caused by protozoa.

Some of Monginot's comments approach those that were later to be made by Torti. He wrote that in order to be relieved of the sickness, it was necessary for the patient to take a certain amount of the powder: "Ordinarily for the cure of each person it is necessary to use an ounce and a half of *quinquina*, or a little more."[61]

It will be shown later that Torti sometimes employed the powder diagnostically. Monginot's ingenuity approached this innovation without really reaching it. He stated that cinchona could be used to detect resemblances among diseases that appear to be different; this could be called a taxonomic or etiological rather than a diagnostic use:

It is at least easy to imagine that, up to the present time, just as *quinquina* has only been used against fevers,[62] it could be intended by Nature for other beneficial uses that have not been tested . . . and if the tests confirmed this idea, one could conclude that most of the illnesses for which it is appropriate differ less in their causes than in their effects, and that the drug destroys equally in all places the same fermentation that might produce different effects.[63]

Monginot's statements show full approval of the bark, and at the same time combine Galenic concepts with fermentationism. They provide a fair sample of the opinions current in his time and reveal, incidentally, that France was beginning to recover from its prolonged retardation in clinical science.

Jean de La Fontaine (1621–95), the fabulist, at the request of his patroness, the duchess of Bouillon, wrote a "Poëme de quinquina," which was published in 1682.[64] It is a didactic composition and reads like a routine command performance, but it claims our attention because it was based on the opus of La Fontaine's friend Monginot.[65] In discussing fevers, the poet, having done his homework, wrote that their hidden location was said to be in the humors. They created a focus that distributed vapors throughout the blood, reached the heart, and attacked solid structures. When the dominant poison is melancholic, the attacks allow two days of remission: "thus speaks the School and all its followers." But their error was put to rest long ago; *quina* has destroyed it, and we follow new rules. Away with humors, whether they are peccant or not; fever is a ferment that exists without them. As soon as a certain acid is dominant in the body, everything ferments. *Quina* rules today, our clever people use it; some still keep, like a matter of religion, the opinion of the school.[66]

An analytical review by J.-B. Fonssagrives, a medical officer in the French navy, deserves mention at this juncture.[67] Fonssagrives recognized that La Fontaine's poem was written during a period when the French public, influenced by persons of high rank, began suddenly to have high esteem for the Jesuits' bark; at the same time, haters of the French medical profession could smirk at the discomfiture of traditionalists who were defeated by a medicament that had been introduced empirically. In commenting on La Fontaine's precision in the description of technical details respecting the fevers and the therapeutic bark, Fonssagrives pointed out that the poet had displayed similar accuracy in explaining the mechanistic doctrines of Descartes.[68] It is to be regretted that the perceptive reviewer apparently was unaware of the relation between La Fontaine and Monginot, since the latter was La Fontaine's source. Fonssagrives incidentally resurrected the fact that La Fontaine's obscure contribution was not the only poem inspired by the new drug: "Poets of the second and third rank sounded their lyre in its honor and directed to it a host of madrigals and ballads."

In a letter dated December 12, 1680, Jacques Spon (1647–85), a member of a Lyonnais medical family, wrote that he had been examining Blegny's book, *La découverte de l'admirable remède anglois* (1680), in order "to see whether the methods of administering it [the Jesuits' bark] were the same I had practised with good success in Tertians, double Tertians, Quartans, and also in continual or malignant fevers *for five or six months* past. In the last of these Fevers, it is not so infallible as in the Intermittents, which it cures in a few days."[69] In other words, Spon had used the bark successfully in Lyon as early as July 1680 and had noticed that the drug worked better in intermittents than in continued fevers.

In 1681, Raymond Restaurand (1627–82), an individualistic or eccentric professor of medicine at Montpellier, issued an instructive essay on the use of "china-china" for the treatment of fever.[70] In the traditional manner Restaurand attributed various fevers to bile, either unmixed or else mixed with other humors. He stated clearly that *China chinae* is, by reason of its efficacy, the most outstanding remedy. To this he added the remarkable comment that the Jesuits in the Indies had noticed that the Indians used the bark to overcome the effects of cold, experienced especially while they swam across rivers. This had led the priests to use it in fevers. They then introduced the drug in Europe.[71] The same narrative by Spanish authors is discussed in Chapter 1.

During the final decades of the seventeenth century mention of the Jesuits' bark, usually designated *quinquina*, appeared with increasing frequency in the French medical and pharmaceutical literature. An example is furnished by Nicolas Lémery (1645–1715), a Protestant pharmacist who studied medicine at Montpellier and in later years felt obliged to become a Catholic. His *Cours de Chymie* contains an extensive discussion of *quinquina*, in which he states that it is the most reliable drug discovered up to now for halting the ferment of intermittent fevers. He points out that the dosage had been changed from what had been in use "for a long time"; unfortunately he gives no dates. He adds that failure to use preliminary purgation might increase the gravity of the patient's troubles by producing asthma, dropsy, rheumatism, dysentery, and amenorrhea. Lémery's *Dictionaire ou traité universel des drogues simples* includes an explanation of the financial profit that the Jesuits gained from selling the drug. Compatibly with his Protestant origins and his training at Montpellier, the same author also wrote a treatise on antimony.[72]

In view of the extensive discussion that the Jesuits' bark received in the writings of Lémery it is astonishing that major works of another noted pharmaceutical writer, Möise Charas (1618–98), fail to mention the drug, especially since as early as about 1677, Charas had presented before the Académie des Sciences a discussion of a new preparation of *quinquina* and its dosage.[73] His *Pharmacopée royale galenique et chimique* first appeared in Paris in 1676 and continued to reappear for seventy-seven years. The original issue does not mention the bark. The edition issued in Lyon in 1704 significantly continues to contain the original approbations by d'Aquin and his archiatric successor Fagon, both of which are dated *1676*. The index of this volume exhibits four columns of entries on antimonials. The text describes two febrifuges, both of which are antimonial, and a third that contains mercury. There is no mention of Jesuits' bark. It is evident that iatrochemistry continued to maintain a firm hold. The successive editions of Charas were not really revisions in the modern sense.

In 1685 a pharmacist of Provence named Alary presented to d'Aquin, the physician of Louis XIV, a secret febrifuge, which on royal order the physician tested and then approved. The nature of the new medicine remains unknown. Alary discusses it in a book (1685) that bears d'Aquin's formal approval. This work received a perceptive review that embodies the opinion of Spon: "In this decade febrifuges have been more vigorously investigated than in all preceding centuries, and not without benefit. For in addition to the astonishing power of the Peruvian bark, so often proclaimed, in quieting the fermentation of fever, various men have produced various things, and among them B. Alary, the Provençal pharmacist, deserves recognition."[74] This statement allows us to infer that the success of the Jesuits' bark had a stimulating effect on research in pharmacology and perhaps on quackery also.

Additional evidence that the Jesuits' bark was in use and under discussion in France during the final decades of the seventeenth century exists in the form of theses. One such document, which appeared in 1684 under the name of Joannes Daval, who was supervised by Pierre Perreau, attacks the "English" method—that of Talbor. A few other French theses (which I have not seen) are mentioned by Delaunay and by Waring.[75]

In 1687 Dr. Francesco Maria Nigrisoli of Ferrara published in Latin four treatises on the proper administration of the bark.[76] These had appeared in France during the preceding six years. They were written originally by Blegny, Monginot, Restaurand, and Spon; each has received attention in this chapter. The significance of the collection is that it evidences widespread acceptance of the bark in France; at the same time it implies also that French medicine at this time was not devoid of prestige. In addition it may be said to represent the consolidation or early maturation of a growing mass of clinical experience. Further, its publication in Italy may have been intended to prevent or offset a possible decline in the use of the drug in that country. The work carries the imprimatur of the Jesuits and that of the Inquisition.

In 1689 the caustic, ill-natured Jean Bernier (1622?–98), a graduate of Montpellier, published the first edition of his *Essais de médecine*. In this work he declared that "if we have some specifics in medicine, this one [Jesuits' bark] is the surest, the most harmless, and the most admirable that has ever been known." The foreigner [Talbor] had learned that the drug had to be given more often and for a longer time than had been customary. He also did not recognize that if the patient's body had not been prepared in advance by the administration of "general remedies"—phlebotomy and purgation—the drug might fail to be effective.[77] In other words, remnants of the old doctrines persisted.

Moreover, Bernier continued, the French had been unwilling to accept under the name of *quinquina* what they received willingly under the designation of secret remedy. The drug, he wrote, is a true febrifuge, effective especially against fevers that have a focus and recur, also against inflammations of the intestines and chest and against malignant fevers. He made the interesting additional comment that at the time that *quinquina* was successful in the case of Louis XIV it had already lost much of its former repute, either because it had become too common and too well known and there was no longer any great mystery about its preparation, or because it had become so cheap that the public could no longer regard it as precious. Bernier's statement becomes intelligible only if it is interpreted as a reference to treatment given to the king, not by Talbor in 1679 or 1680, but by his regular physician d'Aquin in 1688 or thereabouts. If this reading is correct, it points to an additional vicissitude in the history of the bark in France, one that has not been noted by historians. Confirmatory evidence would be welcome.

The distinctly procinchonal tenor of Bernier's presentation gains additional interest in the light of the comment made by Bayle and Thillaye that Bernier had been a leading protagonist of antimony.[78] Not all seventeenth-century conversions were religious.

A further additional indication of fluctuations in the repute of the Jesuits' bark is found in an anonymous book attributed to Guy-Crescent Fagon and first published in 1689 under the title *Les admirables qualitez du kinkina*.[79] This work contains the curious statement that *kinkina*, which was making so much noise nowadays in France, had few advocates in Italy. But we must admit, the commentator continued, that it was not so popular in France as it was after Talbor gave his secret to the king; those physicians in Paris who are distinguishable from the common lot use the drug only for tertians and quartans, only after trying everything else, and only after the chill appears. At present the drug is used very widely. The leading physicians of France and Italy consider the bark a sovereign febrifuge for all sorts of intermittents, as well as for continued fevers that are preceded by chills and followed by sweats. Avoidance of preliminary purgation is justifiable. The best quality of bark is sold at 12 to 20 sols per ounce.[80]

The statements in this anonymous essay repeated the well-known opinion that in 1689 the bark was used widely in France,[81] its popularity being attributed usually to Louis XIV. The allegation of reduced esteem in Italy at about this time is discussed in Chapter 7.

In 1693 the Abbé Bancalis de Pruynes wrote, in a letter that is still extant, that a coarse Dutch physician named Helvetius presented to Louis XIV "an infallible remedy for treatment of all kinds of fevers." Before buying it, the king had had it tested in hospitals, where it did not fail to cure patients to whom it was administered. The treatment consisted of three enemas administered on successive days, each containing an ounce of *quinquina* in tepid water. Although the procedure was more promptly efficacious than oral dosage, it was continued for a few additional days in order to assure a favorable result.[82]

The abbot added that Helvetius usually prescribed at the same time plasters [of unspecified content] to be applied to the wrist, but these were rumored to be nothing more than a trick designed to impede revelation of Helvetius's secret. The king took the enemas and overcame his fever. In the following year Helvetius published his method. In many ways the career, methods, and achievements of Helvetius, a capable man but not a regular physician, paralleled those of Talbor.

An important contribution, obscured by the passage of three centuries, was made by Jacques Minot in a book on the nature and treatment of fever.[83] In this volume, dedicated to Fagon, Minot divides fevers into chylous and sanguine. An acrid blood, he says, coagulates the chyle or thickens it; these are the essential causes of the febrile fermentation and of all the accidents that follow it. Bleeding is not a remedy for fever but only for the symptoms that accompany it. If a fever is not cured by bleeding and purgation, diaphoretics and specifics are used. *Quinquina* is a sure specific (*spécifique assuré*) for the cure of fevers; it cures fevers of all sorts and is also beneficial in pleurisy. The water of the Seine is purgative and likewise is effective in fevers.[84]

However extravagant some of Minot's contentions may appear to the twentieth-century reader, they are significant because *he undertook to test them experimentally:*

In order to be fully convinced that *quinquina* mortifies acids and destroys them, which is quite different from fixating them, I have made new experiments on blood and on fluids analogous to chyle. For this purpose I took two glass vials, which I warmed moderately, and into each I put four or five ounces of the venous blood of a pig. In one vial I had placed two spoonfuls of vinegar and in the other I put about the same amount of wine of *quinquina* such as is given to fever patients. Then I immediately placed both vials in a pot of hot water, in order to have heat comparable to that of blood.[85]

The blood in the vial that contained vinegar was completely coagulated and brownish red verging on black, whereas the blood in the cinchona vial was fluid and beautifully red, almost the color of arterial blood. Apparently Minot was trying to reconcile the use of the bark with iatrochemical doctrine. The experiments show that the origin and the influence of his ideas deserve further investigation.

A few of his obiter dicta should not be overlooked. He found that the bark is beneficial in bulimia, in other diseases caused by acid, and in gout and rheumatism; in this respect he is reminiscent of Morton. In addition, he denounces "the false prejudice" that the bark fixates humors and thereby causes "scirrhi" of the liver and spleen. Evidently splenomegaly and hepatomegaly occurring in intermittent fever were thought to be *produced* by the drug.[86]

That the series of French theses and other writings on the Jesuits' bark continued its forward march from the end of the seventeenth century into the eighteenth is evident in the copious bibliographical compilation of Edward J. Waring.[87]

When we come to summarize the history of cinchona in France during the seventeenth century, we necessarily encounter traits and processes that are shared with other countries or areas and that belong to the general history of medicine. Other traits are special to France. Since the attentive reader will have no difficulty in assigning any individual trait to the general or the local category, I shall attempt instead to follow a topical order and to disturb the chronological sequence as little as possible.

From the moment of its arrival in France, most probably through agency of the Jesuits, the Peruvian bark was obliged to contend with other febrifuges. Of these the longest established were Galenic or post-Galenic botanical drugs. The iatrochemical febrifuges were for the most part much more recent arrivals; among these the antimonials far outnumbered the mercurials in variety and likewise greatly exceeded them in frequency of use.[88] The use of iatrochemical preparations in cases of fever can be attributed to the influence of Paracelsus, which came to France from Germany and Switzerland. In a third group, not to be ignored, were products of folklore, poorly recorded in written or printed documents and hardly susceptible to precise dating.

The oldest drugs were defended by the oldest doctrines, represented by the conservatism of Paris, and were attacked by the newer doctrines acclaimed by rebellious inhabitants of southern and southwestern France, the home of French iatrochemists. The former group were mainly Catholics, the others mainly Calvinists. The geographical division accompanied an epidemiological difference, in that malaria in the seventeenth century had higher incidence in the Protestant domain. Whether the Lutheran Protestantism of Alsace and Lorraine and the Calvinist Protestantism of southern France were associated with any perceptible differences in the use of Peruvian bark or of iatrochemical drugs such as the antimonials is a theme that might well attract an energetic investigator.

The influence of social structure and stratification was no less important but somewhat more intricate. The first of the French Bourbon kings, Henry IV, came from southern France, was Protestant by birth, and was not averse to iatrochemical medication. In the last-named preference he was followed by Louis XIII and Louis XIV. To these monarchs the aristocracy not rarely genuflected. Necessarily the Catholic church played a role in the conflict of influences.

In his youth Louis XIV recovered from a fever after he had been given antimony; this event fortified the reputation of iatrochemical therapeutics. At about the same time cinchona was scarce in France, its use there was either scanty or unrecorded, and its reputation was minimal.

When the century had run three-quarters of its allotted time, the successful treatment of malarious nobility and royalty by Talbor abruptly reversed the fortunes of the Jesuits' bark. Thereafter it never disappeared from the scene, although minor fluctuations occurred. To the extent that a single factor can be isolated, it is the influence of royalty and nobility that produced the enduring acceptance of the bark. This fact is fully compatible with the strong centralization of French government and society. Also, the centralization of French administrative practice is known to have affected the management of hospitals throughout the country and presumably guaranteed the distribution of the bark to these and other public institutions.

During the intricate early career of the Jesuits' bark in France, the role of the French was always one of either rejection or acceptance, but almost never of innovation. Despite the vigorous activity of French pharmaceutical science at this time, no important invention in the preparation of the bark is ascribable to the Gallic intelligence, nor can French clinical medicine be credited with any new observations in this field of medical practice. We must however assign a modicum of recognition to Minot's early experimental approaches, which are scarcely remembered nowadays.

The concurrence of all the factors that have been enumerated, while it assured the survival of the Peruvian bark in France, did not throw the iatrochemical and folkloric drugs into desuetude. But the later parts of the narrative would draw the author and his patient reader beyond the temporal limits of this history.

Antimony in Seventeenth-Century France

Single-minded concentration on the career of cinchona, without concomitant consideration of other febrifuges, incurs the hazard of distortion. For this reason it is requisite and instructive to examine, however briefly, the vicissitudes of the principal rival drug, antimony.[89] Such an undertaking admittedly involves the occasional amplification, or even the partial repetition, of several matters that have been recorded earlier in this chapter.

It is well known that the use of antimonial drugs was furthered by iatrochemical doctrine, of which the most famous partisan was Paracelsus. The earliest French protagonists were mostly Protestants; their strongholds were La Rochelle and Montpellier.

Antimony, believed to have been introduced into France by Louis De Launay of La Rochelle about 1560,[90] was proscribed by the strongly Catholic and conservative Paris Faculty in 1566, also by the Parlement.[91] The Paracelsian writings of Leo Suavius (Jacques Gohory) were published in Paris in 1567 and 1568.[92] The ensuing war of antimony was to last exactly one hundred years. Despite official Parisian disapproval, the physicians of the royal court, among whom graduates of Montpellier preponderated then and later, favored the drug strongly. Antoine Vallot (1594–1671), who held the rank of chief physician to Louis XIV, was an antimonialist, and Antoine d'Aquin, who subsequently occupied the same office, had studied at Montpellier. Concerning the Montpellierians, Jean Astruc later commented: "As to chemistry [i.e., iatrochemistry], although almost all the chemical or spagyric physicians who wished to insinuate themselves into practice in Paris almost two centuries ago took the title of Montpellier physicians, it must be admitted that few genuine physicians were members of that *Faculté.*"[93]

The energetic early advocacy of antimony in France is associated with the activities of devoted Paracelsians—Joseph du Chesne, commonly known as Quercetanus, and Pierre de la Poterie (Poterius). Quercetanus (1546–1609) was born in southwestern France, studied in German universities, and received the doctorate in Basel. In 1593 he went to Paris. Soon afterward he became physician to the first of the French Bourbon monarchs, King Henry IV. Promoting the use of spagyric drugs, especially the antimonials, Quercetanus was involved in polemics with the Paris Faculty, which was led by Jean Riolan the elder. Poterius, also a determined antimonialist, was expelled by the Faculty and took up residence in Italy.[94]

The Paracelsian (i.e., Swiss and German) sources of iatrochemical doctrine, the German and Swiss education of Quercetanus, the impor-

tant southern and Occitanian preponderance among French iatrochemists, and the Pyrenean origins of King Henry IV—all these contributed exotic and partly foreign components to the historical background
of antimony, which can be compared or contrasted with the even more
exotic provenience of the Peruvian bark.

In 1622 a professorship of chemistry, the first in France, was established at Montpellier. The position was occupied by Lazare Rivière
(Riverius, 1589–1665), a native of that city and a graduate of its university. He introduced there the teaching of Paracelsian therapeutics
(and not of Paracelsian philosophy). His noncinchonal treatment of intermittent fever has been noticed earlier in the present chapter. The
strength of his influence is shown by the repeated reissue of his writings over a period of more than thirty years.

The antimonialist activities of Renaudot and the constant opposition of Guy Patin were also mentioned above. Patin's letters abound in
attacks on antimony,[95] a substance he hated but apparently never
tested.

While preparations of antimony were employed for the treatment of
many symptoms and many diseases, their use in fever is what brings
them close to the history of cinchona. In this respect an important
landmark was the case of Louis XIV, who in 1658 was attacked by a
fever—possibly typhoid—and recovered after treatment with the wine
of antimony. In 1666 the Paris Faculty admitted this product as a purgative. Later in the same year the Parlement, on royal order, removed
the restrictions which it had imposed.[96]

The pharmacopoeias of Charas (1676 et seq.) were mentioned
above, and the perceptive reader will have observed that the iatrochemical repertoire of febrifuges included a mercurial preparation as well as
several antimonials.

Comparison with English doings at about this time can be obtained
by examining Salmon's *Synopsis medicinae*. The edition of 1671 mentions as "diaphoreticks" mineral bezoar and diaphoretic antimony but
utters no word about the bark. The edition of 1680 says that when an
intermittent fever seems stubborn and keeps its hold, the "sudorificks
ought to be specifick Antifebriticks, and openers of the Obstructions of
the liver; such as the cortex Peruanus."[97]

Less weighty than the compilations of Charas, but possibly comparable in its widespread use, was the popular recipe book of Mme Marie
Fouquet, widow of the French superintendent of finance. Acting from
motives of piety and charity, the lady issued her compilation at least as
early as 1676; later editions appeared for three decades. The book describes in detail the preparation of diaphoretic antimony but makes no
mention of the Jesuits' bark.

In seventeenth-century France, as far as can be ascertained in the absence of statistical data, antimonials were used much more frequently than the bark for the treatment of fevers, at least until the arrival of Talbor, but no comparative statement can or should be made until the records of Jesuit pharmacies have been examined; the investigation might well be extended to records of other religious orders that conducted apothecary shops.[98] While it is certain that successful treatment of fevered royalty and nobility increased, and indeed established, acceptance of the Peruvian bark, it would be rash to infer that antimonials thereupon fell from grace. On this score suggestive evidence can be borrowed from the experience of other countries. In his remarks on the treatment of quartan fever, the eminent Friedrich Hoffmann of Halle (1660–1742) mentioned the use of cinchona and antimony *in combination*. The use of the two drugs in intermittent fever was reported from Seville around 1698 by Salvador Leonardo de Flores. Editions of John Huxham's treatise on fevers, published as late as 1757 and 1765, praise the use of antimony in *peripneumonia notha*.[99]

Another sign of reconciliation is the use of cinchona by devotees of iatrochemistry, such as Eberhard Gockel (1636–1703), whose *pulvis febrilis*, containing cinchona bark and its Achates, the lesser centaury, were recorded in Jüngken's pharmacopoeia. In Holland, Boerhaave published, as a supplement to his *Aphorisms*, a list of prescriptions used in intermittent fever. Here we find numerous antimonials as well as several preparations of Peruvian bark. From Spain, Francisco Suárez de Ribera, physician to Felipe V, reported in 1724 the successful use of *quarango* (cinchona) bark with flowers of lesser centaury and diaphoretic antimony.[100]

The developments in France during the seventeenth century continued, in France and elsewhere, in the next century. To take a single example, a large treatise on antimony by Nicolas Lémery (1645–1715) had the official accolade of presentation to the Académie Royale des Sciences and was translated into Italian in 1717.

Skipping over the events of the subsequent twenty-seven decades, we observe with interest that the use of antimony has survived to our own time. In the 1940s stilbamidine was employed in the treatment of multiple myeloma.[101] Nowadays tartar emetic (antimony potassium tartrate) continues to be used for schistosomiasis, a newer alternative being sodium antimony mercaptosuccinate;[102] and sodium stibogluconate and other antimonials are under trial in cases of leishmaniasis.[103]

This brief account presents some of the religious, geographical, political, social, and clinical factors that affected the history of antimony in seventeenth-century France. The reader may wish to compare and

contrast them with the factors that influenced the history of the Jesuits'
bark in the same era and region. Absorption with these fundamental
considerations should not cause the analyst to forget that both antimony and cinchona are still alive and active.

An additional aspect requires brief mention. While it is true that in
France and in other countries antimony was the chief rival of Peruvian
bark in the treatment of intermittents, the preference for antimony applied especially to devotees of iatrochemistry and presumably to some
of their patients. For others a leading drug was the lesser centaury,
mentioned in textbooks, casebooks, and pharmacopoeias. Its history,
from Dioscorides to the *Deutsche Arzneibuch* no. 7 (1968), is summarized encyclopedically by Schneider.[104] This plant, like gentian, was
deemed useful in intermittent fevers because it was classed as bitter,
astringent, and aromatic. At times it was used instead of antimony and
Peruvian bark, or in combination with either of these drugs. Its popularity in the seventeenth century is demonstrated by a remark of Sydenham: "I have succeeded better, with this treatment [*pilulae cochiae
majores*, composed of hiera picra, colocynth, scammony, and lavender]
in getting rid of a fit of tertian ague than with the *usual decoction*
[italics added] of gentian root, centaury tops, senna, and agaric."[105]
Supplementary evidence is widely scattered through the medical and
pharmaceutical literature.[106]

Germany and Switzerland

At about the time when the Peruvian bark entered northern Europe, Germany was emerging from the Thirty Years' War
(1618–48). Ferdinand III held the throne of the Hapsburgs from 1637
to 1657. His successor Leopold I (1658–1705) was a very devout Catholic, the son of a Spanish mother. Leopold was followed by Joseph I
(1705–11).

The treaties of Westphalia (1648) formalized the preexistent governmental localism and disorganization that was later symbolized in the
Diet of Regensburg, a body established, with intent of permanence, in
1663. The political and administrative system, characterized by *Partik-
ularismus* (fragmentation), was ineffective, impotent, and almost incredible. It stood or teetered, with its eighteen hundred principalities
and fifty-one free imperial cities, in total contrast to the centralization
of France.

By the middle of the seventeenth century the German population of
thirty million had been reduced by one-third. The survivors could
hardly have been well nourished, but they improved their sustenance
by the innovation of growing potatoes. Many villages were deserted.

Industry was prostrate until a degree of relief was obtained by the arrival, decades later, of Huguenots. Commerce suffered from skilled competition by Dutch and Scandinavian merchants and merchantmen. As an almost inevitable consequence of all these conditions, intellectual life was impoverished.

In medicine and in the nonmedical sciences a sign of revival was the resuscitation of the *Academia Naturae Curiosorum,* which started in 1652, was restored to life by Dr. Philippus Jacobus Sachsius à Loewenheim, and began to publish its *Ephemerides* in 1670.[107] The dedicatory letter of this periodical makes the significant statement that neighboring nations—the English and the French—protected by their kings, had made notable contributions to the world of letters. Their successes had now impelled their German neighbors to emulation.

Slightly later came the creation of the University of Halle, chartered by Leopold I in 1693. Both the *Ephemerides* and the universities were to provide materials of value, or at least of significance, to the historian of medicine and science. The academic contribution is exemplified in the seven volumes of theses published by Albrecht von Haller (1757–60). In this collection the subseries on fevers contains thirty-nine entries, of which twenty-four refer to works issued in Germany before 1750.[108] The clinical writings in the *Ephemerides,* especially those that deal with fevers, are usually short, sometimes speculative, and often anecdotal.

It is appropriate to begin the chronicle of Peruvian bark in Germany with a negative observation, which will serve as a *terminus a quo.* The copious *Pharmacopoeia medico-chymica,* issued in Ulm in 1649–50 by Johannes Schröder (1600–1664), is amply endowed with information about antimonials and other alleged febrifuges but contains no word of the Peruvian bark.[109]

The earliest bit of information available from Germanic sources is discussed in Chapter 3. This is the statement of Johannes Glantz, dated May 5, 1653, that the Peruvian bark had been tried, presumably in the armies of the Holy Roman Emperor Ferdinand III, and had been found useless.

Another early German report is the work of Werner Rolfinck (Guernerus Rolfincius) of Jena, the eminent anatomist (1599–1673). A statement that appeared in 1658 in his treatise on fevers can be paraphrased as follows: To all these things it is appropriate to add the Chinese bark (*cortex Sinensis*), highly commended in tertian and quartan fever. A book issued, under orders of Prince Leopold William, archduke of Austria, by Jean Jacques Chiflet, principal archducal physician, shows that the miracles of this powder are not permanent and that everyone in Brussels who took this febrifuge (including the archduke himself) and through its action was freed from quartans, suffered recurrences; so that it is not suitable for Europeans.[110] Rolfinck added an excerpt from the *Noctes geniales* of Johannes Nardi, discussed in Chapter 3,[111] with the comment that some patients reach convalescence after treatment with the bark but subsequently have recurrences or die because the great heat of the drug ignites the humors and arouses the bile. Consequently, tertian fevers replace the quartans.

To these statements Rolfinck subjoined: "The reverend Jesuit fathers are said to have undertaken patronage of their bark and to have published a defence of it, but this has not yet reached me." From these remarks it must be inferred that by the year 1658 Rolfinck had had no firsthand experience with the Peruvian bark, that he knew of the drug through the predominantly unfavorable opinions of Chiflet and Nardi, and that he had heard of the *Schedula Romana* but had not yet seen it.

In 1663, one Christophorus Rothmann, whose fame, like that of his professor Paulus Ammann, does not overburden the annals of our art, produced a thesis on what he called "the Peruvian antiquartan." Rothmann stated that quartan fever, previously incurable, now yields to the Peruvian medicine, but *no one has yet seen the tree* or even an engraving of it.[112] Since he had had no experience with the drug, he felt obliged to rely on published testimonies. He presented a Latin version of the *Schedula* and emphasized the precautions that are recommended in that document. He referred to Chiflet, Sturmius, and Willis, and emerged with a conclusion favorable to use of the drug in quartan fever. Except for Glantz's letter, this thesis is the second earliest German writing on the bark; hence it implies that the drug was slow in reaching Saxony.

In 1667, Balthasar Timaeus von Güldenklee (1609–67), physician to the Great Elector and comparable to Glantz in rank and function, issued an extensive clinical treatise that made no mention of the bark. In 1668 and 1669, according to evidence found by Schelenz, the bark was price-fixed in Frankfurt and Leipzig.[113]

The encyclopedia of pharmacognosy compiled by and under the direction of Alexander Tschirch includes a chronologically arranged list prepared by Dr. O. Tunmann and gives the German heading *Arznei-taxen und Verwandtes bis zum Jahre 1799* (Prices of Drugs and Related Information up to the Year 1799). The word *Taxen* signifies *valuations*. In the present context it refers to prices fixed by official edict and is not to be confused with the English word *taxes*. Indeed, drugs were not taxed in Germany at this time. The material in Tunmann's summary runs to twenty-six double-column pages, which cover the years 1221 to 1799.[114] This discussion is limited to the period between 1663, which marks the earliest entry that mentions Peruvian bark, and the year 1741, when Torti died.[115]

For this span of almost eight decades there are 145 entries, 32 of which contain announcements concerning the Peruvian bark (usually designated here as *Cortex chinae*) in Germany. In only 16 of these entries are prices mentioned. Most of the individual statements merely show that a sales price had been fixed; hence it can be inferred that the drug was available. The information about prices is considered in Chapter 12; the discussion here is limited to places.

With the exception of Berlin, Leipzig, Jena, and Zerbst, all the German cities that appear in the list are situated in the area designated (until recently) as West Germany. The relative commercial eminence of Frankfurt am Main is suggested by the fact that this city appears three times in the list, while Jena and Berlin appear twice each. The other cities have one mention each.

In the attempt to draw valid inferences from the Tunmann-Tschirch data we must recognize first of all that the number of relevant entries is small. Numerous official pharmacopoeias and unofficial *Arzneibücher*, unconnected with the announcement of prices, were not included. We must consider also that small areas may have issued no formal declaration and, moreover, may have lacked archives from which fugitive statements could be retrieved. Further, since the list is limited to official statements, it excludes private sources and church sources, which might have distributed the drug gratis and without regard to official prices. Military sources also are unrecorded.

The places mentioned in the lists are mostly between longitudes 7°37′E and 13°25′E; this embraces the eastern half of West Germany. With this area there is no distinct north-south difference in intensity of distribution. The principal focus is the center; the entire Baltic Coast, and a large area south of Münster and west of Mühlhausen, are unrepresented. An important feature is the absence of some famous Hanseatic cities; of these, Lübeck fails to appear—it was not listed until 1745—and Riga (1685) and Copenhagen (1672) are not discussed here, since they are outside Germany. It is worth noting that some old centers of trade, such as Leipzig (1669) and Frankfurt (1668), are among the earliest to appear.

With respect to the history of trade Tschirch wrote, "The discovery of the sea route to the East Indies, which made the Portuguese the masters of world trade and Lisbon the queen of the seas, undermined not only the commerce of Venice but also the intermediaries of its northern trade; in this way the great German intermediate markets (Augsburg, Nürnberg, Erfurt) lost their importance as foci of world commerce."[116]

The three cities that Tschirch here specified fail to appear in the list of *Taxen* between 1663 and 1741. However, between the voyage of Vasco da Gama and the earliest date in the list there is an interval of sixteen decades, which witnessed in turn the maritime supremacy of Spain and that of the Netherlands and England. Hence the events of the Portuguese era could be at best only remote predecessors of the German commercial plight that was manifest in the seventeenth century.

We may suppose, but cannot prove, that the relative scantiness of evidence reflects aftereffects of the Thirty Years' War, which is known to have depressed the German economy severely. The inclusions in the list must be attributed to local and administrative factors that are extremely difficult to identify. In other words, the Tunmann-Tschirch *Taxen* are descriptions of governmental actions, which constitute only one factor in the transmission of the drug. Routes of distribution cannot be elicited from this information. We are safe in saying that the inclusion of Peruvian bark in the list signifies not only that this drug was present but also that its use was deemed important enough for official imposition of a price, even when an actual quotation is not given. The number of entries signifies extensive and rather intense dissemination of the drug. It is consistent also with the well-known political fragmentation that existed in Germany after the Thirty Years' War.

In a letter addressed to Francesco Torti from Geneva and dated March 23, 1720, J. J. Mangetus wrote that he had used *le Quin-quina* with great success for more than forty-four years, that is, since 1676 or earlier. His words are: "Il y a plus de quarante quatre ans que je pratique le Quin-quina, avec tant de succès, que je dois être un de ses plus ardents apologistes." [117] This clear statement would establish Mangetus as the earliest recorded user of the Peruvian bark in Switzerland.

From the note on Mangetus in the *Biographie médicale* of Bayle and Thillaye it can be inferred that Mangetus's recollection, being that of a man aged sixty-eight who wrote almost four and a half decades after the alleged fact, is probably inexact, but it need not be far from the truth. Bayle and Thillaye state that Mangetus, born in 1652, studied medicine without teachers and by means of books only. In 1678 he received the medical doctorate and entered medical practice in Geneva.[118] These facts do not negate the possibility that he prescribed the Peruvian bark as early as 1676. Mangetus's letter to Torti is considered in a different connection in Chapter 9.

Using literary or historiographic license, Kurt Polycarp Sprengel declared in his history that the famous Johann Conrad Peyer (1653–1712), a native of Basel and a professor there, was German.[119] Since Peyer was influential in German medicine, we incur no great blame in including him at this juncture. In 1679, during a visit to Paris, he wrote to Johann von Muralt that "to allay fevers, especially quartans, many people here now recommend a bitter fluid that first came from England with doubtful success. After this drug is used, fevers quite often are checked or removed, after a sweat and often a sleep. It is the general opinion that the main ingredient of the fluid is *china chinae.*" [120]

Six years later, in 1685, Peyer wrote in the *Ephemerides* that this drug *had been neglected for a long time and had spread again very recently*, to the plaudits of the English and the French.[121] Imitation of Talbor most certainly proved successful, despite the utterances and writings of opponents. With his report Peyer included simple posologic instructions. In summarizing Peyer's article, Albrecht von Haller was later to state that at this time the bark was hardly known in Germany (*corticem peruvianum, in Germania vix notum*).[122]

In 1689 von Muralt reported, very briefly, four cases of intermittent fever in which recovery followed administration of the Peruvian bark.[123] The first patient had been treated by von Muralt's friend Francesco Redi. In a relatively long *scholium* von Muralt showed that humoral doctrine explained the symptoms of intermittent fever adequately and provided satisfactory rationale for phlebotomy and catharsis, yet von Muralt was skeptical about these opinions. Taken together, the papers of Peyer and von Muralt demonstrate the approximately simultaneous spread of the use of the Peruvian bark from France and from Italy to Switzerland.

In 1687, Johann Andreas Stisser, professor of chemistry at Helmstädt, issued *A New Consideration of the Intermittent Fevers Adapted to Modern Opinions.* He valued the Peruvian bark, although he thought that it worked better in warm climates than in cold. He agreed with Willis and Barbette that a single treatment with the drug produced no profound cure, yet he had observed temporary alleviation of symptoms, and he advocated use of the drug in persons debilitated by repeated attacks. Stisser's essay reveals judicious and unprejudiced use of the Peruvian bark, but the dosages that he employed were later shown to be inadequate.

The long clinical and pedagogic activity and the pronounced pharmacologic preoccupations of Friedrich Hoffmann (1660–1742) make it almost inevitable that his name should appear in a detailed history of cinchona. In 1687 he published his *Thesaurus pharmaceuticus,* which describes febrifuges but fails to mention the bark.[124] In 1693 he became the first professor of medicine at the new University of Halle and in the following year presided over the procinchonal (or procortical) thesis of one Johannes Balthasar Schondorff. This investigator attempted to explain the properties of the drug by microscopical examination of the powder; his concept, like that of his master, was iatromechanical. In discussing abuse of the bark he made no mention of deafness.[125]

In 1695 Hoffmann issued his work on the fundamentals of medicine. Here he stated clearly that the bark is a specific remedy in intermittent fevers; by means of its bitter, earthy, gently astringent, and resinous-balsamic particles it neutralizes the defective quality in the febrile material. In the same work Hoffman vouchsafes the broadminded general comment that "it is always completely necessary to use both chemical and galenical medicines."[126]

While Hoffman was writing these works and supervising the composition of others, additional papers on cinchona appeared in the *Ephemerides* and elsewhere. Krugius (1691) reported the cure of an extremely severe tertian "by the only genuine specific remedy," his *liquor* of china china, administered without emetic, purge, or clyster, in contravention of long-established rules; and G. C. Schelhammer, professor at Jena, wrote of cinchona favorably and in a manner indicative of personal experience. He was aware that it had been used also in lower Saxony.[127] Ledelius (1694) described success in treating quartan fever with the bark, but included in his small series one patient who recovered without it. In a more combative manner Wolfart (1695) of Giessen, writing under the supervision of Valentini, referred to early opponents of the bark as lice. He found the bark to be undoubtedly curative; indeed, it was like an anchor in quartan fever, a disease that was formerly the scandal of physicians.

In 1696, Bernhard Valentini of Giessen (1657–1729) contributed to the *Ephemerides* an essay on the Peruvian bark. In this paper he did not fail to report that the opinions offered by Cardinal Donghi's consultants in Piacenza[128] thirty-five years earlier on the avoidance of the bark in tertian intermittents had now been rendered erroneous and obsolete. Valentini stated that his own experience with the drug was usually but not invariably favorable. He remarked incidentally that the drug had been used earlier in Heidelberg, at an unspecified time, by [Lorenz] Strauss (1603–87) and by Faustus.[129]

Toward the end of the century Valentini's contemporary, Christian Johann Lange (1655–1701) of Leipzig, was writing or rewriting numerous discussions and dissertations, which were published posthumously in 1704. His essay on the febrifugal action of *china china* resulted from the diversity of the opinions that had been promulgated. The article contains a rapid but thorough historical review and, indeed, shows that a confusing plethora of occurrences had already created a need for retrospect, just as the entire essay demonstrates that the drug had achieved acceptance. Less impressive to the modern reader is

Lange's conclusion that the drug is effective, not because it precipitates acid humors that cause fevers but because it overcomes symptoms.[130]

In 1711, a few years after Lange's publication, Berger and Stieler mounted a strong attack on all extant theories. They contended that we cannot detect the powers of *chinchina* by its appearance, odor, or taste. It was a waste of time and oil and labor, they said, to try to assign the powers to degrees of heat and dryness or to unfold them by fire and chemical analysis and to refer them to the preponderance of salt, sulfur, or earth, or to the pounding of acid or alkali, or to the motion of subtle and fiery matter, or to throngs of unknown shapes. Berger and Stieler wished that physicians in all eras had spurned the alleged principles of nature and dubious hypotheses and instead had concentrated their attention on effects and properties of drugs.[131]

To the procinchonal opinions of Hoffmann, discussed above, those of his academic colleague and bitter enemy Stahl provide sharp contrast. This religious, dogmatic, and animistic professor—an ex-Jesuit—was opposed to the use of antipyretics, especially the Peruvian bark, which had become popular.[132] Drugs of this kind, he believed, inhibit the beneficial movements that allegedly take place during fever. He cited unfavorable results and offered the summary statement, "To tell the truth, the *china* is more harmful than all the other things that are ordinarily used to suppress fever."[133] It is not surprising that opinions of this kind are echoed in some of the theses written in Halle.[134]

In the small series of German and Swiss writings that are summarized in the foregoing pages it is difficult to discern a clear or unitary trend. Many record predominantly favorable results with the use of the bark. Krugius in 1691 and Valentini in 1696 reported successful cure of tertians as well as quartans, an outcome mentioned long before in the *Schedula Romana*.

In attempting to explain the action of the drug, Hoffmann in 1695 invoked the familiar particles and at the same time approved the use of both Galenical and chemical drugs. His pupil Schondorff, in an especially attractive contribution, undertook, in the last year of Malpighi's lifetime (1694), to study the bark microscopically; his findings were used in support of iatromechanical explanations. Boehmer (1738), another pupil of Hoffmann, was later to apply chemical methods to the study of cascarilla (*Croton* sp.), a plant used as a substitute for the Peruvian bark.[135] Occasional writers, such as Krugius (1691), disregarded the old rules that required preliminary use of phlebotomy and purgation. Two decades later, in 1711, Berger and Stieler rejected all extant theoretical explanations. Against these authors, most of whom favored the use of the bark, stood Georg Stahl and his school. Yet in 1726 Stahl

commented that the popularity of the drug caused him to fear that it
was being abused.

It is clear that in Germany, as in many other parts of the world, the
Jesuits must have played a role in the distribution of the Peruvian bark,
but the details of their activity in this sphere remain to be discovered,
assembled, and analyzed. The evidence that has been made available
up to the present time is scanty and fragmentary.

In Germany, as elsewhere, the larger Jesuit establishments were
equipped with pharmacies. These were usually managed by a specially
trained brother and often included sick laity among their clientele—a
fact that at times caused hostility among secular apothecaries.[136]
Whatever the Jesuits were able to accomplish with respect to the distribution of drugs was doubtless affected by political and social conditions, including not only those mentioned at the beginning of this
chapter but also, and most especially, the proscription imposed upon
the order in Lutheran Germany. This produced effects that contrasted
sharply with conditions in Roman Catholic Austria.

From a letter of Pietro Paolo Puccerini, pharmacist of the Collegio
Romano, it is known that the Peruvian bark was sent from Rome to
several European countries, one of which was Germany, at some time
between 1647 and 1659.[137] Duhr alludes to other fragments of epistolary evidence and states: "As to *Chinin* for the [Jesuit] apothecary
shops, interesting details are continued in the letters of the procurator
Friedrich Ampringer in Rome, written to father Seb[astian] Grüber in
Munich. See especially the letters of June 15, July 13, and October 19,
1689." [138] Duhr's statement signifies that the route opened by Puccerini
was being followed twenty or thirty years later.

The fragmentary evidences obtained from Jesuit sources represent
the actions of a well-organized international group and in this respect
can be compared with the fiscal and financial reports from Frankfurt
and Leipzig,[139] which can be viewed as local manifestations resulting
from the functioning of international secular commerce. The two kinds
of evidence tell the attentive scholar where he is likely to find additional source material.

Let us now summarize the German developments. We have already
observed that during most of the seventeenth century Germany suffered from war and its concomitants and sequelae. These ills a gro-
tesquely uncoordinated political system did little to alleviate. The Protestant Reformation and the Catholic Counter-Reformation, the latter
furthered by the Jesuits, created an additional division, no less important. Secular intellectual activity, after decades of prostration, began a
late revival.

In view of these events and conditions it is not surprising that the permanent entry of cinchona into the German arena was late; in addition, its use was meager or—an alternative possibility—was meagerly documented. After the first introduction, mentioned by Badus (dated vaguely by Puccerini at ca. 1647–59), and after the isolated report by Glantz in 1653 and the municipal schedules of 1668 and 1669, there is not much in available records. During the next ten years the bark apparently was used little if at all. It reentered the Germanic world at some time between 1679 and 1685, through the agency of Peyer, an illustrious Swiss. From his statement we must deduce that a single man, namely Talbor, was a major efficient cause whereby the drug was restored to active use in three major areas of western Europe: England, France, and Germany.

Late in the seventeenth century, the establishment of the *Ephemerides* and the birth of the university at Halle, accompanied by renewed activity at older academic centers, produced a growing literature in which theses and articles in journals assumed quantitative if not qualitative importance. Associated with the restoration of academic vigor was the prominence of academic physicians, among whom Hoffmann and Stahl were conspicuous and influential, and held widely differing opinions about the Peruvian bark.

Also worthy of mention is Johannes Bohn (1640–1718), professor and dean in the University of Leipzig. He was characterized by Max Salomon as not an epoch-making discoverer but as "one of the most outstanding physicians of all times."[140] Bohn argued vigorously against physicians who allowed the fever to burn out or who delayed treatment. He had used the Peruvian bark successfully, although he occasionally encountered obstinate cases, and he saw no harmful aftereffects. He usually prescribed the drug *in substantia,* that is, unmixed; at the same time he avoided the alternative decoctions and juleps that were popular among "trivial physicians." Exposing as a fallacy the common belief that premature treatment fosters the disease, he recognized that relapse was often caused by adulteration of the drug or by inadequate dosage. His experience with the Peruvian bark was obviously extensive.[141] Another important author, Paul Werlhof (1699–1767), a practitioner rather than a professor, did not begin to issue his major publications on the fevers till 1732.[142]

As late as 1759 Jean Baptiste Senac was to remark: "There are countries in which the celebrated remedy [Peruvian bark] is still in bad repute. Among the Dutch and the Germans, the common people reject it entirely. But all the charges which they bring against it, are to be attributed to an improper method of using it." The reader is welcome to reflect on the differences or discrepancies between Bohn's report and the statement of Senac. The former embodies the conclusions that a skilled physician derived from clinical practice, while the latter describes the opinion current among ignorant laymen. Probably both reports are correct.

Although, as we have seen, the use of antimony as a febrifuge, as well as the iatrochemical tradition of which it constituted an important part, originated, or was promoted, in Germany and Switzerland and was the subject of long controversy, the hostilities associated with its use did not assume the concentrated character that was evident in France. The term "antimony war" is not customarily applied to occurrences in Germany.

6 Russia, the Orient, and the Americas

WE TURN NOW to some developments in the history of the bark in areas remote from the main scene of events, namely in Russia and the Orient. A few occurrences in North and South America are also considered here, although the fragmentary character of the evidence lends itself to impressions that can hardly be assembled into a continuous historical narrative.

Russia

By the year 1650 the Russian domain extended westward from Moscow approximately to the thirtieth meridian but did not include the Ukraine or the westernmost parts of what later became the USSR. Eastward its cold embrace included almost all of Siberia. Economic activity was predominantly agricultural. The immense realm, culturally retarded, thinly populated, and despotically ruled, had long been isolated from the West. Peter the Great, who reigned from 1682 to 1725, was a capable but poorly schooled man whose interests leaned toward mechanical and technical pursuits, not excluding medicine and surgery, but before him the Russian empire was almost devoid of industry.

Trade between Russia and England was established formally in the middle of the sixteenth century by the creation of the Muscovy or Russia Company. Rowell states that "records of the Apothecary Bureau listing plants sent to the physician Matvei Kinfin in 1633 include . . . Peruvian bark." [1] This obviously erroneous statement is probably based on confusion with chinaroot. Appleby, citing Russian and other sources, has written that "from 1660 to 1670 the bulk of medicines [imported into Russia] continued to come from England. An English merchant was commissioned in 1660, and again in 1670, to buy apothecary medicines. . . . In 1661, John, later Sir John, Hebdon, agent for Tsar Alexei Mikhailovich (father of Peter the Great), and the Russia Company, procured large pharmaceutical supplies for the Russians; two years later, he consigned six trunks and two barrels of apothecary goods from England." [2] Appleby has pointed out that these transactions occurred despite the fact that the influence of the Russia Company was then waning and despite the fact that the Dutch also were exporting medicines.

Late in the seventeenth century the tsars undertook the recruitment of trained persons such as physicians, surgeons, and apothecaries, in England, Holland, and Germany. An example is Samuel Collins (1618–70), who was born in England and received the medical doctorate in Padua. After meeting a Russian agent in Holland, he went to Russia, where during 1660–69 he served as physician to Tsar Alexei Mikhailovich. [3]

A second and even better example is Michael Gramann. A member of a German family residing in Moscow, he was sent by the tsar to Germany in 1659 to study medicine. In 1666 he received the doctorate in Jena and then served for many years as medical advisor to the Russian royal family. His doctoral thesis has for its subject intermittent quartan fever. The fact that he studied at Jena well after the middle of the seventeenth century suggests that he is likely to have been aware of the Peruvian bark, whether he favored its use or not. [4]

The text of his thesis, divided into thirty short chapters and introduced by the author's iatrochemical mentor Werner Rolfinck, defines quartan fever in ancient terms as a hot dyscrasia of the heart and the entire body, recurring every fourth day and caused by melancholic humor that collects in the alimentary passages and produces putridity. The author cites the iatrochemists Quercetanus, Joubert, and Riverius, and calls attention to the twenty-year experience of his uncle Hartmann Gramann (previous chief physician to the grand duke of Muscovy), who had treated protracted fevers successfully by purgation. [5] Michael Gramann's thesis, iatrochemically oriented, makes no mention of Peruvian bark.

Less cogent but not negligible is the fact that occasional well-placed travelers and migrants who were conversant with affairs in both Russia and England at this time are likely to have spread word of the bark. An example is General Patrick Gordon (1635–99), a Scottish adventurer and author, who served in the Russian army for three decades, beginning in 1661. He was in England, on an official Russian mission, from

October 1666 to February 1667, and in January 1667 dined with Sir George Ent (1604–89), William Harvey's friend, who at this time was registrar of the College of Physicians.[6]

These bits of information add up to no more than high probabilities that the Peruvian bark was known to a few people in Russia at this time. Convincingly strong evidence is nil.

A Russian scholar named Novombergskiy published a letter dated September 13, 1664, that mentions arrangements for importation of drugs, namely sassafras wood, bark of the "holy wood" [*lignum sanctum*, guaiac], *cassia lignea*, and an item designated as *korenya khiny*, which has been thought to be Jesuits' bark.[7] It is possible that this item was china-root—Smilax, an old favorite—since the Russian *koren'* means root, whereas *kora* is bark. It is of incidental interest, and possibly of significance, that neither *koren'* nor *kora* appears in the copious indexes to the first six volumes of the collected letters and papers of Peter the Great, which represent the years 1688–1707.[8] At the same time it must be remembered that the root bark of the cinchona tree is strongly antimalarial;[9] hence the interpretation of Novombergskiy's document remains equivocal. The use of *khina* for fever allegedly appears also in an order of Tsar Theodore Alekseevich dated 1678.[10] The evidential value of this statement depends on the bibliographer who excerpted it; it is not clear whether the word *khina* appears in the original or is an interpretation. The problem is complicated additionally by the fact that the word *khina* is used nowadays for quinine, a substance that was first isolated in 1820.

In contrast are the negative evidences. Wilhelm Richter's three-volume history includes in its extensive documentary material lists of drugs sold in Russian apothecary shops in 1670–71, as well as a list of drugs ordered from Amsterdam by the tsar's apothecary in 1678, also sixteen double-column pages of recipes written in 1667–74, and various recipes prepared on behalf of the royal family in 1663 and 1673. None of these compilations mentions the Peruvian bark.[11]

Bruce-Chwatt and Zulueta have rescued from oblivion the fact that until the eighteenth century the Peruvian bark was kept in the Kremlin for exclusive use by the tsar and his kin.[12] The reader who chooses to compare this fact with the behavior of Louis XIV will find instructive details in Chapter 5.

At this point two erroneous inferences are possible. First, it would be wrong to deduce that because the tsars attempted to monopolize the drug, it was not in fact distributed, although its date of introduction into Russia remains unknown. Second, it would be unjustifiable to assume that the cold climates in much of Russia necessarily signify absence of malaria.[13] Further, as we have seen, the Peruvian bark was used for a large number of miscellaneous diseases, especially conditions that produce periodic symptoms.[14]

In view of the facts that have been presented and the gaps that have been described, we must judge that, while the Peruvian bark was probably known to a few physicians and occasional laymen in Russia in the seventeenth century, no conclusive evidence has been found that indicates that the drug actually entered the Russian domain during that period.

The advances in naval education which are credited to Peter the Great, for example, the establishment of the School of Mathematical and Naval Sciences (Moscow, 1702) and of the Naval Academy (St. Petersburg, 1715), are unlikely to have affected the availability of Peruvian bark in his domain, since there is no evidence that the drug was sent on Russian ships. The construction of roads, another project favored by the emperor, could have facilitated the distribution of drugs and is likely also to have increased the spread of malaria.

An additional aspect remains to be mentioned, namely the presence of Jesuits in Russia.[15] The facts are fragmentary and interesting, but with respect to the use of Peruvian bark they are inconclusive.

The Jesuits, leaders in the Counter-Reformation—a movement that is examined in greater detail later in the chapter—first appeared in Poland in 1564 and in Lithuania in 1569. They speedily became powerful there. By 1750 they had founded a college in Vilna. At approximately the same time they were active also in another country near Russia—Moldavia.

As to the Muscovite domain, the false Dmitri, also designated as Pseudo-Dmitri I, crowned in 1605, is known to have disappointed the Jesuits by his failure to convert Russia to Roman Catholicism. Somewhat later, their continued and intense efforts to secure for Sigismund III of Poland (king of Poland 1587–1632, king of Sweden 1592–1604), a Roman Catholic, the crown of Russia, gave way to a counterreaction by the Orthodox, which culminated in the coronation of Mikhail Feodorovich, first of the Romanov dynasty (1613). Despite these political misadventures the Jesuits made many converts in Russia, especially among persons of high rank and strong influence.

In 1649, a treaty concluded under Tsar Alexis Romanov excluded Jesuits from Kiev and other cities of the special Cossack area in which Russian schools existed. In 1671 a Moldavian adventurer known as Spafary (né Nicolae Milescu) entered Russia and became leader of a Russian embassy to China. In 1676, he reached Peking, where he participated in the formulation of a treaty with China, the Chinese plenipotentiaries being aided by Father Ferdinand Verbiest and other Jesuit priests who resided in China.

A slightly later phase is described as follows in the charming words of Lutteroth (and his Gibbonesque translator): "Far from obeying the laws which interdicted their entrance into Russia the Jesuits found means to insinuate themselves under divers pretexts; and in 1705 they succeeded in founding a college at Moscow. Peter the Great, on his return from his travels in 1719, closed the college, and expelled the Society."[16] The unexpected restoration of the Jesuits to Russia in 1772 lies outside the temporal scope of this history.

The facts presented in these pages show clearly enough that during the seventeenth century the Jesuits were present in Russia overtly and intermittently. We may surmise that they were also present secretly, and we can recognize that they were intermittently influential. But there is no evidence that they brought the Peruvian bark into the Muscovite domain.

The presence of the drug in Riga at the comparatively early date of 1685 is recorded in the encyclopedic compilation of Tunmann.[17] This date compares favorably with the earliest dates in German lists. At this time Riga was in the domain of Sweden and had not yet fallen to Peter the Great. The route by which the Peruvian bark reached Riga is unknown.

The Great Explorations and the Counter-Reformation

The spread of the Peruvian bark to the Orient, like its transmission from South America to Europe, was a concomitant and consequence of geographical, political, commercial, and religious developments. This inference faces us when we consider the following events. In 1487–88 Bartolomeu Dias sailed southward from Portugal and doubled the southern end of Africa, opening the route to the East. Soon afterward, in 1492–1504, Columbus made his four westward voyages, and in 1497–99 Vasco da Gama sailed from Lisbon to Calicut, on the Malabar (southwestern) coast of India. In 1510, Afonso de Albuquerque designated Goa as capital of the Portuguese colonial possessions. In addition, he established communication with Siam, the Moluccas, and China. In 1519–22 the expedition of Fernando de Magalhães (Ferdinand Magellan), a Portuguese enlisted in the service of Spain, traveled westward and discovered the Philippines, where Magellan was killed. In 1524, Vasco da Gama became viceroy of Portuguese Asia.

Presently two additional groups of actors appeared on the crowded scene. In 1526–30, Babur, a Turkoman descended from Timur and Jenghiz Khan, successfully invaded northern India and established the Mogul dynasty. In 1534, Ignatius Loyola and five companions founded the Society of Jesus. Soon afterward, in 1540, Pope Paul III formally approved the establishment of the Jesuit order. Two years later, Francis Xavier, under patronage of King João III of Portugal, set up a mission at Goa, the Portuguese colonial capital. Then he proceeded to make converts in India, the Moluccas, and Ceylon. Three Jesuit missions from Goa visited the Mogul emperor Akbar between 1580 and 1605. Another functioned at some time during the reign of Shah Jahan, who ruled from 1628 to 1657.[18]

This review shows that while the political and administrative framework was being developed for the increase of commerce and the spread of Christianity in the Orient, as well as for the Counter-Reformation in Europe, a mechanism was being created which was to serve incidentally for widespread introduction of the Peruvian bark.

In the Orient the Iberian initiative did not function alone but was simultaneous with commercial and military activities conducted by England, France, the Netherlands, Denmark, Sweden, Austria, and Scotland. Each of these countries created one or more East India companies. The Dutch enterprise was most successful in the East Indies, less extensive and less durable in India, and least extensive and durable in Japan.

Persia, which is not included in the present investigation, forms the subject of a valuable book by Cyril Elgood (1951). Elgood mentions a "factory diary" of the East India Company, in 131 volumes, as yet largely unpublished but preserved at the India Office in London; in addition, his own book devotes an entire chapter to the East India Company in Persia.

So far as can be ascertained, the spread of Peruvian bark into the immense area that remains to be considered in this chapter, namely, the Orient and the Americas, has failed to attract, even incidentally, the attention of political, social, military, and ecclesiastical historians. Contrary to expectation, the subject proves to have been overlooked by medical historians also. At the same time, occasional allusions, fragments, and hints make it virtually certain that the requisite information exists in governmental, ecclesiastical, and commercial archives, where it awaits discovery by future investigators.

India

As we have already noticed, the Mogul emperor Shah Jahan reigned from 1628 to 1657. The earliest conveyance of the Peruvian bark to India, whether by Jesuits or others, could have occurred no earlier than his reign; another possibility is the era of his successor Aurangzib, who ruled from 1658 to 1707. It must be observed, also, that during the seventeenth century the predominance in European commerce with the mainland of India shifted from the Portuguese to the Dutch, and that in the mainland of Asia and in Ceylon the Dutch were gradually replaced by the English.

Since the great bulk of the Dutch East India Company's records has been lost, for an introduction to Dutch activities in India it would be desirable to examine in minute detail (which I have not undertaken to do) the work of Johan Karel Jakob de Jonge (1828–80), which includes extensive series of documents. Its main content, however, is political, administrative, and commercial. For information about Peruvian bark future scholars will need to consult also the archives at The Hague.

Other Dutch records are represented by fifteen volumes of published selections, held in Madras, which deal mainly with the second half of the eighteenth century.[19] The medical information in these documents is meager. For example, from a report completed in 1781 we learn that items shipped to the Malabar Coast, presumably from other parts of the Orient, included chinaroot (Smilax); there is no mention of Peruvian bark.[20] Another report contains short lists of hospital personnel but no information about the drugs they used.[21]

An elaborate history, either official or officially inspired, of the Dutch East India Company, mentions an admittedly inadequate early hospital in Batavia, replaced in 1743 by one that had on its staff a doctor and six surgeons. This establishment had business relations with a "City Apothecary shop." Peruvian bark is not mentioned.[22]

From records of this kind, the inquirer may turn to the travels of Wouter Schouten (1638–1704), a competent ship's surgeon who visited many places in the Orient during 1658–65. Schouten tells of an ardent fever that broke out after his ship left South Africa and was heading for Sumatra. Immediately afterward there was an outbreak of what appears to have been plague. The report does not state what medicines were used. "Fevers," unspecified, are mentioned as occurring in Goa and on the Coromandel Coast.[23]

Similarly interesting and disappointing are the reminiscences of Monsignor Giuseppe Sebastiani, a highly placed ecclesiastic. Leaving Rome in 1660, he traveled for at least four years in India and other parts of the Orient. He speaks of highly malignant fevers in Goa,

treated mainly by bloodletting, and he tells of his own repeatedly recurring quartan, but he mentions no drugs.[24] It is almost certain that
an important cleric who had been in Rome in 1660 knew of the Jesuits'
bark.

Of the fourteen volumes of Jesuit *Lettres édifiantes*, four (6–8, 14)
are devoted to the Orient. The sixth volume in this series mentions the
dispatch to China of a group of missionaries that included several men
skilled in medicine.[25] This incident, or something similar to it, is discussed later in this chapter. The oriental volumes of edifying letters
have no other medical content.

It would be reasonable to suppose that the English East India Company, which was chartered in 1600 and ended by amalgamation in
1702, took part in early transmission of Peruvian bark to India. The
necessary evidence may exist, but it has not yet come to light, and the
historian's hope is disappointed.

Occasional commentators and annalists have mentioned strong influence exerted on Mogul emperors by English physicians, such as Gabriel Boughton, who treated members of the family of the emperor
Shah Jahan about 1645 and thereby earned large privileges for his
compatriots.[26] In 1717 William Hamilton, participant in an English
embassy to Delhi, successfully treated the emperor Farrukh Siyar and
obtained a firman that granted special privileges to the East India
Company, including exemption from customs duty. There is no evidence that Hamilton administered Peruvian bark to his eminent patient.[27]

A standard compilation of company records, voluminous but not in-
dexed, by John Bruce (1745–1826), makes no mention of the bark but
tells of private traders, designated as interlopers, who "interfered with
the Company's exclusive privileges" by fitting out a ship at Cadiz in
order to convey European commodities to India and to return with
Eastern produce for disposal in European markets. Bruce reports activities of this kind repeatedly for the period 1679–97.[28] The contraband
was taken to Ostend. If the ships started from Cadiz, it would not have
been difficult for the interlopers to include Peruvian bark in their cargoes. However, since the entire process was clandestine, we may doubt
that records, if any existed, are still extant.

The most important of the chartered companies, the East India
Company, which lasted until 1858, is represented by collected records
and by books of memoirs. It is worth nothing that the captains who
served the company were required to file in East India House in London the journal of each voyage; 170 years of these documents are extant.[29]

An impressive series of materials was issued by the Record Office of

Madras presidency. The Dutch records in this collection are discussed earlier in this chapter. Among the English records we may choose for special consideration those of Fort St. George (later called Madras). These documents, prepared for commercial purposes, mention matters of medical interest occasionally and no more than incidentally. For example, deaths and even testaments are recorded, but the cause of death is usually omitted. Closer to our theme is the recurrent mention of lists of medicines requested by surgeons or physicians, without reference to individual drugs. For example, in the contents of a packet, January 1695: "The Shirurgeon his list of me[dicines] to be provided at Fort St. George."[30] And, "The Dʳ complains of the ill Package of Physick Chests and that the list of what is wanted and wrote for is not observed."[31] It remains possible that the original lists of medicines have been preserved.

Indirectly helpful is a letter written from Fort St. George on September 30, 1698, by Samuel Browne, a company surgeon, to James Petiver, the apothecary and botanist (1663–1718), requesting, *inter alia*, thirty-eight "Druggs and Medicines."[32] The list includes twenty pounds of antimony, five pounds of gentian root, and three pounds of lesser centaury; we have seen that all of these drugs were standard items used in the treatment of fevers, especially intermittent fevers. The letter does not mention Peruvian bark. The safest interpretation is that this drug was not used at Fort St. George at the time. Ironically the list of requests includes another Peruvian product—the balsam.

D. V. S. Reddy has found and reprinted a list of supplies dated July 27, 1737, from the surgeons to the president and governor of Fort St. George. This document mentions "Rez Cort Peru oz 7."[33]

Less helpful are the books of reminiscences, such as those of Hedges and Collet.[34] The two-volume diary of Streynsham Master reports an outbreak of fever in June 1676 which appears to have been malaria, but the Peruvian bark is not mentioned.[35]

While it seems obvious that the Peruvian bark must have been known to some or many of the English physicians who reached India before 1700, definitive proof has been scarce. John Fryer (d. 1733), M.D., 1683, traveled in India and Persia for the East India Company. In 1675 he observed in Surat a Brahmin practitioner who prescribed a powder for agues, "which works as infallibly as the Peruvian Bark; it is a preparation of natural Cinnaber."[36]

In view of these hints and fragments it is highly probable that search of the records of the East India Company will reveal abundant and important information about the transmission of the Peruvian bark to India and also to Persia and lands beyond.

The sequel to the story of the East India Company and cinchona occurred after the lapse of more than a century and a half. In 1839, John F. Royle (1799–1858), a surgeon and naturalist employed by the company, suggested that the cinchona tree be transplanted to India. The subsequent resistances and delays, the renewed proposals by Royle (1853, 1856), and the success of the enterprise in 1859, have been related by Sir Clements Markham.[37]

Siam

To write the early history of the Peruvian bark in Siam requires audacity in the writer and the hope of indulgence from the reader, inasmuch as the essential primary information concerning the arrival and distribution of the drug has not yet been disinterred from archival repositories, whereas information about the political, religious, social, and commercial history of Siam is readily available. Hence we have a rich background and no foreground. As to the latter, the historian must limit himself to pointing out such written materials as appear likely to fill the large lacunae.

According to a French ecclesiastical historian, extant letters of Francis Xavier (1506–52) show that the famous missionary had a strong desire to work in Siam, but his wish was never gratified. According to the same source, a few years after Xavier's death several Portuguese ships reached Siam.[38] A much more recent authoritative account states that the Portuguese first established relations with Siam in 1511.[39] The two statements are not necessarily in conflict.

About two or three hundred soldiers from the earliest vessels settled near the capital city and presently obtained spiritual support or guidance from Jesuits, Dominicans, and Franciscans, who set up three small parishes.[40] Other Christians who then resided in or near the capital were Dutch, Japanese, Chinese, and Cochin Chinese.

Of the letters and printed books about Jesuit doings in Siam that are listed in the copious bibliographies of de Backer and Sommervogel, none bears a date earlier than 1664.[41] The Arquivo Nacional da Torre do Tombo in Lisbon is a likely source of information on this part of the problem.

In 1658, during the reign of Pope Alexander VII, the Congregation for Foreign Missions (Société des Missions Etrangères de Paris), a religious institute of secular priests, that is, those not affiliated with the Jesuits or analogous orders, was founded by two French prelates, Bishop Palu and Bishop de la Mothe-Lambert, with the purpose of creating a group of indigenous clergy in the Orient. Under these auspices the congregation sent a small mission to Siam, which was headed by de la Mothe-Lambert and which reached that country in 1662.[42]

The new group, composed of Frenchmen professing fealty to the Holy See, encountered resistance from the Portuguese priests, who were subjects of the archbishop of Goa, primate of the Indies. These and other troubles lasted more than a century. In 1780 priests were expelled from Siam by royal edict. Since 1662 there had been visits to and from Rome and other European centers, as well as correspondence. In addition there were formal diplomatic embassies, such as that sent by the King of Siam to Louis XIV in 1685,[43] and uncounted visits were made to Siam by European naval vessels and merchant ships.

All of these miscellaneous facts signify contact between Siam and Europe—more specifically, between urban and royal Siam and powerful places in Europe. Therefore the opportunities were numerous for the transfer of knowledge about the Peruvian bark, as well as for transfer of the drug and transmission of malaria.

This interpretation is supported by a few medical details. The French clergy built at least one hospital or hospice in the capital city and a hospice in another large urban center ("pour travailler à sauver les âmes, sous pretexte de guérir les corps"). They acted as amateur physicians. In at least one instance ointments were used that had been brought from France. In addition, the king of Siam had a hospital built and placed it under management of the French vicars apostolic. A French surgeon named Charbonneau is known to have served in this establishment about 1677.[44]

Despite these facts and probabilities, the main question is left unanswered: we do not know whether the bark in actual fact ever reached Siam during the period examined in this history.

The Philippines

The Philippine Islands became part of the Spanish empire and are to this day the only large Asian region in which Roman Catholicism predominates. Like Siam, the archipelago exemplifies the scarcity of information derivable from oriental countries on the early history of the Peruvian bark.

The Augustinian friars undertook missionary work in the Philippines in 1565, and the Franciscans were at Cebu in 1567. In 1579 the Dominicans were in Luzon. The first Jesuit expedition to the Philippines arrived in Manila in 1581, while the Real Audiencia de Filipinas was established in 1584. A college of Manila was opened in 1595.[45] In 1601 the Colegio de San José was established under the direction of

Jesuits.[46] It is obvious that by the middle third of the seventeenth century, when the Peruvian bark was being disseminated widely in Europe, the Philippines possessed clerical and secular resources sufficient
for its reception.

A history of medicine in the Philippines, published in Manila in
1953 under academic auspices, makes no mention of Peruvian bark or
of malaria.[47] The darkness of our subtotal ignorance is relieved to a
small extent by the astonishing and little-known achievements of
Georg Joseph Kamel (1661–1706), apothecary, botanist, and lay
brother in the Jesuit order.[48]

Kamel was born in Brünn (now Brno) in Moravia and studied pharmacy in Bohemia. While it has not been established that he ever
received a diploma, it is evident that his scientific knowledge was extensive. In 1682 he became a lay brother in the Society of Jesus. By
1688 he was in the Philippines, where he held successively the titles of
infirmarius, apothecarius, and *botanicus.* He worked at the Jesuit college of San Ignacio in Manila and was the first in the archipelago to
establish a pharmacy on European models. In accord with the habit
of the era, he also practiced medicine. Apparently his clientele was
large.

As if these labors were not enough, Kamel made extensive studies of
the local fauna and flora; the camellia commemorates him.[49] His interests brought him into correspondence with Samuel Brown and Edward
Bulkley, physicians to the East India Company in Madras, and with
famous botanists such as John Ray (1627–1705) and James Petiver
(1663–1718). Ray's *Historia plantarum* includes in the third of its three
volumes two appendixes: one is a syllabus of Philippine plants observed and described by Kamel and one is Kamel's description of trees.
The second volume, *which Kamel is known to have possessed,*[50] contains a description of the Peruvian bark and a discussion of its effectiveness in intermittent fevers (see Chapter 4).

What do these facts tell us? In the last decade of the seventeenth
century—or very slightly earlier—a member of the Jesuit order who
was both an apothecary and a naturalist established in Manila, a city
not devoid of clerical and academic activities, a pharmacy of European
type. At the same time this apothecary was in correspondence with
leading English botanists and possessed at least one book that described the Peruvian bark and advocated its use in intermittent fever.

We are justified in concluding that Kamel knew of the bark and its
febrifugal property. There is no evidence that he possessed the drug or
used it, nor is there evidence that it was used by anyone else in the
Philippines at this time.

China

As we have seen, the obscure early adventures of the Peruvian bark in Russia were based on the deeds of emperors, aided by the physicians whom they had imported form western Europe, and on quantities of medicine imported chiefly from England. Evidence of participation by missionaries in the transmission of Peruvian bark into Russia is absent. With the earliest relevant incident in China the pattern returns to the more usual form of mediation by Jesuits, and once again an exalted personage is included in the cast of characters.

Three decades after the death of Francis Xavier (1506–52),[51] Jesuit missionary activities in China began. From its first site, a coastal island, the enterprise spread, through the labor of a slowly growing group of trained men. By the beginning of the seventeenth century— during the decades that preceded the introduction of Peruvian bark into Europe—the Jesuits were hoping to find an overland route to China, since travel by sea was extremely hazardous.[52] One group managed to reach Macao in 1658; by 1661 they had arrived in Peking and then departed on a long journey back to Europe. These travels, as well as the later participation by Jesuits in the negotiations that in 1689 led to the Sino-Russian treaty of Nerchinsk, have no direct bearing on the fortunes of the Peruvian bark in China but are significant because they demonstrate the extensiveness and intricacy of Jesuit activities in areas in which the bark was sooner or later to appear. Other Roman Catholic orders, such as the Franciscans, had arrived in China much earlier, and also later, than the Jesuits, but there is no evidence that they participated in the transmission of the Peruvian bark.[53]

Especially noteworthy and memorable are the astronomical activities of Jesuits in China, represented by the example of Matteo Ricci, S.J. (1552–1610), who entered the Chinese Empire in 1583 and remained there until his death. In addition to his mathematical and scientific work he founded missions in several districts. Somewhat later came Ferdinand Verbiest, S.J. (1623–88), who served as chief of the Imperial Astronomical Bureau in Peking and also aided in Sino-Russian negotiations. In the words of one scholar, "Appointments in the [Chinese Astronomical] Bureau provided the Jesuits with access to the ruling elite, whose conversion was their main objective."[54]

In the final decade of the seventeenth century, during the K'ang Hsi reign (1662–1722) the emperor, a luminary of the Manchu dynasty, suffered a severe illness, which appears to have been malaria. Two French Jesuits, de Fontaney, a mathematician and meteorologist, and Visdelou, a sinologist credited with having set the foundations for the

famous French mission to Peking, treated the emperor successfully by
means of Peruvian bark. A member of the Jesuit mission, Joachim
Bouvet, wrote the following report, which was first published in 1697:

A large number of sick persons, among whom were many officers of the household and even one of the Emperor's own sons-in-law, were cured by taking
medicines that we had brought from Europe. A short while afterward the Emperor himself fell into a dangerous illness. After having tried without success
the medicines of his physicians, he had recourse to ours, which rescued him
from the danger in which he had been. His physicians wanted to have the
honor of effecting a cure but they were not too fortunate in this respect. The
emperor could be cured only by means of *kinkina*, which Fathers de Fontaney
and Visdelou, who fortunately arrived at that time, had brought with them.[55]

The historical background against which these scenes were played
is depicted in a treatise by Peregrino da Costa.[56] This author, after presenting a mildly variant version of the emperor's name and cure, adds
that in 1714 the senate of Macau (Macao) sent the Chinese emperor a
box of *quinquina*, "together with other drugs in vogue in that century."
The same author points out, significantly, that all the Peking missionaries possessed medical knowledge obtained at the College of St. Paul
in Goa and that emphasis had been placed on their possessing it. It is
not difficult to view their treatment of the K'ang Hsi emperor as similar
or analogous to the famous Jesuit proclivity for becoming confessors to
royal personages.

It would be interesting to discover which drugs were used by the
emperor's Chinese physicians prior to the administration of the Peruvian bark. An old Chinese antimalarial, *qinghaosu* (artemisinin), is
presently under study.[57] It is said to be mentioned in a Chinese book of
recipes dated 168 B.C., in a handbook of A.D. 340, in a compendium of
1596, and in a treatise of 1798.[58]

The Americas

With respect to the transmission of cinchona from Peru
to other South American countries in the seventeenth century, until an
exhaustive search of documents is undertaken, the scarcity of available
direct evidence compels us to rely on probabilities derived indirectly.
We may take Brazil as an example.

In 1580 the crowns of Portugal and Spain were united in the tenure
of Philip I of Portugal, who was recognized also as Philip II of Spain.
The territory of Brazil was part of his realm. In 1640 a Portuguese re-
volt established João IV of the house of Braganza as monarch of Portugal and hence of Brazil also.

In 1621 the Dutch West India Company was founded. The Dutch made extensive conquests in Brazil before 1661, when their power there was terminated.[59] Their comparatively brief incursion into the history of Brazil was disproportionately significant in the history of science, since Prince Maurice of Nassau-Siegen, who became governor of Brazil in 1637 and remained there until 1644, was a notable supporter of science and gathered capable investigators around him.[60] His physician, Willem Piso (1611–78), in a highly regarded book on the natural history of Brazil reported that the country was not lacking in tertian and other intermittent fevers.[61] He does not mention the Peruvian bark, but it is at least possible that the drug was brought into Brazil, even at this early time, by trans-Andean smuggling.

A well-marked feature of Brazilian history during the dominance of the Spanish Hapsburgs (1580–1640) and under the house of Braganza was the activity of the Jesuits, who had established missions in Brazil as early as 1549.[62] While rendering extensive services to the health of the populace, they did not establish hospitals,[63] but they maintained specialized workers of two kinds—nursing brothers (*irmãos enfermeiros*, some of whom were surgeons) and pharmacist brothers (*irmãos farmaceuticos*).[64] Many were Germans, Austrians, or Bohemians.[65] In Brazil they found it necessary to have large stocks of drugs, including many autochthonous products. They also compiled recipe books, some of which are still extant.[66]

A noted nurse-practitioner, Irmão Manoel Tristão (born ca. 1546, died before 1631),[67] is associated with recipes transmitted by Samuel Purchas (1575?–1626).[68] Also recorded is a *Collecção de varias receitas* (Collection of Various Recipes), a miscellaneous work of unknown authorship dated 1766 and said to have been current in Jesuit drugstores in the eighteenth century.[69] In discussing works of this character Father Leite points out that the drugs originated by the colleges or Jesuit practitioners in Brazil included four that were used against fevers, including malaria,[70] but he does not give their names.

A manuscript work titled *Receituário brasilico*, a compilation of 444 pages plus an index of 50 pages, completed in Rome in 1762, has been discussed by Jorge (1937). It is obviously outside the temporal scope of this history; according to Jorge it mentions cinchona. A large and comparatively recent work on the history of medicine in Brazil makes occasional mention of cinchona and repeated mention of malaria but fails to report, or to approximate, the date when the drug first entered Brazil.[71]

Information concerning the sale of the bark by a pharmacy in Lima in 1770 has been presented by Valdizan and Maldonado.[72]

These facts tell us little about the South American spread of the Peruvian bark, but they reinforce the opinion that study of Jesuit records is almost certain to fill gaps in knowledge of the subject. The same expectation applies a fortiori to Paraguay, where the Jesuits maintained an almost autonomous regime for nearly one hundred fifty years until their defeat in the middle of the eighteenth century.[73] With regard to Brazil the examination of Dutch commercial records is more than likely to be instructive.

In 1712, in the city of Mexico, Juan de Esteyneffer (Johannes Steinhöffer, 1664–1716), a Jesuit lay brother designated as coadjutor formal, issued his *Florilegio medicinal de todas las enfermedades*. In 1978, this work, now scarce, was reissued with valuable annotations by Carmen Anzures y Balanos, under the auspices of the Academia Nacional de México.[74] It discusses the use and especially the dosage of Jesuits' bark under the name of *la cascarilla del Peru* but provides no evidence about the date when the drug first reached Mexico. However, it might be used as a starting point for a proper historical investigation. Additional clues are to be found in an essay by Kay (1989), who mentions the Jesuit missionary Father Eusebio Kino (1645?–1711) and several of his followers. Kino is known to have reached Mexico as early as 1681.

In 1681, Lionel Wafer, the peripatetic English buccaneer and surgeon (1660?–1705?), crossed the isthmus of Panama; later he was with Dampier in Virginia. In his book of travels, published in 1699, he noted that he had obtained some of the Jesuits' bark in Arica. He wrote: "I found it to be the right sort, by the frequent use I made of it in Virginia and elsewhere; and I have some of it now by me."[75] This incident, apparently an act of uncomplicated empiricism, can be reckoned an accidental or temporary introduction of the drug into North America. Until Jesuit records, including those of Canada and Louisiana, have been studied completely, it must rank as one of the earliest. There is clear need of a conscientious study, page by page, of the *Jesuit relations;* its extensive indices are not oriented toward the subjects under discussion in this history.[76] Moreover, the arrival of samples or shipments of the bark would not necessarily or invariably be deemed worthy of mention in the original reports.

A hint of public tastes and behavior in eastern North America three decades after the time of Wafer is found in an "almanack" of 1713, which recommends "gension" (gentian) and madder for the ague.[77]

7 Italy and Spain, 1679–1718

WE NOW PROCEED to consider the history of the Peruvian bark in southern Europe in the late seventeenth and early eighteenth centuries.

The attitudes of Marcello Malpighi (1628–94) toward the use of the drug are obviously important, not only because of the great man's undisputed eminence in biological research but because he practiced clinical medicine at the same time. The intricate narrative of his opinions has been given best by Adelmann, who pointed out that "Malpighi seems to have been for some time reluctant to prescribe it [the Peruvian bark] even as a febrifuge." This is shown in a letter that Malpighi wrote in 1679 concerning a case of what was almost certainly malaria. In its list of suggested remedies the letter did not even mention the bark. Adelmann showed also that as late as 1687 Malpighi "was still apparently avoiding comment." In 1691 and subsequently he recommended the drug.[1] His protracted reluctance is not explained by evidence that has come to light thus far. Unquestionably it is a conspicuous if not famous example of resistance to innovation, the more remarkable because it occurred in a great innovator. There are obvious parallels with the attitudes of Sydenham and Willis.

In 1682 the ever-progressive Francesco Redi wrote that *chinachina* is the best, or rather the only, febrifuge that is truly efficacious; so many others that receive great encomia in medical books are unequal to their reputations.[2] How gracefully he disposed of all the rivals! A few years later, in 1687, four French treatises on cinchona, published originally in 1679–82, were collected and reissued in Ferrara by Nigrisoli.[3] These have been discussed in Chapter 5.

As we have already observed, an anonymous author—possibly Fa-

gon—wrote in 1689 that *kinkina,* then popular in France, had lost popularity in Italy.[4] This opinion is expressed also in a work written slightly
later by Adriaan Helvetius [1661?–1727], or under his influence, and
translated into Italian by Carlo Ricani: "It may be accounted not a little
surprising that *kinakina,* which nowadays receives so much approval
for the treatment of an almost infinite number of persons whom it has
restored to health, has so few partisans in Italy, where it began to appear forty years ago under the name of the Spaniard Cardinal de
Lugo."[5]

Ricani's allusion to a decline in the popularity of the Peruvian bark
in Italy is confirmed by a remark of Morgagni, which apparently refers
to his early days as a practitioner (1701–6).[6] Contemporaneous with
Nigrisoli's collection is a significant and charming compilation issued
in Spain and written by Juan de Cabriada (1687). In strongly supporting the use of powdered Peruvian bark this author proclaimed it the
knife that cuts the danger and prevents recurrence, this property being
especially valuable against the threat of the syncopal tertian.[7] To Willisian explanations that invoke ferments and particles he added saga-
ciously: "I shall speak of it as the most powerful [febrifugal] remedy
known up to now. I say 'up to now' because time and experience may
allow us to know others that are still better."[8] Cabriada's book had been
attacked by an author pseudonymously called "Aduanista," who based
his contentions on the alleged maltreatment of a Castilian grandee.[9]
The exalted personage was given the Peruvian bark for treatment of a
simple tertian, which then converted to a double tertian. The title of
the book tells us that this attack was based on "dogmatic and rational"
medicine, a system exposed and condemned in the riposte of another
pseudonymous contestant, Filiatro (1688).

The reader will have observed the resemblance between this minor
war of pamphlets and the more famous conflicts that were ignited by
the fevers of the viceroy Ferdinand and the archduke Leopold and that
are discussed in Chapter 3. Vitriol, anonymous or pseudonymous authorship, and participation of the socially eminent were common to all.
The Iberian controversy evinces growing infidelity to ancient and
medieval medicine, an attitude compatible with its later date.

Several special orientations are observable in another complex of
writings that developed at about this time. Giambattista Giovannini
(Juanini) (1636–91), a Milanese physician who held degrees from
Milan and then—according with the current of European politics—
from Salamanca, published in 1679 a treatise that was reissued in
French in Toulouse in 1685 and was dedicated to Don Juan of Austria.
The French version is titled *Dissertation physique, ou l'on montre les*

mouvements de la fermentation; les effets des matières nitreuses dans les corps sublunaires, & les causes qui alterent la pureté de l'air de Madrid.[10]

That pernicious intermittents producing cerebral symptoms and syncope were especially common in Spain in this era is suggested not only by the writings of major authors such as Ludovicus Mercatus (Luis Mercado) and Pedro Miguel de Heredia, by less famous authors such as Diego Salado Garces, and by the special treatise of Isaac Cardoso but also by incidental comments and observations.[11] Salvador Flores, for example, says, "It is commonly heard that in other times there were not so many syncopes in tertian fevers in Seville."[12] These facts suggest that falciparum malaria was increasing in incidence in Spain. A later chapter relates that a similar development is suspected to have occurred in Modena in the time of Francesco Torti. Here we have a problem in which valuable information might be obtainable by paleoserological research.

The title of Juanini's book shows that the work uses atomist, fermentationist, and iatrochemical concepts; these the author derived from the continuously and widely influential Thomas Willis. The book attempts also to apply the author's ideas to explanation of the atmospheric pollution that allegedly existed in Madrid.

Juanini supports Fernel's old belief that the principal focus of tertian fever is situated in the hollows of infrahepatic organs such as the stomach and intestines. He recognizes the efficacy of Peruvian bark[13] as well as the frequency of paroxysms recurring after its use. Its value in syncopal fevers, a persistent preoccupation among Spanish physicians, he leaves in doubt.

Late-century opposition to cinchona is amply embodied in a treatise by Colmenero of Salamanca. This work, too long and intricate for convenient summary, selects authorities of whom its author approves and rejects the others, including Juanini, who is politely and variously characterized as *agudissimo, eruditissimo,* and *perdocto.* Included with appeals to selected authorities is the empirical argument that the drug often fails to effect a cure. This objection Colmenero ingeniously supports by high-level opinion, namely that of Cicero and Galen, both of whom declared that authority must yield to reason and experience.[14]

Colmenero's attack was promptly refuted by Tomás Fernández, a fermentationist who supplemented his clinical experience by extensive literary quotation, which even included the comments of St. Ambrose on the value of orderly presentation. Fernández asserted that the essence of fever does not consist of heat. He accepted the Willisian contention that fever is inordinate movement and excessive effervescence of blood; heat, he says, is merely a concomitant symptom. The proxi-

mate cause is an acid created in the stomach. The Peruvian bark, which
is alkaline, absorbs acid and impedes fermentation because it contains
an abundance of terrestrial salts. It extinguishes the febrile ferment,
expelling it in stool, vomitus, urine, or sweat. Colmenero, he adds,
erred in asserting that for extinction of the ferment to occur, it must be
fixated or precipitated.[15]

For Fernández's text an introduction was written by Dr. Andres de
Gamez, ex-professor of method at the University of Granada and protomedicus in Naples. His remarks are significant because they mention
the importance of a "secure and rational method" for administration
of the drug. This orientation was to be conspicuous in the work of Francesco Torti.

Colmenero was attacked also by Francisco Suárez de Ribera, who
used much information derived from the influential and repeatedly reissued pharmacopoeia of George Bate (1608–69) and added that Colmenero had denounced a medicine accepted universally "by learned
members of the Apollonian profession." The drug, Suárez asserted,
had the special power to suspend febrile ferments and to rid the patient
of febrile attacks, both intermittent and continued remittent, that start
with coldness of the extremities; hence it is a true vegetable specific.
Further, it opens obstructions and resolves putrefaction. His onslaught
on the use of analogical reasoning may be regarded as a historical curiosity since it is included in a treatise on intermittent fever.[16]

With respect to the Peruvian bark the experiences of Milan up to the
year 1658 have been recounted in Chapter 3; a postscript was provided
in 1661 by the vigorously discussed illness of Cardinal Donghi, who
developed tertian fever in Piacenza and was visited by Milanese consultants.[17] Not long afterward, in 1668, the College of Physicians of
Milan issued its pharmacopoeia, which makes no mention of the Peruvian bark.[18] At the very least this omission suggests that the drug had
not yet received general approval from the physicians of Milan. Doubtless the authors remembered the Donghian controversy.

The second edition of the Milanese pharmacopoeia, issued in 1698,
shows the changes that had occurred in thirty years. The later version
discusses *china chinae* and includes a brief retrospect, which mentions
the Genoese merchant Antonio Bollo as well as Richard Morton. The
bark is characterized as "the celebrated febrifuge of our times, highly
esteemed by the whole world." The note adds that the price of the drug
was high in the early years, when the difficulties and dangers of navigation made it scarce, but at the time of writing availability had increased and the price had declined. The note ends with a laudatory
sonnet.[19]

The eminence of Antonio Vallisneri (1661–1730) in medicine and biological science makes it obligatory to consider his brief dissertation, *On the Usefulness of China China in Fevers.* In this work, which bears the date November 5, 1699, he denounced the doctrine of critical days, the use of cupping, and the like. He highly commended the Peruvian bark, which, he asserted, suppresses fevers "not by long and dire ambiguities, mysterious days, and a fabulous contraption of opinions, but almost in the blink of an eye. . . . The intellects of physicians exert themselves to determine the cause of fevers and may direct their remedy against them; but let the laborious struggles come to an end. *China china* goes far beyond the falsehood of opinions and immediately extinguishes whatever has been the febrile ferment."[20]

Vallisneri refers to many successes in cases of intermittent fever treated with the Peruvian bark. As to its usefulness in malignant fevers, he says that this must be decided by experience rather than by ratiocination. He mentions Morton and Boyle but not the contentious Ramazzini. Vallisneri's dissertation of 1699 reappears in the third volume of his collected *Opere fisico-mediche*, which was issued in 1733. The same volume also includes a few minor remarks about the Peruvian bark, discussions of nomenclature and physical properties, and two consultation notes, one of which records Vallisneri's use of the bark in 1729.[21]

We have already noticed a remark that Morgagni made around 1701–6, to the effect that some physicians of his country—the Veneto, not Milanese Lombardy—had been deterred from using the bark by "fear, and I know not what kind of aversion."[22] Morgagni's reminiscence merely suggests that at this period the popularity of the drug was subject to local variation. In addition, it may imply a contrast between the boldness of a young practitioner and the conservatism of his elders.

In "Letter the Thirtieth" of the *De Sedibus* Morgagni tells of a nobleman in Bologna who had a double tertian fever. The illness, not clearly dated, appears to have occurred about 1689. Morgagni states: "But these things happened . . . at that time, in which they were as yet afraid of using the Peruvian bark, by way of a febrifuge, in the manner that we use it at present, and as it was first made use of at Bologna successfully, by that very ingenious physician Dominic Guliclmini [*sic*]."[23] This tells us not only that the bark was used in Bologna in or about 1689 but also that Guglielmini later introduced an improved dosage.

Guglielmini (1655–1710), a pupil of Malpighi and a teacher of Morgagni, worked on hydrodynamics, astronomy, and medicine. He was professor of mathematics in Padua and then professor of medicine. One biographer states that he was better known in hydraulics than in medicine.[24] Apparently he planned a treatise on fevers, which has not been published. However, his posthumously issued *Opera Omnia*, which contains a biography by Morgagni, includes also a letter addressed to Alexander de Bonis on the Ides of October 1702 in which Guglielmini speculates about the manner in which *quinquina* bark operates.[25]

Guglielmini's summary discussion, devoted to fundamental principles, does not reveal the extent of his experience, nor does it present reports of individual patients. The bark, he says, is useful in periodic fevers only. When the paroxysm is overcome by the bark but returns a few days later, one must deduce that the causative ferment has merely been suspended, not conquered. When the bark interrupts the fever, the patients do not regain healthy color or appetite or strength. This is a very clear sign that some kind of disease remains in the humors and the bark cannot overcome it. [Here we have both a clinical observation and an inference.] At the time of such interruption, Guglielmini continues, this kind of malady can disappear spontaneously or be removed by some other drug. He adds, by circular reasoning, "This is what happens when there are no relapses" [*qui casus iste est, in quo nulli contingunt relapsus*].[26]

Further, it is established by experience that the bark often stops the fever for three weeks or more. Hence it is to be inferred that the action of the drug is exerted against the pyrogenic ferment only. In periodic fevers the ferment is nothing but a certain saline and sulfurous mass, which the ordinary agitation of the blood cannot dissolve.

Guglielmini's letter to de Bonis refers repeatedly to relapses occurring after administration of the bark. It does not reveal what dosage was used, and it does not say anything about the improved system of dosage for which Guglielmini was praised by Morgagni. On chronological grounds it is certainly possible for Guglielmini to have introduced such an innovation after the letter was written.

In 1711, the year after Guglielmini's death, an essay was published by his pupil and academic successor Carlo Francesco Cogrossi (1681–1769), *Della natura, effetti, ed' uso della corteccia del Perù, ò sia china china; considerazioni fisico-mechaniche e mediche* (On the Nature, Effects, and Use of Peruvian Bark or China china; Physicomechanical and Medical Considerations). This publication, cast in the form of a letter to Giovanni Domenico Santorini, is significant rather than important.

Cogrossi says that the Peruvian bark is very effective and that its value is not a matter of opinion: he will try to explain its action. He has already drawn up numerous histories of fever patients whom he has treated. In addition he has tested the powdered bark against the venous blood of one patient in order to find out whether the components of the drug, being bitter and rough, were adapted to mixture with the blood. Cogrossi believed that his conclusions were based on observation.[27]

The largest faction of physicians, he remarks, holds that fever is a disorderly movement and morbid fermentation of the blood. He adds, vaguely, that the febrifuge constrains and fixates the turbulence or ferment or peccant humor. Morton had maintained that the Peruvian bark is an antidote to the malignity of the pyrogenic poisons, but this is specious. Cogrossi, following Guglielmini, proposes to use physical and mathematical concepts. However, his statements contain no hint of quantitative thinking. It becomes evident that his principal source is Sydenham, and a lesser one is Willis. He cites also the experiences of Ramazzini. Using Willis's statements as a basis, he offers a mechanical explanation whereby the action of the bark is made to depend on displacement of its particles from the axial current of blood in capillaries to the concave walls of these vessels.[28]

Cogrossi says that the bark is a mixture composed mainly of saline materials. The power of the febrifuge consists in dissolving rather than fixating. He constructs a largely imaginary pharmacodynamics, according to which the particles of the drug enter venous orifices situated in the coats of the intestine; this is shown by the fact that the drug is effective when administered rectally. A more important channel is provided by the lacteals. For methods of preparing and administering the bark Cogrossi relies on Sydenham.

Cogrossi does not mention Torti, whose *Synopsis* had been issued in 1709 but apparently received limited dissemination. Torti's major treatise (1712) was yet to appear.[29]

Cogrossi's essay depicts full acceptance of the bark and recognition of occasional failures. It also shows that the empirical triumphs of the drug continued to be far beyond what nascent physiology and biochemistry could explain. Moreover, it was still possible and acceptable to propound explanatory doctrines supported by little or no evidence. Cogrossi's devotion, energy, and verbiage obscure the fact that treatment of the fevers had made almost no progress since Sydenham. We may award him a modicum of credit for his implied opinion that his explanations must rest ultimately on clinical fact.

A notable contemporary of Cogrossi was Bernardino Zendrini (1679–1747), a medical graduate of Padua and an admiring pupil of Domenico Guglielmini. A native of Brescia, Zendrini practiced medicine there and subsequently removed to Venice, where he gained high esteem as a physician and also as a hydraulic engineer.[30]

The writing that mainly claims our attention is Zendrini's bipartite book titled *Trattato della chinachina* (Treatise on Chinachina). This work bears the title-page date of 1715 and a censor's approval dated February 3, 1714. A remark in the text reads, "It is now the twentieth year that Venice has not had an epidemic."[31] From the compilations of Corradi it becomes apparent that this is a reference to outbreaks of plague that occurred in the Venetian domain in 1693.[32] Hence Zendrini's book was written during 1712–13. In the first of these two years, Torti's *Therapeutice* made its debut.

Zendrini's "preface" takes up one-third of his book. Describing the various prejudices and false opinions held by physicians and by laymen, he explains and strongly defends the beliefs of the iatrophysical school. Concomitantly he insists on the importance of observation, experience, and mathematics.

The second and larger part of the book could be called the *Trattato* proper. Devoted to chinachina (Peruvian bark), it begins with a historical summary of the objections that impeded acceptance of the drug. This discussion is in effect a sequel to the litany of prejudices set forth in the long introduction. It is to be noted that, despite his progressiveness, Zendrini attributed intermittent fever mainly to corruption of bile. He also invoked the more modern Bellinian *lentor* as a pathogenic force.

Zendrini declared that the Peruvian bark should be administered in the form of the powder, which he deemed preferable to the tincture. This preference was based on his belief that the powder acts within bile in small channels in the stomach and proximal small intestine. The drug, he wrote, need not enter the blood, which in intermittent fever is inert and does not play a primary role.

The powder should be administered promptly, when the symptoms begin. The ordinary dose is two drachms; in severe cases up to an ounce may be given. The dose of two drachms may be repeated as often as necessary. To prevent relapse, the physician should give three-quarters of an ounce divided into three or four parts, administered in one day, beginning at the decline of the last attack. It is usually necessary to add two or three ounces more, divided in the same way, or even divided into six doses per ounce, in order to extirpate the sickness completely and prevent recurrence. In urgent cases it may be necessary to give an entire ounce in twenty to twenty-four hours, dividing it into ten or twelve parts. Subsequent treatment should consist of two drachms per day up to a total of three to four ounces. It is desirable to use bezoar to combat residua. Chinachina, Zendrini adds, is the only drug that is effective against intermittent fevers; there is no suitable substitute. Chinachina is the proof that true specifics exist.

Zendrini says that the drug may be used during health, but then it would do nothing except keep the recipient more fully in good health. He makes no other reference to prophylactic use.

Zendrini's book contains ample practical detail with respect to therapeutics. Although he makes almost no mention of individual cases, his book shows that he was an experienced practical physician. While he refers to "urgent cases," he does not characterize them as pernicious or malignant.

It is noteworthy also that Zendrini makes no mention of Torti. As I have shown, it appears probable that the *Trattato* was being written in 1712–13, whereas Torti's *Therapeutice* came forth in 1712. Torti's *Synopsis*, issued in 1709, may have had a small circulation and hence could well have failed to reach Zendrini, even though the latter was working in Venice.

Much later, in 1741, Zendrini issued a major treatise on hydrology. Here he states that stagnant waters pollute the air "with I know not what unhealthful exhalation," which has depopulated large communities near Venice. Most surprisingly, this book makes *no* mention of intermittent fever, or Peruvian bark, or any other drug, nor does it refer to Lancisi's famous *De noxiis paludum effluviis*, which had been published in 1717.

8 Antonio Frassoni and Francesco Torti's *Synopsis*

Antonio Frassoni

We must now turn to important developments that had their roots in the seventeenth century. An interesting contribution, not widely known, was made by a Modenese physician, Antonio Frassoni (1607?–80), to the history of the Peruvian bark.[1] In a letter dated November 5, 1656, Frassoni wrote to Badus as a reply or addendum to the work Badus (then Baldus) published in that year,

> Know that ten years ago, more or less, I first administered the bark, [giving it] with highly successful result, to the illustrious Count Alexander Facchineti [*sic*], brother of the eminent Cardinal Facchineti [*sic*], who had received it in Rome from the eminent de Lugo. Later I administered it to others with the same result. Later it was sent to me by friends, to whom it was always given by the same de Lugo.[2]

To these remarks Frassoni subjoined that he had discussed the Peruvian bark with eminent physicians at Bologna, including the archiaters of the university, and found that they knew little about this drug and had never used it.

Frassoni's observation about Bologna merely shows that, at this early stage, knowledge of the Peruvian bark had percolated incompletely and irregularly from Rome to other cities. In contrast, his recollection about Count Alessandro Facchinetti and his brother Cesare Cardinal Facchinetti has greater significance.

Cesare Facchinetti (1608–83), member of a papal family, had been created cardinal by Urban VIII on July 13, 1643, at the same time as Juan de Lugo and Gianstefano Donghi, both of whom have figured in this history. The additional fact that Cesare Facchinetti had been papal nunzio in Madrid from 1633 to 1643 indicates that he had knowledge of Spanish affairs and contact with influential Spanish personages but does not indicate that during this period he was acquainted with de Lugo, who had been in Rome since 1621.[3] At any rate, it is highly probable that the two men were acquainted by 1643.

That Frassoni had received the Peruvian bark from Cesare Cardinal Facchinetti, and not from any medical, pharmaceutical, or commercial source, emphasizes the continuing role of de Lugo and of the Catholic Church in the dissemination of the drug. It also points to the role of personal contacts within the Church. Moreover, it provides at least a hint that Frassoni either was receptive to innovations or had found it advisable to yield to the influence of the cardinal. There is no evidence that Frassoni was an innovator or revolutionary in medical matters other than the use of the Peruvian bark.

It should be noted also that even though Frassoni's letter to Badus does not mention an exact date for the treatment of Count Alessandro Facchinetti, even the approximate dating derivable from the letter shows that the incident was one of the early European examples of successful individual treatment of fever by means of the Peruvian bark. There is no mention of relapse. The patient was known to have been an intemperate man, but he lived until 1685.[4]

In addition to the information recorded in the letter to Badus, almost all that is known about the life and work of Antonio Frassoni is to be found in the masterwork of his pupil Francesco Torti and in an article, already cited, by Professor Pericle di Pietro (1952) of Modena. Torti says that when the Peruvian drug reached the West [sic], Frassoni was one of the first to employ it. He began to give it in prolonged quartans, when tired patients and doctors usually resorted to almost any empirical medicine or even to products suggested by old women (*quo tempore tum Aegri, tum Medici taedio affecti ad remedia quaelibet Empirica, atque etiam anilia solent confugere*). When cures were obtained in quartans, he turned to spurious [i.e., mixed] tertians, then to simple and double tertians, benign and not pernicious, and to other intermittents, especially the protracted cases. Meanwhile, Torti continues, almost all the other physicians were reluctant. As long as Frassoni lived, they clamored, so that, in order to avoid their severe censure, the bark, like a refugee or an exile, did not dare to enter the pharmacopoeias but was obliged to hide in nuns' cloisters, where the conscientious physician sought it out in order to administer it to sick persons for whom he was responsible.[5]

Following the instruction in the *Schedula Romana*, at the start of the paroxysm (as was then usual), Frassoni gave adult patients two drachms of the fine powder, sometimes in about five ounces of wine or

in a bolus. By this method he was able to suppress all prolonged intermittents. He had been doing so since the drug first came to Italy, and
was still doing so in 1677, when Torti joined him as a pupil. Not rarely
there were relapses, which Frassoni terminated by giving the bark once
or twice more. By the time of Frassoni's death in 1680, much of the
hostility to the drug had ceased.

Frassoni wrote little. He composed a work on the baths of Montegib-
bio, published at Modena in 1660 and summarized by Di Pietro. In
addition, the Biblioteca Estense contains twenty manuscript consultations by Frassoni.[6] Preliminary examination of these writings shows
that they are undated. Despite this deficiency they are obviously worthy
of further study and analysis, especially since several of them describe
cases of fever.

An additional minutia remains to be mentioned. A letter written by
Malpighi to the duke of Modena on December 22, 1679, reported that
a Count Morandi had been treated successfully by Frassoni for "periodic fevers."[7] At this time, as Adelmann showed, Malpighi was reluctant to use Peruvian bark.[8]

One of the most significant cases in Frassoni's experience occurred
in the year 1678 or thereabouts. From the abundant detail and the dating of Torti's account, the case can be assumed to have passed under
Torti's observation. An obese, middle-aged man named Ottavio Maselli had intermittent quartan fever. The paroxysms began to become
stronger and longer and to be accompanied by tremors, subsultus tendinum, and mental alienation. The patient's tongue was rough, his
urine scanty and thick. Frassoni decided to administer the bark before
the fever became continuous. He had been accustomed to give half a
drachm in a bolus every morning, but a friend of the patient—a physician of higher authority and rank but not of greater knowledge or equal
experience—was horrified at the suggestion and cited many dangers
that might arise. He advocated cardiac remedies and bezoartics instead, in addition to venesection, leeches, and cupping.

These objections prevented Frassoni from prescribing the Peruvian
bark, although he asserted that the outcome would be very bad if it was
not given immediately. The patient's kinsmen insisted that the bark be
postponed until at least one more attack had occurred. Frassoni answered that delay would be dangerous but that he was now unwilling
to give the bark as long as the other physician disapproved and was
openly condemnatory. Meanwhile, despite cardiac drugs and the like,
the patient had an additional attack, which included hiccup; the other
signs did not disappear but were reduced. Frassoni now predicted that
death would occur after two or three further attacks, but the other phy-

sician proclaimed that it was wise to abstain from using the bark, an untrustworthy drug.

Meanwhile, Giovanni Battista Boccabadati (1635–96), a jurisconsult learned in the sciences and a close friend of the patient, privately urged Frassoni to give the bark, ignoring the sophistries of the other physician, since the patient could not be cured by the present treatment and was hurrying to destruction. In Boccabadati's opinion it was unjust that because of medical scoffing or caution or vain courtesies, the man should die. Frassoni answered that the fever had become not merely continuous (although remittent) but malignant and hence could not be overcome by the bark. Asked whether the drug could at least be given without harm, he said that in this case it was harmless and powerless, yet he was unwilling to prescribe it in a doubtful trial. "If such is the case," said the other, "I will give it, and it does not matter if I am called the murderer of my dear friend, who would otherwise die; and it is not beyond hope that he can be saved from certain danger by a safe remedy."

Saying this, Boccabadati departed immediately. He bought two drachms of the bark from the nuns, added wine, and administered the mixture to the patient as a paroxysm seemed to be impending. The new paroxysm did not develop. Unaware of what had happened, Frassoni's rival sang triumphantly, attributing the ensuing improvement to cardiac drugs. Frassoni then prescribed half a drachm of the bark daily in a bolus, pretending that it was merely a confection of alkermes and hyacinth. This pious fraud relieved the patient of all his symptoms in a few days, and he had no relapses.[9]

I have reproduced this case report in detail because, apart from describing prevalent medical customs and procedures, it gives insight into some of the difficulties that accompanied administration of the Peruvian bark in a northern Italian city as late as 1678, when this drug seemed close to final victory. Administration of the bark was opposed by an influential physician and advocated by an obscure one. The drug was sold by nuns and was administered by a learned layman, who used a much larger dose than the physician habitually employed. Further—and this is most important—Torti says that his recollection of this case impressed him strongly when he came to think about a more effective method for using the drug in both intermittent and subcontinuous pernicious fevers. The modern reader is likely to have reservations about pernicious signs ascribed to quartan fever.

In its essentials the tale of Frassoni is one of simple empiricism, unburdened by doctrine and uncluttered by footnotes. Yet it exhibits some of the traits that earlier chapters of this history have revealed again and again, especially the influence of the higher clergy and of highly placed laymen, the less conspicuous participation of the obscure, the tenacity of old opinions, and the intrusion of new.

We shall now return to Frassoni's energetic disciple, Francesco Torti.

Francesco Torti

Francesco Torti[10] was born in Modena in 1658. As a young man he started to study law but changed to medicine. Academic medical instruction being unavailable in his native city, he went to Bologna, where he received the doctoral degree in 1678. In 1677 he became a clinical pupil or assistant of Antonio Frassoni in Modena. This arrangement apparently lasted until Frassoni's death in 1680.

In 1682, Rinaldo d'Este, duke of Modena, reestablished academic teaching in that city, and the first chair of medicine was entrusted to Bernardino Ramazzini, an outstanding practitioner and consultant. Three years later, in 1685, the second chair was given to Torti, who in addition became the duke's physician. The services were poorly recompensed.[11]

Torti's pedagogic duties included the teaching of anatomy. A synopsis of his sixteen systematically arranged demonstrations and lectures, dated 1698 and preserved in the official archives at Modena, has been published by Di Pietro.[12] This outline, limited to normal anatomy, makes no mention of what nowadays is called morbid anatomy, nor does it mention any individual disease such as intermittent fever. However, the sixth demonstration, on the liver, gall bladder, and spleen, includes the ramifications of the vena cava and portal vein, while a supplementary presentation shows a spleen "floating in water and completely depleted of blood." Possibly the last item indicates the influence of Malpighi.

In 1717, Torti was honored by election to the Royal Society of London,[13] and he received many other honors (Fig. 3). He declined the offer of professorships in Turin (1717) and Padua (1720).

He composed four oratorios and several poems and epigrams, some of which appeared in print.[14] The following discussion, limited to Torti's important published work on the intermittent fevers, takes no account of his literary and musical efforts and accords only brief mention to his numerous unpublished consultations.[15] His early essays on the movements of mercury in the Torricellian barometer (Torti, [1695] and [1698]), which point to his position with respect to the Scientific Revolution, are mentioned incidentally in Chapter 9.

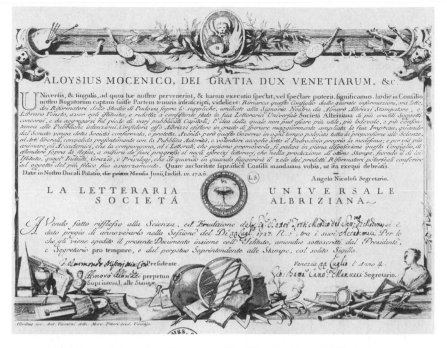

FIG. 3. Diploma awarded to Francesco Torti by the Società Albrizziana, Venice, 1727—an example of Torti's many honors. Mocenigo, member of a famous family, was the reigning *doge*. Courtesy Biblioteca Estense, Modena.

The *Synopsis*

In 1709, Torti issued a four-page statement titled *Synopsis libri, cui titulus, Therapeutice specialis ad febres quasdam perniciosas, inopinatò, ac repente lethales, una verò china china peculiari methodo ministrata sanabiles* (Synopsis of the Book Titled "Special Therapy of Certain Destructive Fevers, Unexpectedly and Suddenly Fatal, but Curable Only by Means of China china Given by a Special Method"). Torti was later to remark, in the *Therapeutice specialis,* that [Giambattista] Davini, an academic and clinical colleague who from time to time called him in consultation, had mentioned or discussed Torti's special method of dosage in *La Galleria di Minerva*, a periodical published in Venice by Girolamo Albrizzi from 1696 to 1717.[16] Hence fear of preemption may have been part of Torti's motive in preparing the *Synopsis*, but this is merely conjecture.

The brief text, which might be called the *editio princeps* of the *Synopsis*, was published by Soliani of Modena; according to Torti's *Thera-*

peutice specialis of 1712 it was also published "in the *Ephemerides* of
Trévoux and immediately afterward in those of Leipzig."[17]

Trévoux, 20 km north of Lyon, was the site of a famous printing
press operated by Jesuits. Neither in the *Mémoires pour l'histoire des
sciences et des beaux-arts, 1701–1767,* printed at Trévoux, nor in its
three-volume index[18] have I been able to find a trace of Torti's *Synopsis.*
It was evident, however, that articles had been contributed to the *Mémoires* by Lodovico Antonio Muratori, Torti's learned friend and biographer.[19] Hence a link between Torti and Trévoux is far from improbable.

As for the "*Ephemerides* of Leipzig," a search of the volumes issued
in this series under various titles[20] between 1697 and 1711 likewise
brought to light no edition of Torti's *Synopsis;* moreover, the lists of authors in successive volumes do not mention his name.[21]

An edition of Torti's *Synopsis* is found in the sixth volume of *La Galleria di Minerva,* which bears the date 1708, but like its Modenese prototype, this edition contains subterminally the words *Mutinae, Typis
Bartolomei Soliani Impress[oris] Duc[alis]* 1709 (Modena, printed by
Bartolomeo Soliani, Ducal Printer, 1709).[22] Since the same volume of
the *Galleria* also contains notices of other books that appeared in 1709,
the printed date of this volume, namely 1708, must be regarded as
merely nominal. It is not improbable that Torti's synopsis appeared in
other periodicals than the *Galleria,* but this detail has not been ex-
plored.

Despite its dual (or perhaps multiple) publication, approximately simultaneous, the *Synopsis* is not well known. The Modena edition, issued as a separate item and not as an article in a periodical publication,
is not recorded in the *National Union Catalog* or in the major European
catalogs, nor is it included among the collections of the Biblioteca
Apostolica Vaticana or those of the Biblioteca Estense of Modena. By
courteous permission of the Biblioteca Centrale Nazionale of Florence,
which has the only known example of the original text, it is reproduced
in full in Appendix C. My English translation follows.[23]

Synopsis of the book titled *Special Therapeutics of Certain Destructive Fevers
Which Are Unexpectedly and Suddenly Fatal But Are Curable by Means of* CHINA
CHINA *Administered by a Particular Method.* Amplified by histories of cures, by
questions and practical observations, and by many other things having to do
with the varied nature of fevers of this kind, and of all intermittent and continued fevers, and with the superiority and action of *China Chinae* and its use and
abuse in different kinds of fever. Intended as a mark of esteem especially for
juniors and candidates in the Art, by the author, Francesco Torti of Modena,
physician to the Most Serene Raynaldo I, Ruler and Duke of Modena, and
Professor of Medicine in the Ducal College.

The purpose or primary intention of this treatise is to convey an uncommon treatment (performed by means of *China Chinae* given by a special method, remote from the ordinary procedure and concept) of certain fevers that are deadly in the extreme of their danger, but the book also contains a discussion and complete examination of every kind of presentation of the said *China Chinae* in every kind of fever, in addition to that recommended by mature consideration and uninterrupted use of this febrifuge for thirty years and more, so that, especially for beginners, who often flounder among conflicting opinions, nothing should be missing for complete practical knowledge of all the fevers in which *China China* is appropriate (especially certain pernicious fevers), and for knowledge of the suitable and useful administration of this drug. For this reason the entire treatise is divided into four sections, summarized as follows.

The first section, more general than the rest, and divided into ten chapters, deals with the ordinary use of *China China* in lasting intermittents and shows how the Peruvian bark first became known to Frassoni, an eminent practitioner and the author's teacher, as soon as it arrived in Italy, and indeed in Europe, and how it later became known to the author himself. The ordinary offering of the drug in the more benign intermittents, and the more preferable prescriptions, are reviewed incidentally. The superiority and harmlessness of the outstanding drug, in the concurring opinions of many distinguished men, are examined, although fear of relapse is not always excluded. The antipathy of those who criminally disapprove the drug is considered at length, the objections are refuted, and reliable methods for preventing relapse are pointed out. Its power is shown to be exercised, quite often but not always, without perceptible evacuation, yet it is not on this account to be mistrusted or refused. The nature of its indescribable power is investigated by various trials, and it is shown that its use, even though it does not produce perceptible evacuations, is consistent with the teaching of the Galenists and humoralists. The more famous opinions of moderns concerning the causes of intermittents are also considered briefly and in all of them likewise the action of the bark has nothing to do with perceptible evacuation. Next, from these widely accepted opinions certain credible general theorems as to the nature and causes of intermittent fevers are brought forth, and according to them the ordinary presentation of the bark is regulated. As to abstruse and profound causes sought hesitantly, an unformed notion is published with which the author himself does not at all agree. After these preliminaries the question is asked whether in the beginning of the same common intermittents, that is, of those in which there is no danger of death, the bark can or must be given, just as is done during their course, and the problem is solved clearly. It is also asked whether purgation or venesection must be administered before the drug is given, and with equal clarity it is answered and shown how little benefit is usually derived in these intermittents (and even less in continued fevers) from bowel movement, especially the artificial but not rarely the spontaneous also, unless the illness is already declining at the same time. This is made obvious, by experience alone, without reasoning and authority, merely by particular cases adduced and described for this purpose. Then to establish the rule for the aforementioned distinctions, for the timely, moderate, and appropriate use of the bark in these ordinary intermittents, some histories are adduced, mingled at intervals with suitable observations, which illustrate and confirm the same aforementioned distinctions in all their parts.

The second section, which includes eight chapters, presents nothing else than the description of these pernicious fevers in general with regard to their nature, being intermittents at least at their onset; although the patient does well on the intervening days, during the third, fourth, or fifth attack they unexpectedly and almost suddenly kill him, or else come close to developing continuity, acuteness, and malignity, with less abrupt but not less serious endangerment of life. Since all of these fevers, at least the precipitous ones, and their appearance, were discussed excellently by one man among the older writers, namely Luis Mercado, who depicted them graphically as full of danger and terror, and by Richard Morton among the more recent authors, although more concisely and somewhat less clearly (but he cured them more successfully, since *China China* had been discovered), the entire little treatise of the first author and a special chapter of the second are reprinted and constitute the greater part of this smaller section. To the work of both authors extended comments have been added, as has seemed appropriate—to the former for correction of the old doctrine and in order to point out certain noteworthy things, to the latter for clearer explanation of the subject and for modification both of the rather liberal use of *China Chinae* and of his hypothesis of the fevers.

The third section, which is the most important, explains in twelve extensive chapters the special administration of *China Chinae* in the aforementioned pernicious fevers, and their nature, habit, diagnosis, and prognosis, according to the author's observation. According to him they are of eight kinds, described individually. The general causes of these pernicious fevers, insofar as they are such, are considered, as well as their different behavior in the three regions of the body. To this is added the treatment by means of an unfamiliar use of *China Chinae*. A special method is unfolded, based on certain rules, methods, and precautions drawn from rational practice by means of which many persons have manifestly been saved from death and saved repeatedly, obviously cured, not only before matters had rushed to catastrophe (for them any method, even a common one, is acceptable if only it is used promptly) but even (and here is the most important part) after the patient's life would seem to have been lost unless it could be drawn out for about twenty-four hours longer. In such circumstances the cure cannot be hoped for otherwise, unless occasionally by chance, from any other drug or even from *China China* given by some other method. For that reason this method is compared generally with the more famous methods of others such as Talbor, Helvetius, and even Morton himself. His method, although closer to mine [one word blurred] yet is not a little different, since the method invented by the author is surer and more active and was practiced before the works of Morton were printed in Geneva. The same method is examined carefully, as are its superiority, usefulness, and whatever unusual and new it may contain in comparison with others, since it may convey something new to foreigners as it did in the author's fatherland, where it was previously known to nobody, whether we consider the special management and administration of the drug or the alleged special ability of fevers to thwart its power and to reject it, or the otherwise deadly circumstances in which never-theless it is used very successfully. And thus it is defended against easily con-trived objections and from popular witticisms, and at length the circumstances are determined in which it has a place and in which it has not. For this reason a faithful and candid description is given of all the unfortunate cases, few as these are, in which *China China* could not help. In contrast there are added many of the very many truly wonderful cases that agree fully with the eight kinds of pernicious fever, representing each order and variety, which have been cured by this method up to the present time, beginning with the year 1695, when the method was first devised by the author and put into practice success-fully and was openly communicated at once to many medical men for public use. Finally the sections close with the difficult question, very weighty in prac-tice, whether when pernicious fevers of the eighth class, or the like, degenerate into essential and malignant continued fevers, and do so immediately in the very beginning—this phenomenon is not rarely encountered in practice—it is advantageous or permissible to interrupt their course immediately by adminis-tering the Peruvian bark and to suppress the febrile effervescence, which per-haps purifies, just as when this occurs gradually and during their course, al-though fevers of this kind do not threaten certain and precipitous death as do pernicious fevers of the other kinds, but only threaten a doubtful and later dan-ger, which is the same as asking whether the life of an endangered person should be saved during the uncertain suspicion of a new sickness or should be left in danger. The problem is examined seriously and is not solved distinctly. However, it is considered in a useful manner while it is investigated analyti-cally, and several successful examples are presented in which patients have been, at the very onset of such fevers; even then, because of the intensity of the symptoms, fever preponderated heavily over hope. These instances can give the learned and judicious physician a degree of confidence—although not without great and watchful caution—with regard to this problem.

　　Finally the fourth section, standing as a sort of corollary, divided merely into six chapters, all the kinds or varieties of continued fevers having been consid-ered incidentally to a degree sufficient for the purpose, answers several ques-tions about the use of the Peruvian bark, such as whether it may be given with benefit and appreciable usefulness in putrid continued or nonremittent fevers, both primary or essential, and symptomatic or concomitant, such as inflam-matory fevers, for example, and among them both the malignant as well as simply the acute. This is answered in the negative, and even more so in true hectic fevers. However, several successful cases known to the author and de-scribed apparently show that in what are called the puerile hectics, or rather in slow fevers that resemble hectics, the *China China* can be beneficial. It is also asked whether the drug should be given in fevers that have become continuous through subintrant attacks, also in what are called complicated fevers such as hemitriteans, etc., and this is affirmed. However, in fevers simply called contin-uous or proportionate continued fevers—that is, not indeed the continent fe-vers but those that recur and remit periodically—a distinction is made. And here Morton is explained and partly defended; otherwise, his contention, im-moderate in many other cases that have to do with the bark, clearly cannot be admitted. Finally, in considering generally all the cases in which *China China* may or may not apply, the general class of fevers and their variable metamorphoses, which sometimes warrant the drug and sometimes do not, are discussed. Finally it is inquired whether the same drug is appropriate in other diseases, especially periodic diseases, apart from the fevers, and this is given little credence. Also, it is asked whether, when the drug is injected in enemas or applied to the wrists, it is of any use in the treatment of fevers, and practice of this kind, however feeble, is not entirely condemned.

By a bibliographic mischance that has matured into an ineradicable tradition, the year 1709, which is the date of the *Synopsis,* has been cited repeatedly and erroneously as the date of the *Therapeutice specialis,* which did not make its debut until 1712.[24]

When the text of the *Synopsis* (1709) is compared with that of the *Therapeutice specialis* (1712), a curious difference is observed. According to the *Synopsis* the work was to be divided into four major sections, containing respectively ten, eight, twelve, and six chapters, which add up to a total of thirty-six. In the *Therapeutice* it is evident that the third of the four projected sections has been divided into two, each containing six chapters. Hence the text of 1712 has five major sections, but the total of thirty-six chapters is unaltered. This is a minor editorial change and does not affect the content.

An undated letter,[25] probably written by the astute Ippolito Francesco Albertini, states that cases of severe intermittent fever had appeared recently in Modena and that Torti had succeeded in curing the patients by means of the Peruvian bark, administered according to a special method that he does not describe in the printed synopsis (*quale nella stampata sinopsi non espone*) but reserves for the book that he will print. This observation is correct: the *Synopsis* announces the problems that are to be discussed but omits details of administration and dosage.

It would be rash to declare that Torti was aiming at deliberate concealment, especially since he was soon to complain in the *Therapeutice specialis* that his procedure was not widely known. It is at least possible that, since Torti habitually used an intricate manner of expression, he felt that a compendious synopsis would be inadequate as a presentation of an intricate and important subject.

9 Torti's *Therapeutice Specialis*

In 1712, three years after the *Synopsis*, the *Therapeutice specialis*, Torti's classic work, appeared. Its complete title, twice as long as that of the King James Bible, conforms to the habit of its era in that it is almost equivalent to a table of contents. In English translation it reads as follows:

Special treatment for certain unexpectedly and suddenly fatal pernicious fevers, curable only by *China China* administered by a particular method; amplified by histories of cures, by questions and practical observations, and many other matters that have bearing on the varied behavior of fevers of this kind and also on the character of all intermittents and indeed of continued fevers likewise, and on the superiority and actions of *China China*, and its use and abuse in individual kinds of fever and in many other diseases, especially those that recur

As will be shown, this title does not reproduce Torti's arrangement of subject matter; instead, it directs attention to the major purpose of the book—therapeutics. It has the additional virtue of calling attention to the emphasis on *pernicious* intermittents and to the suddenness with which they may kill.

Torti's literary style is one of baroque elaboration, comparable to the most exasperating passages in Morgagni and occasionally outdoing them. In both authors a diagnostic clue is the Latin word *inquam* (English: *I say*), used in a sentence that has an exordium long enough to make the reader and author lose track of the subject, so that the theme must be recalled to mind by a rhetorical device.[1] In the fourth chapter of book 5 *inquam* appears three times in two pages (639–40). The intricacy of Torti's style being matched by the complexity of his taxonomy and by the occasional elaborateness of his descriptions, it must be referred to personal idiosyncrasy as much as to the literary or scientific habits of the era.

It would be grossly unfair to assert that Torti's elaborate treatise is unsystematic. On the contrary, it is systematic, but the arrangement differs markedly from our current practice. In a book, or even a chapter, devoted to a single disease or group of diseases—especially a work that is to include students and beginners in its readership—we expect the author to discuss, in clearly demarcated subsections, the definition of each disease, its etiology, pathogenesis, morbid anatomy and patho-physiology, symptoms, diagnosis, prognosis, and treatment. Torti's less evolved method is well exemplified in the eight chapters of his book 2. Here he presents pernicious intermittents and their treatment as de-scribed by Mercatus and Morton; to long excerpts he adds original scholia. This exposition, obviously medieval in its style, is supple-mented by the six chapters of book 3, on pernicious fevers, including the intermittent and the subcontinuous, in an original description based on Torti's personal experience, including the treatment of these diseases by a special method. The differences between Torti's arrange-ment and that of our contemporaries cannot fail to multiply the diffi-culties of the modern analyst.

From time to time the reader is astonished and cheered by the un-dogmatic character of Torti's text. For example, in discussing the ma-lignant and destructive tendency of pernicious intermittents, a subject theretofore considered by not very many authors, Torti says that any-one who holds a different opinion should be free to believe what he wishes (*liberum sit ei sentire quod velit . . . me quidem hic loci minimè reluctante*).[2] Expressions of this kind stand in bold contrast to the con-tentiousness of more than a few writings described in this history, many a treatise on Peruvian bark being as bitter as its subject. Indeed, the benignity that Torti manifested in the *Therapeutice specialis* yielded later, at least temporarily, to the vitriol of Ramazzini, which is discussed in Chapter 10.

A valuable feature of Torti's style and method is his use of original case reports. This is exemplified in book 1 of the *Therapeutice*, in which nine chapters dealing with fundamentals are followed by a tenth chap-ter headed, "The foregoing doctrine concerning the bark, [that it is] to be administered on some occasions and not on others at the beginning of intermittents, is confirmed by the histories of various cures." This part of the book contains sixteen detailed case reports and refers inci-dentally to several others. Torti here points out that he is excluding or-dinary cases—routine cases of intermittent fever—which he evidently

judged to be uninstructive. In this respect, as in many others, he followed the lead of Morton.[3]

Torti's case reports, probably valuable to his contemporaries,[4] are
certainly valuable to the historically oriented reader and can be con-
templated with edification by the harassed practitioner in our own busy
era. They mention the opinions of patients, kinsmen, and physicians,
including the fears (592, 627–34) and pressures to which each group
was subjected. The intricacies of medical consultation—even the occasional use of guile, stealth, or secrecy—are not omitted (185, 441,
456, 482–83, 498). One report describes dissension among bystanders
(133), while another contrasts the methods employed by a conservative
or ignorant old practitioner with those of the more progressive Antonio
Frassoni (185). In addition, Torti says that he has been careful to include all of his fatal cases (365–84), and in a separate chapter he sets
forth all reports to him by friends (501–24). A few of his case reports
were recorded or mentioned previously in a collection of manuscripts
included among the papers of Malpighi; a striking example is a case of
puerperal fever in which Torti was summoned in consultation. The
husband insisted on administration of the bark. The fever subsided
after the uterus emptied itself.[5]

Torti found part of his impulse for the writing of the *Therapeutice
specialis* in Francis Bacon's *De . . . augmentis scientiarum*, which includes in the scope of its discussion some comment on current deficiencies in pharmacologic knowledge.[6] The significance and relevance
of this passage are suggested later. Torti also cites the twenty-second
line of Horace's *Ars Poetica*, which is a plea for simplicity! Whether
Bacon and Horace really influenced Torti or whether their alleged influence was merely an imaginative reconstruction, they at least described what Torti considered to be some of his fundamental beliefs
and motives.

In attempting to explain the fact that his therapeutic method was not
known widely, Torti remarked that "there is hardly enough commerce
with more distant cities for me to have investigated this matter properly" (xxi). This explanation could apply to difficulties of travel, to im-
pediments produced by wars, to the political barriers that separated
Italian principalities from one another and from foreign countries, or
to the paucity of up-to-date publication in medicine.

An important additional part of Torti's motivation for the writing of
his book was derived from the residual opposition that the Peruvian
bark was encountering. Torti says that by the time of Frassoni's death
(1680) almost all hostility to the drug had ceased, "so that nowadays
[ca. 1709–12] nothing is better known in medicine than that intermit-

tent fevers are dispelled by the bark" (5). But he also wrote, somewhat awkwardly, that there was still "no lack of fearful or prejudiced persons—although these are few—who mistrust the China china even in benign and prolonged intermittents" (xix). He stated further that "there are those who, against the experience and concurrence of the whole world, curse the bark as if it were arsenic or [corrosive] sublimate" (18–19).

Other persons, says Torti, had overestimated the power of the drug, using it indiscriminately in various fevers and in other periodically recurrent diseases; this was true especially in France (xxii). Much of what has been said about its cure of continued acute inflammations and malignant fevers is false or doubtful, as practice reveals. One man, Richard Morton, came close to the truth.

Torti states that he wanted to establish a rationale, so that future use of the bark would not be a matter of mere empiricism; the drug should be used selectively (xx). At this point a logician might wonder whether Torti's laudable effort to introduce rules based almost entirely on experience can be designated as abandonment of empiricism. Finally, Torti adds that his book is intended for students and beginners (xv, xix–xx). This statement is an optimistic departure from reality.

Contents of the *Therapeutice Specialis*

Since the verbosity of the *Synopsis*—an English translation appears in Chapter 8—is not at all points favorable to rapid comprehension, the reader may welcome the following summary of the *Therapeutice specialis*, which is based on the first edition (1712). This work, logical in its structure, discusses first common intermittents, then pernicious intermittents, and finally continued fevers. The order of battle is as follows:

Book 1, ten chapters: the excellence and effectiveness of the Peruvian bark; a defense of the bark; its systematic use in *common* intermittent fevers. (Much historical information, as well as analyses of diverse opinions.)

Book 2, eight chapters: pernicious intermittents as described and treated by other authors; excerpts from Mercatus and Morton, with thirty-three scholia by Torti.

Book 3, six chapters: pernicious fevers, including the intermittent and the subcontinuous, an original description, based on Torti's own experience (*ex propria observatione*); treatment by a special use of the bark; difficulties; narrative of the first significant case.

Book 4, six chapters: *pernicious* fevers affecting the three major regions of the body; case reports; the special problem of malignant subcontinuous fevers that threaten to become continuous.

Book 5, six chapters: *continuous* fevers; their classification; use of the Peruvian bark in some of those that are recurrent; use in hemitriteans, in
pregnancy, puerperium, and childhood; use in periodic nonfebrile ail-
ments; the tree of fevers.

Torti's Problems

Appraisal of Torti's work requires, at the very least, a
brief review of the main problems that confronted him. It has already
been stated that residual opposition of physicians and laymen to use of
the Peruvian bark was one of Torti's principal motives for the writing of
his book. Fear, in addition to prejudice, formed an important component of the opposition. We know that this was true when the patient
was an eminent person such as Archduke Leopold, whose illness was
discussed in Chapter 3. Several of Torti's case reports, not all of which
recount the annals of the eminent, include mention of his own fears
(627–34). In occasional cases, whether he approved or not, he administered the bark at the insistence of laymen (627).[7] This fact is surely of
historical significance because it shows that, despite fluctuations in its
popularity, the drug continued to have the respect of some nonmedical
persons, as had been evident since the days of de Lugo.

Some of the more important causes of opposition to the bark came
from ancient doctrine and have been noticed on preceding pages. A
principal cause, which Torti designated as *princeps oppositio* (33), was
that the drug produced no perceptible evacuation. This is a reference
to the Hippocratic concept that acute illnesses, especially those that are
accompanied by fever, are resolved by coction—cooking or digestion—
of the causative humors. In favorable cases this phase was followed by
crisis and the discharge or evacuation of the residues.[8] The apparent
absence of crisis after the use of the Peruvian bark, violating a basic
principle of medicine, necessarily elicited a long discussion by Torti
(33–48), which is considered later.

A second cause of opposition to use of the Peruvian bark was expressed in the Hippocratic aphorisms, namely that intermittent fevers
are not dangerous (4.43, 7.63)[9] and that an exact tertian (*tritaios ak-
ribēs*) reaches a crisis in seven periods at most (4.59). These important
pronouncements had bolstered the opinion, held by authorities such as
Plempius, that the Peruvian bark was unnecessary (see Chapter 3). Obviously it was impossible to reconcile the ancient dicta with the reports
of Mercatus, Morton, Torti, and others, who described intermittent fevers of utmost malignity.

In discussing this vexatious contradiction Torti mentions some early
dissents and, as already observed, presents extensive quotations from

Mercatus and Morton, plus his own comment (194–244). That some
tertians are lethal, he remarks, is a violation of Hippocratic doctrine,
but the fact is undeniable and many physicians have been deceived.
With respect to the normal and abnormal distribution of humors Mercatus had made some errors because he was necessarily unaware of the
Harveian circulation, but he had distinguished six kinds of pernicious
tertian fever, not all of which are deadly, and had described their signs.
Torti had even found that some *quartans* may be pernicious (201). It is
probable that in such cases the term *pernicious* refers to cases complicated by edema or ascites.

In the light of modern knowledge the benignity of intermittent fever
reported or alleged by Hippocrates has led to the inference that *Plasmodium falciparum* may have been absent or rare in ancient Greece.
The facts are summarized as follows in the authoritative book by
Bruce-Chwatt and Zulueta: "There is overwhelming evidence in the
Hippocratic collection for the existence in Greece towards the end of
the fifth century B.C. of *P. vivax* and *P. malariae*. The evidence in favour
of the existence of *P. falciparum*, is on the other hand, far from conclusive. All that can be safely said is that, if it was present at that time it
must have been a rare infection."[10]

Grmek, in an attempt to describe the evolution of malaria in the
eastern Mediterranean region, has concluded that the disease was hy-
perendemic in the neolithic period and again in the Roman era. He
writes: "It seems reasonable to admit as a working hypothesis that a
correlation exists between the frequency of cranial porotic hyperostosis
and the degree of malarial infestation."[11] I see no justification whatever for using cranial hyperostosis as an index to the incidence of malaria. Moreover, it is well enough recognized that correlation is not
proof of causal relationship. Further, Grmek adds that according to his
table of frequencies "*malignant* [emphasis added] forms of malaria"
had invaded "during the mesolithic period and again during the classical period"; however, he presents no evidence to show that the alleged
correlation of hyperostosis with malaria can be assumed to have extended to malignant malaria. Further, it may be noted that in the encyclopedic Henke-Lubarsch treatise on pathologic anatomy, the section on skeletal disease—published in seven parts totalling 4,215
pages—*makes no mention of any gross skeletal lesion ascribable to malaria*. Nor does the elaborate discussion of malaria mention hyperostosis.[12]

Upon perplexities emanating from ancient doctrine discussed by
Torti were superimposed the newer problems that attended introduction of the Peruvian bark. First was the observed fact that the fever

sometimes recurred after the bark had been given (19). This difficulty was not overlooked by early observers. For example, Badus quoted a letter written in 1658 by his Genoese colleague Antonius Gibbonus, who stated that he had used the drug successfully in about three hundred cases of intermittent fever and had encountered only a few relapses, most of which yielded to additional doses.[13] On this point Torti observed that relapses occurred when the Peruvian bark had been given only once and that they were usually milder than the original attack (7).

In addition, as has been stated above, Torti felt that misuse of the Peruvian bark was widespread. Indeed, in France it had been prescribed for fevers of any kind, and much of what had been written about its use in continued, acute, and inflammatory fevers was false or doubtful (xxii). Clearly there was need for an exact classification of fevers. In other words, taxonomy was to be an indispensable guide to therapy.[14]

Torti's Taxonomy of Fevers

These perplexities take us to one of the most demanding parts of Torti's book—his taxonomy. The difficulties result from a combination of causes, some of which were not to be clarified or overcome for two hundred years: the inherent intricacy of the problem, insoluble in the absence of precise etiological knowledge; the frequent inadequacy of available or published clinical histories; the complexity and unreliability of physical signs unsupported by laboratory methods; the defectiveness of methods for clinical measurement, especially of body temperature; the vagueness of nomenclature, especially the scarcity of clear definitions; and the scantiness of statistical thinking (in clinical medicine) and of usable statistical methods, with consequent overemphasis on single cases or coincidences or tiny series.

Torti held that it was necessary to classify the fevers in order to understand them and to state clearly which were overcome by the Peruvian bark and which resisted it. His purpose was clearly practical, not theoretical, completeness and logical rigidity being sacrificed to necessity. His arrangement, he admitted, is not complete in all details, "although to complete it altogether in accordance with scholastic rules would be useless and disputatious, it will at least be sufficiently convenient, especially for the purpose for which we shall use it, and it will be taken largely from the older authors but at the same time it will be adapted sufficiently to modern rules; and the sound of the old terms, especially those that are better known, will be retained, particularly in the more general members [categories], even though these for the most part were based originally on false suppositions, which I do not at all accept" (578).

Part of Torti's taxonomy is not presented in the form that is usual in our own time, namely a series of indented categories usually separated by superintended subcategories. Instead, it is set forth as a verbal description spread out over fourteen pages and interlarded with discussions and *obiter dicta*. Torti usually describes entities instead of defining them.[15] His taxonomic account is supplemented, to a degree, by an arborescent diagram, the clever but somewhat bewildering Tree of Fevers (*Lignum Febrium*), which is preceded by a separate introduction (664–66).

Torti's taxonomy of fevers was not intended to include all major varieties. While mentioning incidentally the so-called simple fevers (together with subgroups), it concentrates on what were called the putrid fevers, believed to occur in the blood (see Appendix A), and it suppresses another major ancient category, that of pestilential fevers, which were sometimes given the confusing label of malignant. Torti's statement, a fair sample of his reasoning, can be paraphrased as follows.

The ancients divided all fevers into simple, putrid, and pestilential or malignant. We omit the pestilential because it contains nothing that is not in fevers of the first two categories and because its entire distinctiveness consists of nothing but a poisonous quality—putridity—that is added to putrid or simple fevers. Hence the inclusion of this category would be a redundancy. Because the malignity of the pestilential is a trait superimposed on fevers that are curable when they are benign, these fevers can be cured by the bark even though they are malign. (578)

In what may be regarded as an aside, Torti says that he will designate simple fevers as ephemeral, and that they are divided as follows:

Ephemeral
   Synochus
   Hectic
      Primary
      Secondary

Of putrid fevers he says that the meaning of such terms is generally known (*quorum terminorum nota est significatio*), hence no definition need be given (579–80), but the ancients classified them as follows:

Putrid
   Continued
      Continent (or *synochi*)
      Proportionate (also called periodic)

Regrettably he does not trouble to discuss the difference between periodic and intermittent.

After these preliminaries Torti explains that he has accepted two broad categories, namely the continued and the intermittent. At the same time he recognizes a subordinate category, *proportionate fevers derived partly from the continued fevers and partly from the intermittents*, not by metaphysical arrangement but by physical and practical arrangement and without disrespect to the schools (*non ordine quidem plane metaphysico, sed ordine physico, ac practico, absque ulla etiam Scholarum injuria*). A further consideration, not altogether easy for the modern reader, can be paraphrased as follows:

We divide the continued fevers, not directly into continent and proportionate, as is customary, but into the continent and, in a certain manner, the remittent, just as we divide the intermittent into discrete and subintrant (although the subintrant strictly cannot be called intermittent). Then we say that the continued proportionate or periodic fevers are made up from continued fevers that remit in any manner . . . and from subintrant intermittents. (580)

To this comment Torti adds, significantly, that since the continued proportionate or periodic fever is of a nature intermediate between the continued fever and the intermittent, it is not inappropriately set up as a third entity, made up by combination of the intermittent and the continued fever, or if you prefer *resulting from mixture of their ferments* and sharing the nature of both. This remark gives clear expression to Torti's fermentationism. In addition it contains the suggestion that taxonomy might reflect etiology.

Torti says that intermittent fevers are divided, according to the paroxysms, as separate (i.e., legitimate), or subintrant, or false. The fever is subintrant when a new paroxysm begins before its predecessor has ended. Characteristically, he adds a complicating feature: if the ending of the previous paroxysm is very near or has occurred immediately before the subsequent one, the fever is merely called *communicating* or *coalternating*[16] and retains the nature of a true intermittent. A subintrant can metamorphose gradually into a proportionate continuous fever.

A discrete intermittent has clearly divided paroxysms. It may be irregular (erratic) or regular (periodic). The latter may be quartan, tertian, or quotidian, as well as legitimate or spurious. In addition, it may be single, double, triple, and so on, and may be involved in various kinds of mixture, exemplified by the semitertian. Further, it may undergo degenerations and transmutations into subintrant, continued, acute, slow, cachectic, or marantic fevers. Also recognized are corruptive and depurative or perfect intermittents, but these are said to be difficult to distinguish from one another (132–33, 530).

After these troublesome intricacies we come at last to Torti's main subject, the pernicious or malignant intermittents. Malignity, he says, occurs in all kinds of intermittent fever, either intrinsically or because of some additional noxious symptom, which simulates a very severe disease, but it occurs especially in tertians, to which any kind of malignity is easily added (582–83). Similarly, quartan fevers not rarely add lethargy, and any other intermittent may acquire continuity—that is, it may become a continuous fever—and then malignity. Moreover, the malignity may be either colliquative or coagulative; that is, the blood may liquefy or it may clot.

The principal categories and subcategories in Torti's taxonomy of the intermittent and the continued fevers can be tabulated as follows:

Intermittent fevers
    Tertian [occurring on the first, third, fifth . . . days.]
        Benign
        Malignant
            Solitary (*solitariae*) [unaccompanied]
                Subcontinuous
            Concomitant (*comitatae*) [accompanying]
                Becomes concomitant suddenly because some fierce and special symptom is added; this is worse than the disease it mimics and the fever it accompanies
            Colliquative [liquefying]
                Choleric, subcruent, cardiac, diaphoretic
            Coagulative [clotting]
                Syncopal, algid, lethargic
    Quartan [occurring on the first, fourth, seventh . . . days]
            [Torti does not provide separate taxonomy for quartans but assumes that the reader will supply one by analogy. For example, when he mentions solitary malignant tertians, he adds, "the same for quartans etc."]
    Continued fevers (*febres continuae*)
    Continent (*continentes*)
            No exacerbation or remission from beginning to end, whether the course is level or ascending or descending; the descending are called putrid synochous (*synochi putridae*). ("The ancient classification of the continent fevers has been superseded," he says.)
      Essential or primary
            Caused by inborn universal disease of the fluids, with no accompanying localization to any part of the body.
        Solitary (also called synochi)
            Caused by dyscrasia [bad mixture] of fluids alone, without accompanying or important disease of solid parts

Acmastic [continuous]

Epacmastic [coming to a crisis]

Paracmastic [past its climax]

Concomitant (*comitatae*)

Combined with a separate disease that it has produced, or at
least with some serious symptom which imitates a real
disease

Colliquative (*colliquativae*, caused by liquefaction of fluids—
e.g., blood)

Diabetic [transient?]

Diaphoretic [causing sweats]

Dejective [causing excrement]

Coagulative (*coagulatoriae;* produce stagnations or concretions
in various parts of the body and thereby cause other disease)

Morbilliform [taking the form of measles]

Variolar [taking the form of smallpox]

Scarlatinal [taking the form of scarlet fever]

Catarrhal and the like

Inflammatory or erysipelatous

E.g., pleuritic, arthritic, anginal—*provided that the inflammation has come from the fever and not vice versa*

Symptomatic (*accidentales seu secundariae*)

Attached to a disease and caused by the disease

General (*officiales*)

Caused by damaged behavior of a part whose function is
for the whole body

Lactational

In puerperal women

White or pallid fever of chlorotic maidens

Limited (*privatae*)

Caused by sickness of a part whose function is directed
to itself alone

Fixed (*fixae*)

Emanates from a definite structure as its root, but could
come from various sicknesses in any part of the body

Inflammatory

Pustular or nodular

Ulcerative

Sluggish

Migratory (*vaga*)

Attached specially to no part of the body and to no special
kind of fever but come from preexisting disease of several parts of the body with general or local functions
and travel repeatedly through various parts

Verminous

Venereal

Scorbutic

Remittent (*remittentes*)
> These do not have a single continuity but have several indistinct exacerbations, occurring in no order, and have several indistinct remissions. Their uneven course appears dependent on external causes.

Proportionate continued (*continuae proportionatae, seu proportionales*)
> These come from subintrant and the aforementioned remittents. Resemble intermittents at onset, continued and acute fevers in their course. Are designated according to differences in their period.

Continued quotidians	⎫	single,
Continued tertians	⎬	double
Continued quartan	⎭	etc.

It is amusing that, after a passage discussing his points of terminological agreement and his points of dissent with Morton, Torti was able to write: "Up to now I have abstained from multiple subdivision [of continued fevers] as being useless for our purposes, and I continue to abstain deliberately" (609).

Torti's taxonomy differs somewhat from Morton's, especially with respect to the continued and continent fevers (601, 607), and embodies also several further innovations. The most conspicuous, apart from its strong orientation toward treatment—specifically, treatment by means of the Peruvian bark—is Torti's establishment of what he called the proportionate fevers as a separate entity, a composite derived conjointly from the intermittent and the continuous fevers. Obviously this entity represents his experience with fevers that were difficult to categorize; in explanation he suggested the possibility of a hybrid cause, namely mixture of two kinds of ferment. This supposition afforded at least partial understanding of fevers that passed from one category to another.

Torti also felt obliged to account for the fact, real or apparent, that in at least occasional instances a fever was resistant to Peruvian bark at some times and susceptible at others. He was aware that his use of mixed categories might draw the reproof of logicians, but this did not inhibit him. He states that whether proportionate fevers are malign or not is of little importance; what is truly important is their susceptibility [or resistance] to the Peruvian bark; this depends on the nature of the predominant ferment in the pathogenic mixture of ferments (610). His important comment signifies that the bark could be used *both* therapeutically and diagnostically.

Torti adds that the bark is therapeutically effective in cases of proportionate fever in which the periodicity is essential [basic] and the continuity is accidental [incidental or secondary]. In contrast, the bark is ineffective when continuity is essential and periodicity is accidental. He says he had learned this distinction by using the bark and observing the effect, and that to make the differential diagnosis in advance of the therapeutic trial is not easy (*id quidem dignoscere a priori non ita facile*) (615). In modern terms his proposition could signify that the bark is useful in what we now call malaria but is ineffective in typhoid fever, sepsis, and subacute bacterial endocarditis, despite the fact that these three nonmalarial infections may produce recurrent chills.

No doubt the difficulties of the taxonomist and the diagnostician were also augmented by the facts, well known nowadays, that in simple tertian malaria the periodicity may be indistinct or variable early in the course and that tertian periodicity may exist early in infections that later prove to be examples of pernicious malaria caused by *Plasmodium falciparum.*

In his discussions and in his classification Torti occasionally uses adjectives in such a way that the modern reader cannot always determine whether they are intended merely as qualifiers or descriptors or whether they are meant to designate subcategories. Examples are *corruptiva* and *depurativa*. The separation between technical terms and ordinary literary or medical expressions is not always distinct. Moreover, some of the ultimate subcategories, especially those that appear at or near the ends of twigs in Torti's tree, represent single traits, for example, *lenta, diaphoretica,* and they are used as the names of taxa. Such categories are not always explained in Torti's text, but the reader apparently was expected to understand them.

Another peculiarity, most conspicuous in Torti's Tree of Fevers (see below), is the repetitive use of some adjectives and some series of adjectives. Thus, the terms *quotidian, tertian,* and *quartan* appear among the intermittents and also among the proportionates and the continued fevers. This fact, attributable to difficulties in diagnosis and to ignorance of etiology, tends to produce despair in the modern reader.

The Tree of Fevers

The fanciful and artistic parts of Torti's character, revealed in his poems and oratorios, may be credited also with the famous illustration found near the end of his book. This shows the so-called Tree of Fevers, which was designed to depict the taxonomy of fevers as a large, ramose and leafy tree (Fig. 4). As we have seen repeatedly, Torti regarded taxonomy as a major fundamental of therapeutics.

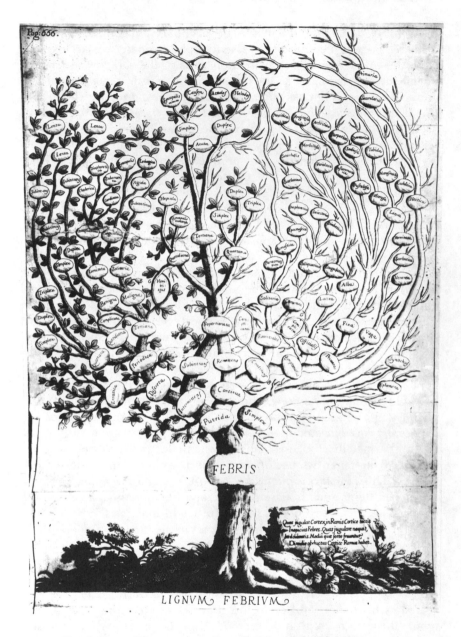

FIG. 4. Torti's Tree of Fevers, 1712. Branches covered with bark represent fevers curable by Peruvian bark. Denuded, leafless branches represent fevers not curable by bark.

It must be remembered that at the time of his first, second, and third editions only the bark was known in Europe. The identification of the cinchona tree was the work of the botanist Joseph de Jussieu (1704–79), whose memoir of 1738[17] was given to his fellow-traveler C. M. de la Condamine. The latter had observed the tree in 1737, four years before Torti's death.[18]

One outstanding feature recommends Torti's taxonomic fever-tree to the reader's attention: fevers curable by the Peruvian bark—the intermittents—are represented by branches covered with bark. These branches have leaves and occupy the left third of the picture. To the reader's right are leafless branches devoid of bark; these represent the continued fevers, not curable by the Peruvian drug. At the center are trunks and branches partly covered by bark; these correspond to what Torti calls the proportionate fevers. In this category, susceptibility to the bark depends not on the presence or absence of malignity but on the nature of the predominant ferment (610). As has been noted above, Torti held that the Peruvian bark is successful in cases of proportionate fever in which the periodicity is essential and it fails when the periodicity is accidental. In the same way his fever tree, which can be mistaken for a display limited to nosologic taxonomy, attempts to indicate therapeutic efficacy of the bark as well.[19]

In Torti's opinion, inherited from antiquity and discussed in several parts of this history, a fever might change from one category to another (Fig. 5). He believed also that this change is reversible. Such occurrences are shown in the diagram by branches that anastomose and in some instances form a closed figure, which Torti compared to a circulation (665). For example, at the very top of the diagram the letter *a* signifies the transformation of the *causon* into the hectic, while *b, f,* and *g* denote other combinations.

Torti says that the unnamed engraver of the picture, a man not ignorant of Latin, inquired about the slow fever (*febris lenta*), which at that time afflicted the engraver's brother, and wanted to know where this kind of fever was indicated on the diagram. Torti replied that probably it was represented by a barkless branch, not curable by the drug (660–61).

Having considered Torti's taxonomy of fevers and his tree of fevers, we may ask ourselves what has become of his taxonomic system. What part of it do we use? Nowadays we are not greatly concerned with the taxonomy of disease. The problem is no longer discussed with medical students, nor do they often ask about it. In contrast, taxonomy was a major concern of the eighteenth century and its predecessors. By the end of the nineteenth century the great taxonomic systems had disap-

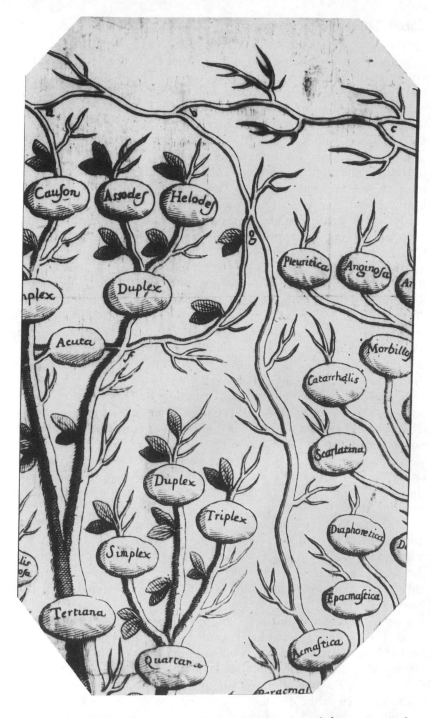

FIG. 5. Torti's Tree of Fevers, 1712. Anastomoses (*a, b, c, g*) denote cases of fever which have changed from one category to another.

peared, interest having shifted to etiology, which is one pillar of such taxonomic notions as we still entertain in our efforts to understand disease.

Of the categories that Torti employed we still recognize the major division between intermittents and continued fevers—a distinction that long preceded him—and we do not spend a thought on whether the intermittents are to be regarded as one disease or many. Beyond this we retain nothing of his elaborate taxonomic construct. Yet our shift toward an etiological system enables us to do what he advocated, that is, to use etiology as a practical basis for treatment. The single effective febrifuge that Torti possessed has now been joined by a host of recent innovations.

Torti's Methods of Examination

Nowhere in the *Therapeutice specialis* does Torti describe his methods of examination, nor was such a description demanded by the purposes of his book. We are therefore limited to observations that appear incidentally in his discussions, especially in his case reports, which are sometimes lengthy but yield no great harvest of methodologic detail.

Unlike many physicians of his time, Torti rarely mentions the patient's habitus or temperament, unless the case is serious and demands elaborate description (e.g., 384). He rarely makes note of pallor; possibly this fact signifies that most of the malarious infections that he treated were recent. Yet he paid great attention to other details of the general appearance. Thus, one report mentions, as Hippocrates might have done, the patient's shallow eyes, sharp nose, and collapsed temples (402).

It is observable also that Torti rarely mentions the spleen. In one patient, seen in 1708 by both Torti and Ramazzini, the reader is told that the spleen had begun to swell, *iam lien illi coeperat nonnihil intumescere* (177–78), and it is implied, but not stated overtly, that splenomegaly is among the indications for administration of the bark. Here Torti makes the curious comment that in cases accompanied by swelling of the abdominal viscera, when the patient had obtained relief by means of the bark and the enlargement had disappeared, Torti could assert that such details, being trivial and obvious, could be bypassed in silence. Another report mentions abdominal percussion in ascites concomitant with quartan fever (378). In severe or malignant cases of fever he mentions tremors, subsultus tendinum, mental alienation (183), and lethargy (472–92). Indeed, one of his clinical virtues was early recognition of pernicious symptoms and signs. This was extremely important because prompt and vigorous action was necessary. As he puts it, in circumstances of this kind there should be no hesitation (*in talibus circumstantiis minime haesitandum est*) (547).

With respect to deafness, familiar to the modern physician as a symptom of cinchonism, Torti was acquainted with Morton's comment.[20] However, his own remarks are contradictory: at one point he says that he had not observed cinchonal deafness (15); on another page he says the opposite (467). In cases of intermittent fever no systematic examination of the patient's hearing was done, nor is it done routinely nowadays.

Incidental remarks indicate that the urine was inspected, at least in the more serious cases, in order to judge the character, severity, and progress of the illness, and to determine whether or not coction had occurred. Today's physician—in the United States, at least—derides the venerable practice of urinoscopy; he is apt to order his office assistant or his hospital junior to send the urine to the laboratory but is not likely to confront it personally. He may, or may not, see the report that emanates from an electronic oracle.

A reference to the stool is of terminological and historical interest: Torti says that one of his patients had melena,[21] *which the ancients called atrobiliary* (412).

The presence of fever was recognized by examination of the pulse (a procedure that sometimes caused confusion between fever and tachycardia) and by inspection and palpation of the skin,[22] with special reference to sweating. Torti's case reports, like those of his contemporaries and predecessors, not infrequently specify the location of the sweat. Recurrence of fever was sometimes detected or confirmed by the observation that sweat had reappeared.

Here are a few of the observations recorded in the first chapter of book 4:

> Shallow eyes, sharp nose, collapsed temples
> Very intense fever, universal burning, obstinate insomnia, collapsed face, sudden thinning of the flesh
> Cold extremities, [later] still almost frigid, [later, with incipient improvement] body a very little bit warm
> Very cold all over; flesh almost dried up
> Subfrigid, with small sweats about the forehead (402, 408, 412, 413, 415)

While the mention of thirst is not surprising, this symptom is prominent in many of the case reports (446, 458), perhaps because fluid was withdrawn from the body not only by sweating but also by bloodletting and purgation. The reports commonly fail to state how much fluid was administered.

Thermometry

Torti's book contains no reference to the measurement of body temperature because his training was received, and the major part of his work was done, during a hiatus of development in this part of medical science. It is well established that thermometry began in Italy in the early seventeenth century, although whether priority belongs to Galileo, or Santorio, or others, remains unknown. It is recognized that at an early stage Santorio used some form of thermometer in physiological experiments and in his medical practice.[23]

Thermometers were fashioned and thermometric trials were made by the Accademia del Cimento in Florence, which existed from 1657 to 1667, and at the private academy of Ferdinand II, Grand Duke of Tuscany, which was established in the Pitti Palace and functioned for fifteen years before the official academy. The collections in the Museum of the History of Science in Florence include several clinical thermometers that belonged to one or other of these two societies.[24]

Such thermometers as were available to Torti were used meteorologically and not clinically; thus they followed in the direction of the Hippocratic *Airs, Waters, Places* rather than the *Aphorisms* and *Prognostic*. Torti's colleague Bernardino Ramazzini mentions a thermometer of his own in 1692, used for studies of the weather.[25]

That Torti was actively interested in meteorology is shown by his early writings on the movements of mercury in barometers.[26]

Equally impressive evidence of Torti's interest in the relation between climate and disease is found in book 2, chapter 4 of the *Therapeutice specialis*. Here, in a scholium on Mercatus, he says that in the present century the air has been forced to undergo examination by thermometers, barometers, and hygrometers, and by the Torricellian tube and the apparatus of Boyle; the art of medicine has been enriched and has begun to establish better use of the air itself, which has become known more thoroughly (220–23). A similar statement was made by Ramazzini in 1710 in his essay on preserving the health of princes.[27]

The interest displayed at this time by practitioners in vicissitudes of the atmosphere and their effects on human beings is exemplified in an undated letter written by one of Torti's contemporaries, Vincenzo Antonio Pigozzi (1629–1729), a member of Malpighi's circle who practiced medicine in Crevalcore. This letter is titled *Iatrophysical Reflections about the Method of Protecting Oneself against Gout*. Pigozzi wrote:

The temper of the air cannot be as well proportioned as would be desirable, since, according to the prevalent opinion, the atmosphere in which we live is essentially a fluid composed of heterogeneous particles or atoms variously shaped, or it is accidentally altered by effluvia raised up from waters, fossils &c and salts of various kinds transported by winds and disseminated into it. Consequently, compelled to inhale this elemental air, we experience perceptible effects and changes, which correspond to its daily alterations. That which we observe in thermometers with respect to the primary qualities of heat and cold, and in barometers with respect to secondary qualities of moist and dry, is manifest in living beings to a much greater extent through the intimate mixture of air with the tiny components of their fluids.

And so, since the air cannot be so equilibrated in itself that it does not depend on one of the four qualities mentioned, when heat and moisture prevail, the humors melt. . . . On the contrary, when cold and dryness prevail, transpiration being hampered, they are concentrated.[28]

From available evidence it does not seem highly probable that, although Torti was interested in meteorological thermometry, earlier development of practical *clinical* thermometry could have exerted much influence on his taxonomy of the fevers. The resumption of progress is attributable to Boerhaave, Torti's contemporary, who measured body temperatures of fever patients before 1708, that is, a short time before the publication of Torti's *Synopsis*.[29] Further progress is credited to Boerhaave's pupil, de Haen. But the general adoption of clinical thermometry did not occur until the work of Wunderlich and Allbutt, more than a century later.[30] In Torti's era it was still true that physicians were likely to be interested in the temperature of the air as a factor in disease but were unlikely to measure the temperatures of their fever patients.

Torti's Opinions

I have stated that disappointment awaits the reader who expects to find completely clear and completely consistent expositions in all parts of Torti's large treatise. No acceptable analysis can conceal the occasional vagueness or the occasional contradictions. Yet it is both necessary and instructive, even at the risk of repetition, to attempt a summary review of Torti's principal opinions, as presented in the first edition of his book.

With regard to ancient doctrine in general he says, concisely, that *humoralism* has been universally rejected (29).[31] He remarks also that it is sufficient to acknowledge those humors that we detect and that moisten us, and not those that were imagined in the metaphysical abstractions of the ancients (60). This statement points to the elementary distinction, sometimes overlooked or misunderstood in our era, between the four standard humors of classical antiquity and all other humors, which are bodily fluids of any kind.

The shift in concepts is readily illustrated. Torti agreed with Mercatus's statement that in cases of pernicious fever it is necessary to thicken the causative *humor* and to keep it from flowing and putrefying (219), but to Mercatus this remark almost certainly referred to diseased yellow or black bile, whereas to Torti it must have meant the ferment, not as yet definitively identified, which causes pernicious fever.

Torti's dissent from ancient dogma necessarily extended to therapeutics. Hence it is not surprising that, being antihumoralist, he objected to the use of purgation in fevers. Despite this statement his case reports show that he occasionally employed purgation, and also venesection, in cases of intermittent fever; doubtless he did not always have complete freedom of choice. This problem is considered at greater length in the discussion of Torti's therapeutic methods.

Torti modestly characterized his concepts of *etiology* as conjectures (621). With regard to pathogenesis of the common intermittent fevers he agreed with Borelli[32] that the cause is a juice (*succus*), small in amount, perhaps only a spoonful, poured into the blood intermittently and able to excite it to febrile movement (45). This pathogenesis is more or less compatible with Torti's fermentationism; reconciliation between the differing concepts is made possible by assuming that the ferments are liquid or are dissolved in liquids.

Torti says that by examination of diverse opinions he has derived a series of theorems, as follows: The ferment of continued and of intermittent fevers is in the blood. It probably comes to the blood from outside and produces injury immediately during the chill and fever until it is overcome and excreted at the time of despumation. It reaches the blood by way of the lymphatics that enter the subclavian vein, (i.e., through the thoracic duct). Moreover, it is difficult to believe that the febrile ferment hides in the intestines and passes from them into the lacteals. Never, or almost never, whether a paroxysm was remote or impending or incipient, had Torti known the febrile matter to leave the body by vomiting or defecation, either spontaneous or induced. This observation, he adds, is derived from experience and not from "false speculations," and it is one of the reasons why he abstains from using purges and emetics in these fevers. In order to be effective, the bark must be given at least four to five hours before a paroxysm of intermittent fever is expected. This observation, also based on experience, is additional evidence that the causative ferment does not lurk in the intestinal lumen but in deeper structures such as chyliferous channels (83–89).

Torti's opinions or hypotheses on pathogenesis receive additional attention in book 3, chapter 2 on the character of pernicious intermittents (esp. 314–16). He says that in order to formulate a crude but useful concept for treatment of these fevers, we should at least imagine that their ferment, although lodged in a special place such that it is inaccessible to the power of cathartics and emetics and cannot be eradicated, nevertheless has close or remote communication with the alimentary canal and especially the chyliferous ducts. Whenever the ferment bursts forth from its little repositories, it can go up through these same channels. In this way, he remarks somewhat less than clearly, it will become easy to understand the action of the bark against the febrile ferment through direct contact between these two, especially if, in addition to the path of the bark through the intestines, we consider the inevitable advance of particles of the bark into the lacteals and the rather long delay of the particles in them.

Torti points out, as Morton had done before him (see Appendix A), that since the various benign intermittents are overcome by Peruvian bark, and this is true of the pernicious intermittents also, the nature of the causative ferments is similar (311).

It is highly probable, says Torti in his habitually undogmatic style, that the ferment of the intermittent fevers arises and lingers outside the blood and flows into it from time to time, whereas the ferment of continued fevers arises within the blood mass (610).

Torti was obliged to cope with the widespread opinion mentioned repeatedly in this and other chapters, that administration of the drug was not followed by perceptible evacuation. This belief caused no schism among enemies of the bark, since traditional humoralists could contend that the drug allowed diseased yellow or black bile to remain within the patient's body whereas fermentationist enemies, as Torti noted (33), could assert that the pathogenic ferment was retained.

In Torti's view, Borelli was not warranted in stating that no perceptible evacuation follows the ingestion of bark; case histories show that considerable evacuations sometimes occur. But ordinary evacuations may suffice (33–34, 56). In addition to rejecting the dictum of Borelli, Torti declined to accept Hoffmann's suggestion that the bark precipitates febrile matter (39). He accepted Mercatus's belief that in pernicious cases it is necessary to thicken the causative humor and to keep it from flowing and putrefying; such restraint should be applied before the paroxysm. For this purpose Torti, before he had learned the power of Peruvian bark, used to prescribe boli of theriac, hyacinth, absinthe salt, and laudanum, given two to three hours before the attack. As we have seen, he later came to disapprove the use of these medicines.

According to another opinion widely held in Torti's time, epidemic fevers were caused by either coagulation or dissolution of the blood. On this point an opinion was solicited from Torti and several other physicians in connection with a large outbreak of undetermined character that took place in 1716 in the town of Cagli, near Urbino. Torti's undated reply, not included in the *Therapeutice specialis*, is recorded in a manuscript at the University of Bologna.[33] Torti tactfully evaded giving an opinion on the special troubles of Cagli. Instead, he wrote, "It is not yet certain that the entire mechanism of the theory of malignant fevers and their symptoms can be made to turn merely on the two poles of coagulation and dissolution of the blood."

The age of scientific pharmacology having not yet dawned, it is not surprising that Torti's statements about the bark are presented mostly in terms of its clinical behavior. Accordingly these statements are discussed in a later section that deals with his methods of treatment.

Torti knew that, contrary to an opinion held by many observers, the bark was *not* devoid of effectiveness in all continued fevers (book 5). This observation was exactly compatible with his insistence on taxonomy as a pillar of rational therapeutics.

In his attempt to understand the action of Peruvian bark Torti undertook experiments in which he added the drug to various fluids (48, 50). He concluded that the bark does not impede coagulation of fresh blood. Unable to explain the antipyretic property, he concluded that his experiments were unsuccessful and that the mode of action of the drug and the cause of intermittent fever are alike unknown. He remarked also that Morton was much better at using the bark than at explaining its action (*vir longe felicior in usu remedii, quam in explicanda ejus actione* [70]).

Torti wrote that the bark is useful and harmless (29); in this he duplicated exactly the report of Gabriele Fonseca, who was one of the earliest in Italy to subject the drug to clinical trial (see Chapter 2). Torti did not deny that occasional bad effects may occur from unsuitable or untimely administration because the bark must be given according to certain rules (36). His comment on cinchonal deafness has been discussed on a preceding page.

Whereas Morton had been compelled to raise the dosage of the bark from two drachms to two or three ounces because his supplies were weakened by adulteration,[34] Torti says that he had never encountered this problem (121–22). His statement is surprising since Cardinal de Lugo had complained of adulteration as early as 1659[35] and the same problem is mentioned in a Venetian manual of pharmacy issued as late as 1740.[36]

While it appears probable that Morton's samples were obtained from Dutch traders, we have no direct information about Torti's suppliers. In his time the main northern Italian entrepôt for drugs was Venice. A hint of this is found in an undated letter written, probably by Albertini, about a sufferer from amenorrhea. Albertini recommended balsam of copaiba (a Brazilian and Antillean drug) and added, "Probably it is

available from Venice."[37] While differences in trade routes may well
have produced differences in the purity of the Peruvian bark, it is difficult to contrive a satisfactory reason for Torti's failure to encounter
adulteration.

It is hardly surprising that Torti, a fermentationist, opposed iatrochemistry. He wrote that antimony, arsenic, vitriol, and mercury are
poisons and do not deserve the name of febrifuge (21). Further, he in-
veighed against the prevalent excess of useless drugs and he agreed
with Sydenham in disapproving most of the additives, "cardiacs," hya-
cinths, and alteratives that were commonly given with the Peruvian
bark (130–31), but he believed that other drugs, which provide symptomatic relief, are not to be despised.

Torti's Methods of Treatment

As we noted in Chapter 8, Torti learned the use of cinchona from his teacher Antonio Frassoni, who followed the procedure
described in the *Schedula Romana* (see Chapter 2 and Appendix A),
applying it "to the more protracted common intermittents" (*in vulgari-
bus intermittentibus diuturnioribus* [115]). Apparently the bark was not
employed regularly in the mildest cases.

When he felt that the bark was needed, Torti administered two
drachms of the powder[38] in wine "at the time that the fever was attacking," that is, when the paroxysm was about to begin. For a double tertian, the dose was given on the day of the stronger paroxysm. In such
cases Torti had noticed, or thought he had noticed, that if the dose was
given on the day when the lesser of the paired paroxysms was expected,
this attack was suppressed, but the greater attack was not; hence the
double tertian was converted into a single tertian. But if the bark was
given on the day of the greater attack, the greater was suppressed and
a lesser attack followed immediately. The next of the smaller attacks
was suppressed also, and no further attacks occurred; the entire double
tertian had been deleted. If the tertian was simple, there was of course
no opportunity for such an observation.

Recurrences were frequent. Grieved at this (*aegre ferens*), Torti devised a supplementary method, which consisted of administering, after
the main series of doses, half a drachm of the bark daily for eight days.
Then, after an interval of fifteen days, more or less, he would give one
scruple every morning for six days. He was still using this procedure in
prolonged cases when he wrote his book.

Torti adds that many other physicians, employing a milder method,
would give as little as half a drachm daily for many days. He himself
used this dosage in protracted mild fevers in delicate people. He felt,

however, that if the cause of the fever was strong and obstinate and there was fear that dangerous symptoms impended, or if for any other valid reason it appeared appropriate to suppress the fever, it was best to give the entire dose of two drachms at the beginning of the treatment and then to proceed gradually to smaller doses. This system he judged to be quicker and more reliable than systems of constant low dosage.

Torti had found that six scruples (equal to two drachms) of the bark distributed over six days are not equal in power to the same amount given at one time. This is why one physician, using six drachms, or even a whole ounce, cures any prolonged intermittent fever and also prevents relapse, while another physician can scarcely attain this result with three or four ounces. In the same way, he adds, one pound of water is enough to extinguish a fire in a heap of coals, but two pounds, falling drop by drop and at long intervals, can hardly produce the same result over an extended period of time.

It is not difficult for the modern reader to see in these comments the observations that in later times would develop into quantitative understanding of blood levels and blood concentrations.

Torti states that Talbor's method, which employed a weak infusion of the bark, was successful because the doses were given often. Moreover, a clear infusion, such as Talbor used, is inferior in potency to a turbid infusion because, in the preparation of clear infusions, the process of filtration yielded dregs that were discarded even though they were potent.

In reviewing currently popular preparations of the bark (127–31), some of which he considered objectionable, Torti noted that Morton, a "vigorous doser" (*strenuus administrator*), gave as much as a drachm every three to four hours on days when fever was absent; this exceeds the need in benign intermittents but is often inadequate in pernicious fever.

As was stated in Chapter 4, Morton remarked that the initial dosage recommended in the *Schedula Romana*—two drachms of powdered bark in four ounces of generous wine—proved to be inadequate because the samples available to him were adulterated. Hence he had been obliged to prescribe much larger amounts.[39] Torti himself had not encountered this problem.

Much better known was Sydenham's dosage, which is set forth in the epistle to Dr. Robert Brady.[40] The method consisted of administering an ounce of finely powdered Peruvian bark, made into an electuary or a pill and divided into twelve parts, one part being taken every four hours, beginning immediately after the paroxysm. Sydenham found that "a quartan takes an ounce of bark to cure it; whereas the others [such as tertians and quotidians] are either cured or relieved by six

drachms." To counteract relapse the entire treatment might be repeated three or four times.

Torti emphasizes that he was reluctant to prescribe the bark automatically and indiscriminately at the start in all cases of simple intermittent fever (142). He also considered the so-called depurative or perfective fevers, now called exanthematic fevers, such as measles and
smallpox, in which it was believed that the emergence of the eruption
purified the blood. These sicknesses, Torti wrote, should not be treated
immediately with the bark, nor should phlebotomy be used, but the
patients should be left to Nature. But if the fever appeared to be corruptive—that is, if the blood or a viscus appeared to be diseased—the bark
should be used even at the time of onset (132–33).

The tenth chapter in book 1 of the *Therapeutice specialis* contains
sixteen case reports intended to demonstrate when the Peruvian bark
should or should not be given at the onset of a common intermittent
fever (160–88); the mildest routine cases are not included in the recital. From these and other parts of the book it is apparent that, where
danger was not apprehended, three chills were allowed to occur before
the drug was given.

*Suppression of chills by means of the bark amounted to a diagnostic
procedure.* This important principle had an ancestor in a precinchonal
doctrine attributed to Avicenna and allegedly accepted by later authors
such as Sydenham.[41] It distinguished depurative or perfective fevers
from corruptive fevers. This has been discussed on a preceding page.

The distinction between depurative and corruptive fevers—according to Torti it was apt to be difficult at the beginning of the illness
(530)—seems to have rivaled the distinction between coagulative and
dissolutive fevers. The latter dichotomy has also been discussed above.

The use of a drug such as Peruvian bark for diagnostic purposes has
another possible precedent, which occurs in a statement made by Gabriele Falloppio (1523–1562). In the seventh chapter of his *Treatise on
Ulcers* this eminent physician and anatomist had discussed ulcerated
cancer and had written: "You may add also a sign based on the action
of the medicine [*ex ratione medicationis*], for if it happens that the physician has applied a drug which might sting insufficiently, such as *unguentum Isidis* or the like, and the inflammation becomes greater and
the pain becomes very intense, you may take it as a reliable sign that
the ulcer is cancerous."[42]

In August 1695 Torti was treating Count Bailardino Nogarola, a
fleshy man, fifty-three years old, who was thought to have a simple intermittent quartan fever (384–98). After six cycles the paroxysms began to triple. The patient now developed tremor, forgetfulness, and
then somnolence, hiccough, and a continuous fever. He appeared to be

dying. At this perilous juncture Torti remembered the case of Ottavio Maselli (see Chapter 8), in which a layman had rescued an almost moribund man by giving *two* drachms of powdered bark in a single dose.

Torti, judging that Nogarola was worse off than Maselli, administered *four* drachms of the bark, in a tincture and, an hour later, an additional ounce (*eight* drachms). Recovery was evident within twenty-four hours. Thereafter, diminishing doses were given for several days. There is no mention of relapse.

The case of Count Nogarola marked the turning point in the development of Torti's methods for the treatment of pernicious intermittent fever. The narrative is captioned with the words, "a special history, which very fortunately provided the first occasion for the discovery of the method that is transmitted" (*Historia peculiaris, quae primam occasionem inventioni Methodi traditae auspicatissime praebuit*). Since this case report appears in the third book of the *Therapeutice specialis*, a book devoted to pernicious fevers, it is evident that in Torti's usage the word *pernicious* applied to all severe or dangerous cases of intermittent fever, including the worst of the acute quartans. Nowadays the term *pernicious* is limited to estivoautumnal malaria caused by *Plasmodium falciparum* and is regarded as obsolete or obsolescent. Although Torti's terminology makes no completely clear distinction between pernicious and malignant, his text provides a good clinical description of pernicious intermittent fevers and an impressive series of case reports, the principal trait being the sudden and unexpected emergence of violent symptoms—especially, but not invariably, cerebral—and great risk of fatal outcome.

In book 2 of the *Therapeutice specialis*, the first chapter heading reads: "The malignant character and generally wicked nature of pernicious fevers of this kind [intermittents] is pointed out" (189).[43] Farther on, Torti says that "fevers of this kind constitute a delimited species within the genus of intermittents" (192).

Torti recognized seven main kinds of pernicious intermittent fever, classed according to the most conspicuous or menacing symptom (286–88). Cases in which cerebral symptoms such as lethargy were prominent made up the seventh group. To these Torti added an eighth group for cases in which a pernicious intermittent fever became continuous. Well aware of the difficulties and limitations of classification, he remarked that the Styx is reached by many routes (*mille sunt viae, quibus ad Stygem itur*) (282).

To the procedure that he devised in 1695 for the treatment of pernicious intermittents, such as befell Count Nogarola, Torti gave the name *methodus valida*, the strong method. In later years he employed a range of dosages, not always sharply demarcated, extending from the mild, *mitis*, to the very strongest, *validissima*. He recognized clearly that not all pernicious intermittents had to be treated by the same method (321).[44] He recalled that in 1696 he had saved himself from death by taking six drachms of the bark in one drink (10).

When the paroxysms were somewhat mild, as in benign cases, two drachms usually sufficed, though it might be useful to give an additional drachm on the next day. In a severe case, in which the patient is almost moribund, at least six drachms should be administered in divided doses. In very urgent cases an entire ounce should be given. Then, to prevent relapse (in pernicious cases), the physician should prescribe a drachm a day for three days. Thereafter the patient should be given a total of six drachms additional, in divided doses. Then, after a free interval of six days, half a drachm should be given daily for six days. This comes to a total of twenty drachms (two and a half ounces), if the initial dose was a full ounce. In cases of less extreme severity the total usually was two ounces given over a period of three weeks (324–32).[45]

Torti considered it very important to use large doses at the start of the treatment; smaller doses were given later. He says that by this method, and the use of two ounces of the bark within a period of three weeks—including days of rest—a pernicious fever is strangled, instead of it strangling the patient, whereas by the feeble methods that other physicians employed, a benign intermittent is hardly dispelled by four or five ounces (333).

Physicians in Torti's time continued to debate the use of cathartics and venesection in intermittent fever, especially as preliminaries to the administration of Peruvian bark. Sydenham had written that these procedures weakened the bodily economy, predisposing to recurrence of the fever and to a host of dangerous symptoms. Torti wrote that he himself expected no benefit from purgation in these cases (150–55). He had found that the bark could be given safely in the absence of an antecedent purge. Yet, in order to escape slander (*ad evitandam calumniam*)—also to provide at least some assistance to the body and perhaps to induce a more favorable acceptance of the bark—he did not deny that it might be appropriate to loosen the bowel and to open a vein. Indeed, this, he says, was almost a ritual with him, yet occasionally he omitted it—especially the purge—if the fever, according to Torti's partly unclear statement, showed that purgation should not be used or the intensity of the fever constituted a counterindication.

Torti remarks that he did not object to ordering a mild preliminary purgation supplemented by an enema or two, but only when these measures were required by other special tendencies of the patient's body. The decision regarding these treatments was influenced also by the season. For example, greater care was needed in the summer than in the spring, because the condition of the body fluids varied with the seasons. Different cathartics were needed, and in the summertime phlebotomies should be small or should be omitted altogether.

It is interesting to observe that Torti, although he rejected ancient humoralism, could not rid himself of humoralist procedures, despite the powerful example of Sydenham. It is equally interesting to notice that Torti's partial and grudging retention of old methods was simultaneous with a vigorous progressiveness and originality in advocacy of the new.

Torti's discussions of therapeutics are limited almost entirely to the dosage of Peruvian bark. He says nothing about the appearance of the drug or the judgment of various samples according to color or other traits. He makes brief mention of the drugs that the bark supplanted and, as stated above, he expresses concise detestation of the metallic drugs of iatrochemistry. His attitude toward preliminary venesection and catharsis was discussed earlier.

In dangerous cases he insisted on immediate extreme unction before he would prescribe the bark.[46] It is at least possible that he feared both the disease and the drug. It is difficult to understand why, in a strongly Catholic country, so many seriously ill patients had failed to receive last rites *before* the arrival of the doctor.

About his entire therapeutic doctrine Torti attempted to maintain a constantly critical attitude, even in successful cases. He says that the physician should always take care not to flatter himself and give undue credit to the drug if the case has turned out favorably; he should see whether the recovery is due to the drug he has given or to another, or to nature, for it is easy to fall into what is called paralogism (question begging), the assertion that a noncause is the cause (636).

10 Torti as Seen by His Contemporaries

IN PREVIOUS CHAPTERS we have considered Torti's life and works, up to and including the first edition of his *Therapeutice specialis*, which appeared in 1712. It is now necessary to examine the opinions that were held, and the contributions to knowledge of the Peruvian bark that were made, by four of Torti's most important contemporaries, Ippolito Francesco Albertini, Giovanni Maria Lancisi, Bernardino Ramazzini, and Nicolò Cirillo (Fig. 6).

Albertini

As Morgagni has shown, Ippolito Francesco Albertini (1662–1738), a kinsman of Malpighi and a professor of medicine in Bologna, was a remarkably perceptive clinician.[1] His fame rests upon his understanding of the relation between dyspnea and lesions of the cardiovascular system, which he presented, in a monumental combination of clinical acumen, anatomical observation, and correct reasoning, before the Bolognese Institute and Academy of Arts and Sciences in November 1726. The presentation was published in 1731 in the first volume of the institute's *Commentarii* and was reprinted in 1748. The same volume contains another work by Albertini, his *De cortice peruviano commentationes quaedam* (Some Comments on the Peruvian Bark), presented before the Bolognese Institute and Academy on December 11, 1716,[2] only four years after the first edition of Torti's *Therapeutice specialis* appeared.

In his second essay Albertini states that *quinquina* is a very reliable safeguard (*certissimum praesidium*) against intermittent fevers and also against continued fevers that have the character of intermittents.[3] He

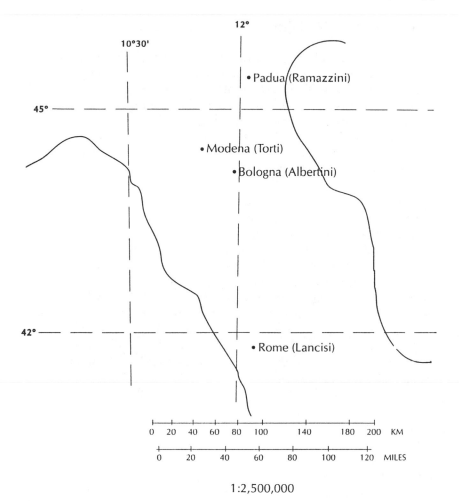

FIG. 6. Northern Italy, 1700. Locations of four physicians prominent in this history.

disagrees with those who assert that the drug dispels fevers without causing any evacuation; he had seen no one who convalesced perfectly after taking *quinquina* without having, soon or later, critical evacuations similar to those that follow fevers treated by other drugs or cured spontaneously. When the evacuations occur late, they are likely to be overlooked by physicians who discontinue their vigilance at the end of the [acute] illness; it is necessary to observe also those patients who are convalescent and also those who appear to have been restored to health. In prolonged fevers that require repeated doses of febrifuge, the evacuations may be difficult to distinguish from natural excretions (406–17).

Transpiration, Albertini continues, follows the taking of the drug and may be perceptible, not merely insensible. It may be evident in foulness of halitus. This fact, unobserved by previous physicians, is shown by the case of a nobleman afflicted with autumnal tertian fever; the history is given in detail (407).

Labial pustules [herpes] are not inherently critical but are signs of crises that are present or that will occur subsequently. The Peruvian bark produces no constant kind of crisis. Sometimes it causes transpiration, and sometimes it produces discharges of sweat, urine, stool, or sputum, which appear at no regular time and may occur after the patient, emerging from convalescence, has returned to his usual work. When the discharge is delayed, it may be overlooked (410–11).

Toward the end of this essay Albertini refers to an experiment made by Torti, who had concluded that there was no reason to believe that the drug interferes with the coagulation of freshly drawn blood.[4] Like Torti, Albertini judged that *experiments have thrown no light* on the action of the Peruvian bark; in whatever way the drug is administered, it is effective (412).

With these discussions Albertini presented four detailed case reports, intended to show the danger of using the bark in intermittents accompanied by suppression of some habitual excretion.

Toward the end of his discussion he remarked that the bark alone is effective specifically against the juice that produces intermittent fever (*adversus eum succum, qui febrem intermittentem facit*); it holds this juice ensnared for many days. If the pathogenic juice does not emerge from the body by crisis, it liberates itself and must therefore be repressed again by a new dose of febrifuge until a subsequent crisis reveals that it has been expelled (416). If we merely replace the term *juice* by the term *plasmodia*, Albertini's concept shows a degree of similarity to the modern belief.

But, says Albertini, the situation has further complexity, since the specific power of the drug does not act against the juices that are emitted in habitual evacuations. If such juices become mixed with the pyrogenic juice and remain in the body, unexpelled in crises and unrestrained by the bark, they produce dangerous diseases.

To readers of Albertini's essay on the Peruvian bark it becomes evident that he applied extensive observation, as well as his large observational powers, to support Hippocratic and Galenic concepts of crisis, coction, and critical evacuation. These he did not trouble to define, probably because they were well known to his Bolognese auditors and readers and were accepted by many of them. At the same time the failure to delimit these concepts relieved both author and audience of the need to question whether a delayed evacuation occurring in convalescence was assignable to a recent fever or to the return of normal bodily function.

In demonstrating, or attempting to demonstrate, that the use of the Peruvian bark was indeed followed by critical evacuation, Albertini aimed to dispel the astonishment that had been experienced by almost all previous observers of the drug, and probably had inhibited not a few from prescribing it. If his contentions were correct, a physician could administer the drug without committing anti-Hippocratic and anti-Galenic heresy.

To Albertini's credit it must be noted that, unlike many a practitioner in his day and ours, he paid ample attention to the reporting of refractory or unsuccessful cases and also that he tried to continue his observation into convalescence and beyond. His skepticism about the applicability of experiments to clinical medicine, warranted in his time, need not be abandoned nowadays.

Albertini's essay, like the Tortian *Therapeutice specialis*, demonstrates persistence of the need to consider Hippocratic concepts, such as that of critical evacuation (which here involved him even in a discussion of labial herpes) and that of perilously suppressed critical evacuation which he also mentioned but like his contemporaries, did not trouble to define. He also mentioned, and accepted, Santorian insensible perspiration. A positive feature is the hint that it is instructive to observe patients during a period of "follow-up" after treatment has been completed.

Yet even when these things are said, the reader who expects to find in Albertini's essay on Peruvian bark a counterpart and equal of the essay on dyspnea suffers disappointment. The lightning did not strike twice.

Lancisi

The famous book by Lancisi (1654–1720), *On Harmful Emanations from Swamps, and on the Remedies*, devotes attention predominantly to epidemiology, climate, and terrain. Relatively little space is allotted to therapeutics.[5]

Lancisi says that two defenses have been found to be very useful in cases of intermittent fever, namely vesicants and Peruvian bark. When employed properly, both can be called specific medicaments for pernicious fevers of this kind. They have saved many people.

Vesicants, he says, are beneficial for two reasons: they cause sluggish

fluids in the body to move more rapidly, and by increasing the tension
in the muscles, they assist expulsion of the dangerous seeds of disease.
It should be noted that, in a treatise dated 1694, Giorgio Baglivi had
discussed the action of vesicants, basing his opinions on clinical and
experimental observations explained in accordance with iatromechanical doctrines.[6] The stimulant effects of vesication had been considered
still earlier, and also on iatromechanical grounds, in Lorenzo Bellini's
On Urines, Pulses, and Bloodletting (1683).

Lancisi says that the Peruvian bark should be used unadulterated.
In pernicious tertians it should be given before the third or fourth day;
if it is given later, the patient may die. In fevers of this dangerous kind
not all formulas are equally effective. Moreover, the medicine must be
adapted to individual differences in habitus and to the symptoms. Patients who have languid forces, cold limbs, phlegmatic temperament,
and no coma or delirium should be given, in equal parts of pure wine
and water of scorzonera, a total of up to three ounces of the bark in
individual doses administered twice on days of paroxysm and once on
intervening days. Gracile patients who have cerebral signs are given the
drug in waters of *carduus sanctus* and scorzonera, with drops of Mat-
thioli's scorpion oil.[7] The dose of bark on single occasions did not exceed two scruples to one drachm. Boli were given until the ninth day,
twice on odd days and once on even days, and then once a day until the
fourteenth. It was marvelous with what success the fever, like the hydra
killed by Hercules, was slain by the boli, for the Peruvian bark, with its
bitter and tart alkali and its volatile oily balsamic particles affected by
the scorpion oil, acted simultaneously as a febrifuge, anthelmintic,
stomachic, and vulnerary.

After these weighty pronouncements in favor of the bark, Lancisi
says that he had seen many patients who because of algid fever were
hurrying toward death but were saved by the use of theriac alone,
mixed into wine (218). He also praised other medicines, such as soup
containing scorzonera, contrayerva, and hartshorn, likewise, simples
given with diaphoretic antimony and antimoniated niter.

In the study of Lancisi's treatise several observations and problems
come to mind. Incidental remarks show that Lancisi had had large
clinical experience with malaria. The relative frequency of his comments on cerebral symptoms suggests that many *falciparum* infections
had come into his ken.

While it is reassuring to read that the Peruvian bark was marvelously
effective, a problem lurks nearby. Why is it that many patients given no
other medicine than theriac in wine did well also? Included in this
happy subgroup were some who had been very seriously ill, *ad necem
properantes* (218). And how is it that vesicants, simples, and antimoni-

als also appeared to be beneficial? Probably the explanation lies in the absence of controlled clinical trials and in the absence of precise observational methods, clinical, hematological, parasitological, and statistical, which would have permitted accurate discrimination of various kinds and various intensities of fever and would have rendered instructive accounting of therapeutic results.

Also to be considered is the fact that if autopsies had been done in failed cases, the revelations would have helped little when the cause of death was malaria, since in this disease acute infections do not yield much by way of gross anatomical change. Morgagni would later write that "after violent fevers, or those that kill unexpectedly soon, scarcely any thing, and sometimes nothing at all, is found, which might bear any correspondence to . . . their violence or impetus.[8]

Ramazzini

It is probable that Bernardino Ramazzini is more widely remembered than Albertini by nonspecialist devotees of medical history, and it is probable also that he is better remembered than Lancisi. Especially among laymen Ramazzini's high reputation rests principally on his classic treatise *De morbis artificum diatriba* (A Treatise on the Diseases of Workers, 1700) and little if at all on epidemiological writings, such as his account of a bovine epizootic and a series of reports that describe the meteorological and climatic phenomena ("constitutions") and concomitant sicknesses of single years or series of years (1716). Yet each of these writings must be considered in any serious attempt to plot the course of Ramazzini's opinions on the Peruvian bark.

The discussion of Ramazzini differs from those of Albertini and Lancisi in that personal and psychological factors are more conspicuous in his life, and the narrative, especially in its final phase, is much less pleasant. Like Torti, all three men were undeniably illustrious.

Ramazzini (1633–1714) was twenty-five years older than Torti, and Torti survived him by twenty-seven years. Since Ramazzini died two years after the first edition of the *Therapeutice specialis* was published, he did not live to see any of the later editions. Moreover, Ramazzini's most controverted work, the *De abusu Chinae Chinae*, was written when its author was blind, and presumably embittered, in the ninth decade of life.

Ramazzini was born in Carpi, situated in the domain of the Este dynasty, 17 km north-northeast of Modena. He received the medical doctorate in Parma in 1657.[9] From 1682 to 1700 he served as primary

professor of medicine at the reconstituted University of Modena. As
was stated in Chapter 8, in 1685 the second professorial chair was
given to Torti, who also became physician to the ducal family. That this
circumstance produced rivalry and hence hostility between the two
men is not certainly known.

In 1700, Ramazzini, aged sixty-seven, became professor of practical
medicine at Padua. Here he spent the remaining fourteen years of his
life.

What may have been the earnest of a contentious tendency in Ramazzini became apparent in 1679 in a reply that he issued in response
to an attack by Dr. Annibale Cervi of Modena. Tiraboschi's biography,
after politely mentioning Ramazzini's "amiable and gentle manners,
which made him dear to everyone," states that the contest originated
in the illness of a woman who had been in the care of Cervi and whom
Ramazzini was suddenly requested to visit. A difference of opinion having arisen, Cervi circulated in manuscript "a pungent script against
Ramazzini," who responded with the *Exercitatio iatroapologetica*
(Medical Explanatory Tract).[10] Cervi then wrote an additional treatise,
to which Ramazzini prepared a reply, but the regnant Cesare d'Este
suppressed the continuation of hostilities.

Another Ramazzinian controversy concerned the death of a partur-
ient marchioness. This incident led to an elaborate pamphlet war between Ramazzini and several other combatants.[11] Both the melee and
the patient's high rank were characteristic of medical squabbles of the
era, as has been noticed before in this history. When beggars died there
were no comets seen.

Still another controversy concerned movement of the mercury in barometers and involved Ramazzini with Gunther Schelhammer (1649–
1716), professor of medicine in Kiel, a scholar who had seen the cities
and known the achievements of many men. The debate, initiated with
barometric observations that Ramazzini had made in 1694, is represented also by a treatise issued as late as 1710.[12]

The published record reveals many instances of contact between
Torti and Ramazzini. In the *Therapeutice specialis* Torti reported several cases in which patients had been seen by both physicians. In 1696
Ramazzini was among those who treated Torti for what was later characterized as "diaphoretic pernicious tertian fever." In 1707 Torti was
summoned as consultant in the care of "a very skilled lithotomist of
this city" who was afflicted with pernicious intermittent fever and almost moribund. Torti intended to order a phlebotomy, to be followed
immediately by doses of the bark. Ramazzini, hearing of the case,
stated "courteously, as is his usual manner" (*humaniter, ut illi mos est*)
that he had high regard for Torti's opinion but that the desperate illness

was suitable for priests rather than physicians. The patient, given the bark in large doses, was rescued.[13]

Incidental remarks of this kind, unlike the pamphlet wars that have been mentioned, describe little more than gentlemanly interchanges between two practitioners who also were academic colleagues. Torti and Ramazzini must have met almost daily until 1700, when the latter accepted a professorship at Padua, 110 km from Modena.

Information about Ramazzini's opinion of the Peruvian bark, as already stated, resides in his epidemiological and climatic reports, designated as [meteorological] *Constitutiones,* and in his lectures. In describing the epidemic constitution of 1690, Ramazzini wrote that the Peruvian bark was used by most practitioners (*major pars medentium*) with little success. The drug was dangerous, producing temporary alleviation of the fever followed by violent recrudescence (120–55, esp. 128). This statement contrasts with the almost universal experience of earlier authors, who had found recrudescences to be milder than primary attacks. Further, Ramazzini remarked, the drug worked better in rural patients than in town-dwellers. It was effective also as a vermifuge.

Under the date of 1691 Ramazzini wrote that the use of china china [cinchona], which had been harmful during the climatic "constitution" of the previous year, was now found to be very beneficial, meteorological conditions being totally different. Many patients with quartan fever were restored completely to health, while a few who suffered relapses became healthy soon afterward (156–81). He added,

I infer that the use of china china is safer when the humors need to be reined in rather than goaded. In the past year, because of the cold and damp constitution the entire humoral mass, being thick and sluggish, needed to be stimulated and roused to move, whereas during the summer it was subject to spasm, unable to stand still, and in need of restraint. This the Peruvian bark supplied wonderfully well by repressing the onslaught of the humors. (149)

This passage, taken in conjunction with the passage immediately preceding, shows that as late as 1691 Ramazzini was not prejudiced against the Peruvian bark but was making an objective attempt to determine the conditions of its usefulness. A somewhat different impression is gained from passages in the *Therapeutice specialis* in which, after an interval of a decade, Torti discussed the Ramazzinian *Constitutiones.* Torti wrote that the treatise on the (climatic) constitutions of 1690–94 was erroneously thought to refer in some manner to Torti's subject (*argumentum meum . . . aliquo saltem modo tractasse*)—that is, malignant and pernicious fevers. Further, in discussing the constitution of 1690, Ramazzini had stated that the Peruvian bark is harmful

in all pernicious fevers. Moreover, Ramazzini's opinions were complex
and had at last become favorable to the bark.[14]

Additional insight into Ramazzini's opinions about the bark and his
opinions on other important matters is gained by reading his public
and his academic addresses. The *Oratio secunda secularis* (second secular oration), delivered in 1700, contains a concise history of medical
science, with emphasis on recent developments (15–29). In addition to
praising "the very famous Harvey, whose name shall stand as long as
blood flows and is driven in a circle," Ramazzini praised the new pharmacy, including iatrochemical drugs as well as botanicals, and he referred also to the recently introduced microscopical examination of
plants. He added that "recently a bark was brought to us from Peru,
clearly a divine remedy for exterminating the ill-born race of fevers,"
and he did not fail to mention the new antidysenteric drug, ipecacuanha (27; see also Chapter 13 below). In his broad non-nationalistic
review the progressive and well-informed old man also included a few
words about scientific societies and about the periodical literature.

Ramazzini's important fourth oration (1702) is devoted to the theory
of fevers and to practical aspects, "including matters which need to be
reconsidered" (45–55). He says that in the recently ended [seven-
teenth] century the Galenic opinion had been supplanted. No longer is
reliance placed on comment and on interpretation of old writings. By
diligent attempts to approach the secret inner recesses of Nature, new
foundations have been created, wonderful huge structures have been
built, and fever has come to be very differently regarded—rightly or
not—than heretofore.

Ramazzini expressed skepticism toward the profusion of recent doctrines concerning fever and toward new nomenclature of fevers. He regarded the Peruvian bark as being easily the chief (*facile princeps*) over
all the antipyretics that had been contrived by antiquity and by the
chemists. This unique drug, he continued, which acts especially in periodic fevers, has obtained for us the benefit that *we can make a correct
distinction between intermittent fevers and those that are truly continuous* and also between their foci of origin. No more are all fevers,
whether gastric or venous, treated by one method—that is, by refriger-
ants and moisteners and repeated phlebotomy and purges that weaken
the human body instead of strengthening it. Only fevers that belong to
the family of intermittents are removed by drinking a little of the powder dissolved in wine; thereby they are either suppressed or thoroughly
eradicated (53).

The introduction of the Peruvian bark into medicine, Ramazzini
continued, resembles in its results the introduction of gunpowder into
military science: the catapults and battering rams had to be thrown

away. This memorable statement has at least two predecessors, which were not necessarily its sources. In his *Apologetico discurso*, Diego Salado Garces (see Chapter 1) compared innovation in pharmacy to innovation in artillery. He cited a remark made by "Carlos Vallesius" in a commentary on the Hippocratic *Prognostic*. The passage, quoted by Salado Garces, is as follows: "Excellent discoveries are rejected because they are new and were unknown to the ancients. This reasoning would debar all drugs discovered by the Arabs and applied to medical use, and all spagyric remedies, and whatever things were brought from the Indies a few years ago, and would debar from warriors the military engines that were not known to the great captains of antiquity."[15]

In his widely ranging fourth oration Ramazzini included also predictions that the nature of intermittent fever would be discovered, that chemical analysis of the Peruvian bark would be made, and that botanists would find some indigenous febrifuge of comparable power. As we have observed, Ramazzini pointed out also the usefulness of the Peruvian bark in differential diagnosis. By this statement, made in 1702, he deserves praise for an advance that has been credited to Torti and the *Therapeutice specialis* of 1712. We have already noted that Richard Morton stated a similar opinion in 1692. This readjustment will appeal to those who are smitten with the importance of priorities in history. Such persons should be urged to ascertain whether a revelation comparable to Ramazzini's and Morton's occurred even earlier to any of the numerous physicians, apothecaries, and laymen who used the drug.

Of at least equal importance is the fact that Ramazzini expected the bark to throw light on the different bodily foci from which different fevers were believed to originate;[16] the drug might prove decisive in studies of pathogenesis by acting like what we nowadays call a "tracer." Further, Ramazzini foresaw the work of pharmaceutical chemists, which would be done more than one hundred years later, and also the search for additional febrifuges. His prediction about indigenous plants (*ad Plantam aliquam indigenam . . . reperiendam*) was hardly confirmed by the reintroduction of the exotic qinghaosu.[17]

In the case of a patient seen in 1707, Ramazzini disagreed with Torti's advocacy of the bark, but the disagreement was courteous. The senior physician is described in the index to the *Therapeutice specialis* as *auctori vel dissentiens, semper humanus*, disagreeing with the author but constantly polite. Somewhat later, Torti praised Ramazzini's essay on preserving the health of princes, which was issued in 1710.[18] It should be noticed that this work makes no mention of Peruvian bark. The omission is especially strange since, as most of the preceding chapters of this history have shown, royalty, nobility, and ecclesiastics in Italy, France, Spain, and England had suffered from intermittent fever. But latent hostility is a common cause of overt omission.

The writings reviewed and described up to this point show Ramazzini to have been a man of wide knowledge, great acumen, and continued progressiveness, able to survey all of medicine and much of natural science. His early contentiousness is unlikely to have disappeared, but it is not clearly evident in the writings of his mature years, even in the debate with Schelhammer. His mention of occasional successes and occasional failures with the use of the bark shows no rooted bias for or against this drug. Nor is hostility to Torti evident in the other writings that he published as late as 1710, or in his correspondence, issued in our own era by Professor di Pietro.[19]

As the reader is well aware, Torti issued his *Synopsis* in 1709 and his *Therapeutice specialis* in 1712. In July 1714 Ramazzini, eighty years of age and blind,[20] published his epistolary treatise on the abuse of *China chinae* (*De abusu chinae chinae dissertatio epistolaris*). I have not been able to trace a separate original edition of this troublesome essay; it is probable that no such edition exists. The work appeared, and is available, as an addendum to what is designated as the second edition of Ramazzini's collected constitutions. The full title of this book is *Constitutionum epidemicarum mutinensium annorum quinque. Editio secunda. Accedit dissertatio epistolaris de abusu chinae chinae ad D. Bartholomaeum Ramazzini.* The dedication is dated Padua, July 20, 1714, and this date is found again at the end of the volume. The date of official approval is June 23, 1714.

The treatise reappeared in Ramazzini's *Opera omnia, medica, et physica* of 1716 (218–38); which is the edition cited here. Another edition is incorporated in Torti's rebuttal of 1715, which is discussed later in this chapter.

Ramazzini opened his essay by remarking that use of the bark has become so frequent that if a patient dies after the drug has *not* been tried, this is considered a great crime (*pro magno piaculo habeatur, remedium istud non fuisse pertentatum*). In addition, Ramazzini's nephew Bartolomeo, a physician, had asked whether the drug could be used prophylactically, that is, whether it could be given during the summer and autumn, before the periodic fevers usually make their attack, so as to prevent formation of the ferment that arouses fevers of this kind (218). In other words, prevention of intermittent fever resolves itself into anticipatory suppression of the causative ferment.

Ramazzini is candid in describing the fluctuations of his own opinions. In youth and young manhood he had held the Peruvian bark in high esteem and used it as a panacea. Later, schooled by experience, he prescribed it only with the greatest of care. As Terence had remarked, changes of opinion are not limited to medicine. Ramazzini says that he does not hold the bark in contempt, but it is more easily admired than understood. Its application is not rational but empirical, and the authors of treatises about it are in disagreement. With the advance of age, Ramazzini has reduced his dosages. He considers it a great abuse to prescribe the drug indiscriminately for persons of all ages, sexes, regions, tempers, temperaments, and constitutions. (Some of these categories are still in use by epidemiologists nowadays.)

The old febrifuges, Ramazzini continues, are slower than the bark but are safer, and the bark should be prescribed by physicians only, not by surgeons, druggists, quacks, and women (226, 232). Perhaps the usefulness of the bark in malignant intermittents would be greater if these sicknesses were recognized at onset. Some of the continued or essential continent fevers are deceptive, but exceptional rescues should not lead to indiscriminate use (228–29).

Ramazzini tells of one very sick patient whom he was obliged to see, about 1704, while he was on vacation from professorial duties in Padua and was trying to avoid consultations. Another physician on the case, "a great advocate of the bark [Torti?]" had begun to shout about using the drug. The patient's condition improved after the bark was discontinued. The tone of this short narration is insulting to the other physician.

Ramazzini alludes to other unfavorable experiences and cites a few from the writings of Ettmüller, Sydenham, Lower, and others. Using traditional techniques of the partisan, he does not overstrain the search for reports favorable to his opposition. He cites in addition six Modenese enemies of the bark; none of their names is readily recognizable, yet this little list contradicts Ramazzini's initial statements about the popularity of the drug. In addition, he notes that the bark is not in great demand in Bologna. This observation is compatible with statements in Chapter 7.

Ramazzini denied that the use of large doses was new, supporting this contention by citation of Brady's letter to Sydenham; it is easy for the reader to suspect that Ramazzini was avoiding mention of Torti, whose name fails to appear. Yet, Ramazzini adds unconvincingly, "Let no one conclude that I want the bark to be expunged from the book. . . . Let it have its uses" (236).

As to prophylaxis, Ramazzini remarks that this term can signify either prevention of recurrence or prevention of a disease that the patient has not had previously. While he considered it permissible for the drug to be tested in a moderate dose for a limited period every morning before the arrival of the summer and autumn fevers, the impression gained is that he is not clearly favorable to prophylactic use.

What does the *De abusu* tell us, and what does it fail to tell us, about
Ramazzini, about Torti, and about the history of the Peruvian bark? If
Bernardino Ramazzini's introductory remarks are to be taken as literally true and not as a rhetorical device, Bartolomeo Ramazzini, his
nephew, to whom the essay is dedicated, had inquired whether the
drug could be used prophylactically; this inquiry, as we have already
noted, furnished the second of the two motives that impelled the older
Ramazzini to compose the essay. His reply, which appears at its very
end (238), shows that the old man was not totally and automatically
opposed to new ideas.

With regard to the therapeutic use of the drug Bernardino Ramazzini reports that his opinions have changed in the course of years, and
especially that youthful enthusiasm in favor of the drug had been replaced by growing conservatism and caution. He writes: "According to
the different ages that I have been indulged by Divine Providence, I felt
differently and diversely about the Peruvian bark; in youth and even in
maturity, I confess, I held the china china in high esteem and I used it
freely, preferring it to all other drugs as if it were a panacea" (218). This
retroactive reconstruction is not accurate; it overlooks the fluctuations
of opinion that Ramazzini recorded in his *Constitutiones* of 1690–94
and that we have discussed. However, the reports in the *Constitutiones*
are not limited to Ramazzini's personal opinions but include also the
opinions and practices that were prevalent in a succession of years.

Torti tells us a different story. In the *Therapeutice specialis* he cites a
case of malignant fever (1707) in which Ramazzini recognized the importance of early diagnosis and early use of the bark, but he says that
in 1695 Ramazzini had not recognized its use in such cases.[21] Indeed
Torti specified 1695 as the date of one of Ramazzini's turning points
and commented also on the complexity of Ramazzini's opinions.

The opinion that Ramazzini presents in the *De abusu* is predominantly negative toward the Peruvian bark. His complaints against the
bark are couched in rather general terms. In addition to this objection,
already cited, against indiscriminate use in patients of all ages, he
states that in children and adolescents the fevers that occur in the summer are usually spurious tertians. In these cases he has observed the
bark to be of little use; although modest improvement may occur when
the drug is given, very often the fever recurs and may persist for many
months. In women the bark is less likely to succeed than in men, and
the results in nuns are not good. Greater success is obtained in nobility
and rich potentates (220–21). These comments have the timbre of
firsthand clinical experience. Ramazzini says that excessive doses have
been given, but he does not reveal the dosages that he considers appro-

priate, and he does not mention tinnitus or deafness. He believes that untimely use of the bark impedes maturation of the humors. He says also that the drug is suspect because it produces no evacuation (233). It is interesting and significant that this old objection, encountered as early as the time of Badus—that is, at the beginning of the historical development—was still being used. Several of Ramazzini's statements, quoted above, suggest that, in addition to being animated by personal hostility, Ramazzini was nettled by failure to excogitate a rationale for the use of the bark.

As to Ramazzini's personal difficulties, it is known that, when his light was spent, his three nephews served him as amanuenses.[22] The burden of old age combined with that of visual impairment could explain a renewal of his earlier cantankerousness.

A reference to the *De abusu* occurs in an undated and unsigned copy of a letter attributed to Albertini because of strong internal evidence.[23] The author of this communication discusses his sister's fever, "which belonged to the race of the intermittents and therefore warranted cinchona," but no evacuation had been observed and recovery had not taken place. Indeed, the writer adds, despite continuation or repetition of the drug, sometimes the desired effect fails to occur. In discussing the further treatments that might be undertaken in this difficult case, the commentator says: "Moreover, I think that Signor Ramazzini was not entirely wrong when he wrote against some uses of the bark." He then describes the preposterous use of the bark in a case of puerperal sepsis. Cases of this kind, as he noticed, lent support to Ramazzini's objections. The modern reader can perceive that they contain only a modicum of rationality.

More than a century after Albertini, another highly perceptive clinician, Armand Trousseau, wrote: "One regrets to include Ramazzini and Baglivi among the opponents of cinchona, but today these two clinicians would probably blush at what they wrote under the influence of wicked emotions (*sous l'influence de quelques mauvaises passions*)."[24] Torti's response to Ramazzini's attack is discussed later in this chapter.

As we have noted, Ramazzini's *De abusu* was approved by the authorities of Padua on June 13, 1714, and was issued in that city on July 20 of the same year as a postscript to the second edition of Ramazzini's *Constitutionum epidemicarum mutinensium annorum quinque*. Torti received the combined publication at the end of October 1714 in Modena. On November 5, 1714, Ramazzini died.

Almost a full year later, on October 15, 1715, Torti issued his reply. In English translation the title is: "Medical and defensive rejoinder of Francesco Torti, Modenese physician, to the critical dissertation on abuse of the Peruvian bark that is falsely charged to the physicians of Modena by that eminent man, the late Bernardino Ramazzini." The chapters of Torti's counterattack have the following titles:

Prelude to the entire discussion; the reason for writing (1–9)

Disagreement between the eminent Ramazzini and me; a summary [in two parallel columns] (10–17)

Disagreement between the eminent Ramazzini and himself; a comparison [in two parallel columns] (18–14)

Ramazzini's inconsistencies, excerpted from the distinguished man's texts, already cited, and his remarks; or, the changeable color of the peacock's tail [in two parallel columns] (25–28)

Comments on the title that the eminent Ramazzini prefixed to his *Epidemic Constitutions* (29–30)

Comments on the dedicatory letter . . . (31–34)

Medical and defensive replies to the dissertation proper, divided into paragraphs, this entire series making up *De abusu* [in fifty sections; the entire text of Ramazzini's diatribe is reproduced, and comments by Torti are added, paragraph by paragraph] (35–191)

Torti's reply is approximately twelve times as long as Ramazzini's original. The hostile tone of the rebuttal, suggested in the main title, becomes fully evident, together with Torti's habitual intricacy of style, on the second page:

There is one thing, beyond all others, that I have been unable to wonder at sufficiently or to pass in silence, namely, that the distinguished man whom a short while ago, on pages 637 to 641 of my *Therapeutice*, I asserted to be no longer unfavorable to the Peruvian bark—as was stated a long time ago in his *Epidemic Constitutions*—from this assertion, openly and publicly promulgated by me in that very place, has deviated in this recent dissertation, to the extent that not only whatever item adverse to the bark that he brought forth in those same *Constitutions* he has confirmed in this *Dissertation*, but in addition [he has brought forth] this [essay] as an annex to those items [i.e., to the *Epidemic Constitutions*], which have been recently reprinted, as if it were something clearly belonging to them, and he has sprinkled it with further bitterness against the medicament and against my procedure, improperly represented.

To this pronouncement Torti added that he shuddered strongly at Ramazzini's shameful comments. Since a complete review of the allegations and refutations would be intolerably burdensome to both the reader and the present commentator—indeed, Torti later advised beginners not to weigh themselves down by reading them[25]—a few examples must be made to suffice.

According to one of the excerpts reproduced by Torti, Ramazzini had accused him of stating that the Peruvian bark could cause harm because it might produce untimely suppression of fevers and also because the drug contains a hidden evil. Torti is alleged to have said, but never to have proved, that the evil exists. Further, because the febrifugal property of the bark is occult and its mode of action is secret (since it produces no evacuation), and because nothing analogous to it is found in the vegetable kingdom in Europe, Torti is accused of having concluded that the use of this bark cannot be rational but is empirical and nonmethodical. Further, says Ramazzini, although Torti does not distinctly disapprove the experiments that have been set up to explore the drug's febrifugal property, Torti considers them subject to many misinterpretations; hence no one can derive anything useful from them (10–11).

Torti disagreed with this description of his statements and opinions. He says he had written in the *Therapeutice specialis* that the Peruvian bark, like all other very choice medicaments, can sometimes be harmful if it is used at the wrong time; that is, if it halts fevers that should be allowed to run unrestrained. He does not agree that the bark causes harm attributable to a hidden evil ingredient or because its febrifugal property is secret (*ob malitiam occultam quam habet vel ex eo quod arcana sit virtus febrifuga*). Moreover, in the *Therapeutice* he had tried, by means of reasons, authorities, and experiments, to demonstrate the opposite opinion (10).

By using paired parallel columns of text, Torti exposes a series of Ramazzini's self-contradictions. For example, at one point Ramazzini had stated that the Peruvian bark is not as harmless as the public believes, but elsewhere he had written that the bark is clearly a divine drug, granted to us by the kindness of God, and that it is easily the best of antipyretics (25, item 6). On one occasion Ramazzini had remarked that it ranks far below the older febrifuges, which are safer; elsewhere he wrote that it is greatly to be preferred to the old febrifuges, which are weaker (25, item 3).

It will be remembered that the conflict between Ramazzini and Torti occurred when the Peruvian bark had been known in Europe for less than eighty-five years and when, as has been shown in Chapters 7 and 8, opposition to its use was not extinct. Ramazzini's terminal diatribe shows that the dying serpent of hostility was sometimes venomous.

Yet it is true that the Peruvian bark was abused and continued to be abused. We have already taken note of a letter attributed to Albertini, which states that Signor Ramazzini was not entirely wrong when he wrote against some uses of cinchona.[26]

Torti's rejoinder was considered important enough to be reprinted. It reappeared, together with the *Therapeutice specialis*, as late as 1821 (see Appendix D). Nowadays it is read only by hopelessly conscientious historians.

Cirillo

Nicolò Cirillo (1671–1734), another contemporary of Torti, was a pupil of Luca Tozzi and succeeded him in the professorial chair at Naples. He was expert in botany and Cartesian philosophy and is remembered as both a devoted teacher of medicine and a busy practitioner. His four centuries of collected consultations (1738) show that he had seen patients not only in Naples and its vicinity but also in places as far afield as Rome, Genoa, Vienna, Ragusa, Messina, and Malta. Included in his published series are only about ten cases that were probably examples of intermittent fever. In these Cirillo used Peruvian bark without evident hesitation or opposition and usually with good result. His reports are notably free from the controversies that befell Torti.

Of special interest is the case of a man whom Cirillo treated in October 1733 (438–41). The patient had had "a fever" (unspecified) in August, then a quartan that became continuous. After taking the bark he recovered from the fever and from incipient cachexia. His physician feared that a recurrence might supervene. Cirillo felt that, in order to prevent this unhappy sequel, preservative treatment (*la cura preservativa*) should be given by repeating what had been administered previously, that is, Peruvian bark with rhubarb or nitrous magnesia. This should be followed in a few days by the prophylactic treatment (*la cura profilattica*), namely, a mild purge followed by martial wine containing absinthe, senna, rhubarb, and Peruvian bark.

It is evident that in Cirillo's terminology prophylaxis consisted of preventing recurrence of a fever that had been dispelled in the past. His reports say nothing about prevention of fever in a person who had never had an attack. The reader may observe that this concept tallies exactly with that enunciated by Torti.

Mangetus

In the annals of hostility to Peruvian bark the tale of the vexed and vexatious Ramazzini is paralleled by the more agreeable story of Johannes Jacobus Mangetus (1652–1742) of Geneva, medical practitioner and encyclopedist, and honorary physician to Frederick III, Elector of Brandenburg.[27]

The second edition of Ramazzini's collected works, published in 1717, includes a two-page prefatory address to the reader. This statement, prepared by Mangetus at the request of the publisher, contains a number of significant comments.[28]

Mangetus writes that Ramazzini's *De abusu* had been received rather sharply by Torti. "If I had had the opportunity," Mangetus continues, "to read Torti's *Therapeutice specialis*, it might be easier for me to understand why Torti was driven to this kind of [contentious] writing, but since this book has not as yet reached me, I shall limit myself to general remarks."

Mangetus observes that in Ramazzini's *De abusu* blame is directed toward the very free and perhaps unsystematic use of the bark among the physicians of Modena. But accusation is made also against prudent users and a few other colleagues; in Geneva excessive recourse to the drug is reproached, hence we avoid such excess as much as possible. The same is true of Torti, who in *Therapeutice specialis* discusses the precautions that must be respected, as Mangetus had noticed in the excerpts that Torti included in the *Responsiones jatro-apologeticae*.

Mangetus now comes to a major issue. "Indeed," he writes, "I do not at all agree with Ramazzini as to the nature and effects of the bark, or the manner of giving it, or the dosage. I have never found any malignity in it. I have always given large doses and I have usually seen the fever dispelled; and no recurrence or sickness of any kind has followed. . . . I never gave the bark alone, but always together with various deobstruents and nerve medicines."

The Mangetan preface closes with a few soothing words: "Henceforth I shall be more careful in the management of a drug whose bad effects, if not permanent, appear at least occasionally. The constitutions and temperaments in which they are perhaps inescapable are shown in good faith by a highly skilled man [Ramazzini]." In the opinion of W. C. Wright, Mangetus's note was written "to conciliate the Modenese physicians attacked by Ramazzini for excessive use of quinine [*sic*]."[29] The facts that are now to be presented give no more than incomplete support to Dr. Wright's evaluation.

The Abbot Girolamo Tiraboschi, whose statements I have not been able to complete or to verify *in toto*, offered a slightly more complex version of the tale (5:276). He wrote that the biography of Ramazzini, which is prefixed to the 1717 edition of Ramazzini's works, and the favorable opinion of Mangetus with regard to Ramazzini's dissertation (the *De abusu*), provided Dr. Ferranti Ferrari with the occasion, in the year 1719, to publish his book, which is titled *Mutinensium medicorum methodus* (Method of the physicians of Modena).

Torti was displeased at the renewal of the contest, and on February 25, 1720, wrote Mangetus a letter in which he reviewed the history of the difficulties and stated that he had been injured severely and unreasonably by the elder Ramazzini (*me a seniore Ramazzino praeter rati-*

onem grauiter laesum). Mentioning his own love of harmony and his disapproval of useless combat, he expressed the desire to have the polemic terminated.[30]

In his frank but courteous reply, couched in the elegant French style of the era, Mangetus explained that at the instance of Bartolomeo Ramazzini, the publishers, Messrs. Cramer and Perachon, had requested Mangetus to contribute a few prefatory lines for the new edition of Bernardino Ramazzini's complete works. At this time, Mangetus writes in his letter to Torti, he had read no work of Torti's other than the *Responsiones jatro-apologeticae*. More recently, on receiving Torti's letter, he had read the *Therapeutice specialis*, attentively, Torti having favored him with a copy. As a consequence, Mangetus continues, he is now strongly in agreement with Torti's views and he has so high an opinion of the incomparable *Therapeutice specialis* that he considers it to be one of the most perfect masterpieces in its field. Far from contradicting it or speaking of the book with any sort of doubt, he can express only admiration for it with regard to the manner, the precautions, and the attention to the character of the fevers on which Torti bases his decisions with respect to the administration of the drug.

Mangetus adds that he had used the *quin-quina* with success for more than forty-four years and considers himself one of its most ardent defenders.[31] The drug is discussed in Mangetus's large pharmaceuticomedical compend, in a note that draws on the writings of Charles Spon and others.[32] It should be noted also that Mangetus's collection of medical writings reproduces, from the Leipzig *Acta* of 1712, an anonymous review of Torti's *Therapeutice specialis* of 1712.[33]

It is surprising that Mangetus, an encyclopedic reader and compiler resembling his greater compatriot Albrecht von Haller, did not read the full text of Torti's *Therapeutice specialis* until eight years after this important work was published. Instead, Mangetus admitted to having read no more than the excerpts that Torti had included in the *Responsiones* of 1715. In 1720, as we have seen, Torti favored Mangetus with a copy of the *Therapeutice*. Perhaps the original press run was too short for Mangetus to have found a copy earlier.

This account of the incident involving Ramazzini, Torti, and Mangetus is necessarily replete with detail that verges on antiquarianism. It shows clearly enough that the fine Italian hand of Ramazzini had inflicted on Torti an injury that caused pain for six or more years; this fact is recalled additionally by the inclusion of Torti's *Responsiones* with each succeeding issue of the *Therapeutice specialis*. But bitter conflicts of this kind were not limited to the eighteenth century, to Italy, or to medicine.

With regard to the Peruvian bark the details of the Ramazzinian controversy, like those of acrid controversies described in previous chapters, increase the depth if not the width of our understanding of processes that were involved, directly or collaterally, in the history of the drug and at the same time augment the embarrassment of those who regard medical history as a continuously harmonious and triumphant procession.

11 Torti's Place in History

OUR ESTIMATE OF TORTI's place and rank in history can be presented as the sum of three components—his scholarship, his originality, and his influence.

Scholarship

On the score of Torti's historical scholarship the principal evidence is to be found in his major opus, the *Therapeutice specialis*, and is conspicuous in the first two books of that work. Book 1 presents ancient notions of fever and their displacement in more recent times. Likewise, it describes changes in opinion about Peruvian bark. The historical orientation is unmistakable.

Another interesting historical analysis appears in book 2, where Torti considers Morton's description of pernicious intermittent fever. Here he mentions earlier authors such as Mercatus and authors cited by Mercatus; to these he adds several whom Morton had omitted. Unhappily, these additions consist only of names, unaccompanied by detailed references, hence verification is often impracticable if not impossible (254–56). Torti concluded that Morton deserved credit for proposing the cure and not for contributing a description (256).

Supplementary evidence of Torti's scholarly procedure and proclivity is to be found in the *Responsiones jatro-apologeticae*. Here Torti undertook a meticulous paragraph-by-paragraph dissection of Ramazzini's *De abusu* and a parallel-column commentary on it. That later generations of readers and publishers valued this kind of contest is shown by the reprinting of Torti's *Responsiones* in several editions of the *Therapeutice specialis* (1732, 1743, 1756, 1821).

The total impression produced by these details is that Torti was a liberally educated scholar-physician, representing a form that nowadays deserves inclusion in the catalogue of endangered species. A hint of Torti's relation to the history of science—and more specifically to what we now call the Scientific Revolution—is to be found in comment included in the preface to the *Therapeutice specialis*. Torti says:

Long ago the notion of preparing a treatise of this kind, along with the confident anticipation of its usefulness to the public, was formulated by the very wise [Francis] Bacon in book 4, chapter 2 of his *Advancement of Learning*. He said that it would be of great importance if some physicians . . . would prepare a work on medicines tried and proved beneficial in particular diseases. The great man was of the opinion that such a special therapeutics was still lacking in medical art and would be very useful to it. (xvi)

Originality

Since the main thrust of Torti's activity as displayed in the *Therapeutice specialis* was an effort to restore the health of persons suffering from the pernicious forms of intermittent fever, and since he held this effort to necessitate a systematic understanding of the major fevers generally, it is appropriate to consider at the outset the original elements that are included in his chosen scope. Like many of his predecessors, Torti recognized, and mentioned repeatedly, that the Peruvian bark overcomes some fevers—mainly the intermittents—but is of little or no value in others, such as the continued fevers and various indeterminate forms. Hence, intelligent and effective use of the drug required the establishment of an exact taxonomy, the purpose being predominantly and clearly practical. In brief, Torti wanted to understand what he was doing.

He recognized that his taxonomy was imperfect, also that it was not impeccable according to scholastic standards. His system has three salient characteristics: (*a*) retention of two of the ancient categories of fever, namely the intermittent and the continued; (*b*) retention of the ancient opinion that some cases of fever undergo a change of character, which can be represented as a change of category; and (*c*) fusion of some intermittents with some continued fevers to form a new and hybrid category, which Torti devised and which he undertook to designate as that of the proportionate fevers.[1] He wrote that some fevers in this category are cured by the bark, whereas others are not. Those proportionate continued fevers in which the character or ferment of subintrants is dominant are easily overcome by the bark, while those in which the nature or ferment of the remittents is dominant are very resistant (615).

This part of Torti's taxonomy is original but it has been overtaken and overcome by nineteenth- and twentieth-century advances in parasitology.[2] In the cool, uncharitable light of retrospect it can now be viewed as a combination of taxonomic error and clinical confusion. In this context the word "confusion," derived from the Latin *confundere*, to pour together, is exactly applicable. But before we allow Torti to be belittled by such considerations, we must recall his important and perceptive remark, already noticed, that whether or not the proportionate fevers are malignant is of little importance. What counts is their susceptibility to the bark.

Torti's tree, for which I find no published precedent, is a clever and slightly bewildering novelty. It can be assumed, but has not been proved, to have had didactic merit, and it has not been dismissed as valueless. Its absence from the two-volume *Therapeutice* in the edition of 1821 indicates its demise. At the very least the tree offers a conspectus of the way in which Torti envisioned the fevers that are discussed in his text.

Having considered Torti's conspectus and perspectives, we must turn to his clinical innovations. In addition to making the observation, usual in his era, that the bark overcomes intermittent fever and is resisted by the continued fevers, Torti took the further step of recognizing that the drug could be used for differential diagnosis (610). In addition, he astutely remarked that it is not easy to distinguish between intermittent and continued fevers in advance of the therapeutic trial (615).

Despite these sagacious Tortian comments I have been unable to find in the *Therapeutice specialis* any clear-cut report of a case in which Torti administered the Peruvian bark *as a test* in order to ascertain in which category a given case belonged. Whether or not Torti ever used the bark in this manner, it should be noted that Ramazzini mentioned this method in his *Oratio quarta*, which was presented publicly on November 6, 1702, and was published in his *Opera omnia* of 1716.[3] A decisive statement as to Torti's use, or his failure to use, the bark in differential diagnosis would require study of his numerous unpublished consultations. This I have been unable to undertake. Here is a lacuna that should attract investigators.

Another innovation that has been credited to Torti is the use of the Peruvian bark in high doses. Before awarding a medal for this important advance in therapeutics, the historian must ponder the facts very carefully, inasmuch as batches of Peruvian bark were known to be adulterated, or were validly suspected of adulteration, on many occasions, even as early as the days of Badus and de Lugo. Especially memorable in this regard is the experience of Richard Morton, already cited.[4]

Since no real standardization of the bark was possible before isolation of quinine by P. J. Pelletier and J. B. Caventou in 1820, earlier reports necessarily yield no exact knowledge of how much *active* material was given to any patient or to any series of patients.

It is possible, however, that in an extensive run of fever patients who were treated with samples of bark derived *from one and the same shipment,* it might be possible to establish relative quantitative notions as to the effectiveness of the bark in various kinds of fever. Such considerations could have applied to the very large group treated in Genoa by Badus and his colleagues (see Chapter 2), if one could be certain that all the samples administered had the same origin. But even for this purpose the necessary data are not available. Indeed, the samples used by Badus had been obtained from de Lugo and Puccerini, and, as we have noticed repeatedly, de Lugo had complained that the drug was adulterated. Hence the evidence derived from the Genoese experience is no better than a qualitative impression, albeit a very valuable one.

Two pieces of evidence reveal to us how Torti came to use the Peruvian bark in larger doses than those that were prescribed by his colleagues. The first was the desperate case of Ottavio Maselli, treated in 1678 by Frassoni, with decisive intervention by a layman, who rescued the patient by daring to administer two drachms of the bark instead of half a drachm. This incident was almost certainly witnessed by Torti, who at that time was Frassoni's assistant, and who later recounted it in the *Therapeutice specialis* (394–98).

In the second major case, that of Count Nogarola, treated in 1695, Torti, mindful of the earlier incident, administered an ounce and a half of the bark within two hours and obtained a successful result (394–98). Both cases were dramatic and at least one of the two patients—the count—was a person of high rank. Torti's description of these two cases reveals the strong impression that they had made on him.

Torti's use of high doses refers only to pernicious cases, the principal subject, but not the sole subject, of the *Therapeutice;* his book explicitly excludes what he called "ordinary" intermittent fever (160). The cases of both Maselli and Count Nogarola were clearly pernicious. For such cases Torti strongly emphasized early diagnosis and prompt treatment with high doses of the Peruvian bark.

The clinical histories and treatment of pernicious intermittents form the subject of Torti's book 4. The reports are arranged according to the bodily region that appeared to be chiefly affected. Most of the textual divisions are subdivided. Almost every bodily part or region is represented. The third region of the body is accorded only one category, which consists of lethargic cases, Torti being fully cognizant of their dangerous character. The modern reader has little difficulty in recognizing these, and also some of the reports in the other categories, as probable examples of *falciparum* infection.

With the aphoristic tendency that was common from the time of Hippocrates almost until our own, Torti summarized this part of his experience by remarking that in pernicious cases most of the trouble is at the beginning. One great difficulty consisted of early recognition. Another was inherent in the urgency of the illness. Still another arose when Torti instituted large dosages—a practice that was often vexatious because colleagues, consultants, and influential bystanders not rarely objected. The patients were almost always those in whom Torti insisted on extreme unction as a preliminary to medical treatment.

Early diagnosis and immediate high dosage of Peruvian bark saved lives. Together they were two major components of Torti's fame. The third was the rational arrangement of the fevers.

Pernicious cases as a definite group had already received ample recognition in the work of Mercatus and less conspicuous notice in the writings of several earlier authors whom Torti also cited. The administration of large doses, given promptly, appears likewise in the writings of Morton but reached its apex—or, more accurately, a high plateau— in the work of Torti.

In mild cases, especially those that were benign at onset and occurred in the spring and the early autumn, Torti almost never used the bark at all, unless severe symptoms appeared (147). This clinical differentiation based on season is likely to have had a double origin: part of it reflected the continuing influence of the Hippocratic *Airs Waters Places*, and part of it can be attributed to the early influence of Ramazzini on Torti.

With regard to possible prophylactic use of the Peruvian bark, Torti made no comment in the edition of 1712, and Ramazzini, in his abusive *De abusu*, expressed tepid opposition.[5] Torti's comments, intercalated in the edition of 1730, are discussed earlier in this chapter. In 1717, a date intermediate between Torti's first two editions, Lancisi issued his *De noxiis paludum effluviis*, in which he advocated prevention by drainage of terrain. Prophylaxis of intermittent fever by means of Peruvian bark was to appear several decades later in the experiences, and then in the writings, of James Lind. In 1762 Lind wrote, "I have . . . been confirmed in my Opinion of the Success to be expected from the Use of the Bark, taken by way of Preservative, by many Considerations and Facts" (54). In 1768 he issued his book on tropical medicine, which states, in an appendix on agues: "For farther prevention, a wine glass of an infusion of the bark and orange peel in water, or what will prove more effectual, a table spoonful of a strong tincture of the bark, in spirits, diluted occasionally with water, may be taken every morning before breakfast" (286). Lind's preventive method was taken up by Edward Ives, who extended it to include ipecacuanha.[6] Whether Lind and Ives had any predecessors, naval or other, in the prophylactic use of the bark I have not undertaken to inquire; at this juncture interesting discoveries may reward the diligent investigator.

As for what may be designated as nascent laboratory medicine, Torti made a small effort to learn the properties of Peruvian bark by adding the drug to various fluids. He did not find that it impeded coagulation of fresh blood and he concluded, appropriately, that his experiments had failed to explain its therapeutic action (48–58).

In endeavoring to judge the originality of Torti's contribution to medicine we cannot avoid the task of comparing his work with that of the valiant Richard Morton. Far from attempting to conceal or belittle Morton's achievement, or to launch a flight of polemic pamphlets against it, Torti quoted it and also described and analyzed it fairly. For example, in book 2 of the *Therapeutice specialis* the eighth chapter is headed, "The noxious character of pernicious intermittent fevers is intimated again, according to Richard Morton's description, extensive comments being added . . . for clarity" (245).

Usually gracious in his comments about Morton, Torti nevertheless could not resist remarking, accurately, that Morton was better at using the bark than at explaining its action (80). As we have already noticed, and will observe again, Torti's own explanations fared no better.

The candid examinations by Torti permit a reliable judgment of relative priorities. Morton's *Phthisiologia* first appeared in 1689, and the first part of his *Pyretologia* in 1692. A volume titled *Opera medica*, first published in Geneva in 1696, contained writings by Morton, Sydenham, and others (see Appendix A). In the extensive preface to the *Therapeutice* Torti says that "one man, namely Morton, came close, and without my being aware . . . preceded me in this matter." Torti then cites Morton's Geneva edition of 1696, "whereas I had used my method in pernicious fevers with great notoriety (*plurima cum notione*)" in 1695 (xxiii). This corresponds to the date of the Nogarola case, already mentioned, and offers the closest possible approximation to a dating for Torti's method of early diagnosis and high dosage. Torti says also that the writings of Morton had reached him about twelve years before the completion of the *Therapeutice* (i.e., ca. 1700), but he had read them carefully only about three years before (i.e., ca. 1709). Both in the text and in the *Synopsis* (see Appendix C), Torti mentions Morton's Geneva edition of 1696 and never any preceding version. Torti remarks that Morton's statements had much in common with his own—*non pauca est cum meis symboleitas*.

With respect to originality and priority these chronological facts yield a double judgment. From the viewpoint of actual discovery Torti's work comes close to being simultaneous with Morton's, or minimally later. But if, according to rules observed nowadays, we limit ourselves strictly to dates of publication as the decisive criteria, Morton has a clear priority of twenty years. But the applicability of this more recent measuring stick to the Morton-Torti era is an *ex post facto* misfeasance.

Influence

An estimate of Torti's status can be assembled readily from the list of his honors.[7] In the journal books of scientific meetings of the Royal Society of London it is recorded under date of November 15, 1716, that "Dr. Torti's Desire to be a Member of the Royal Society was referred to the Council." A roster of the society dated 1717 and issued during the presidency of Sir Isaac Newton includes the name of Torti and that of his close friend Lodovico Muratori. Torti was offered, and declined, medical professorships in Padua and Turin. He occupied several positions of honor and responsibility in Modena.

The editions of Torti's *Therapeutice specialis*, discussed in several preceding chapters and listed in Appendix D, tell us that this book, first issued in 1712, was amplified in 1730 to make a version that became the prototype for a series of later editions, the most recent being that of 1928. If we exclude from this reckoning the edition of 1928 as representing historical or antiquarian interests rather than clinical purposes, we can recognize that the *Therapeutice* was being used by physicians and their students for at least 109 years in at least three countries, and probably in many more.

The last edition, an Italian translation issued in 1928, is clearly connected with historical appreciation, since it is part of a series named *I classici della malaria*, which is tantamount to a pantheon. The only recorded edition in a modern language, it reflects the gradual disappearance of Latin from the ken of medical historians.

The catalog in Appendix D reveals that the *Therapeutice* was often issued with other writings. For example, the valuable biography by Torti's friend Lodovico Muratori first appeared in the edition of 1743, two years after Torti's death, and became a constant component of later editions. Another passenger or stowaway is Torti's *Responsiones jatroapologeticae*, which first appeared in 1715 as a separate publication. It reappeared, as a bedfellow of the *Therapeutice*, in the editions of 1732 to 1821. While this fact may hint at the intensity of Torti's reaction to the venom of Ramazzini, it shows also, and more clearly, that readers and publishers considered the controversy worth remembering. A few of the editions fortunately include Torti's barometric tracts of 1695 and 1698; the original editions of these essays are scarce. Another respected inclusion consists of three letters from Torti to Muratori, one of which contains the reasons for his retirement from medical practice.

The distributional symbols included in the entries of the *National Union Catalog* (not reproduced in Appendix D) show, surprisingly, that in the United States the first edition of the *Therapeutice* (1712) had the widest recorded distribution in libraries. The Italian translation of 1925, based on Venice, 1755, had the poorest.

The estimation of Torti's influence encounters a difficulty that doubtless arises when any clinical writer is judged: the majority of the readers whom he principally influenced—the practitioners—probably wrote little or not at all; their reception of his book must be gauged mainly by the editions and reprints that it received. In the case of Torti, as we have seen, the editions were numerous, extending over more than a century.

Another category of evidence comes from the readers who left written impressions. Here some unexpected observations greet us. A search of Lancisi's malariological classic, the *De noxiis paludum effluviis*, published in 1717, reveals no mention of Torti. The explanation probably lies in a difference of interests, Lancisi having worked in the direction of epidemiology and preventive medicine, while Torti was strongly oriented toward clinical practice. A similar disparity is noticeable in the large epidemiological compilations of Alfonso Corradi, who mentioned malaria but not Torti; and the same omission is noticeable in the epidemiologically oriented classic work of Pringle.[8] Noticeable also is Torti's absence from the capacious indices of Morgagni's *Opera omnia* (1764). But, although Morgagni repeatedly declared himself to be a physician and although he had an ample consultation practice, it would be difficult to assert that therapeutics was at the center of his wide interests, especially during the later decades of his life. It is certain, however, that Morgagni owned Torti's *Responsiones jatro-apologeticae* and the second edition of the *Therapeutice* (1730).

Torti was well known in foreign countries. Although he failed of mention in the pyretology of the well-read Huxham and in the aphoristic clinical lectures of Boerhaave,[9] the deficiency is more than annulled by the summary of the perceptive Albrecht von Haller, who wrote that Torti was

among the greatest medical clinicians of the century, to whom the art owes very much. He established the outstanding usefulness of the Peruvian bark in intermittent fevers so firmly that it can hardly be put back into doubt by anyone in the future. In addition he very appropriately extended the use of the bark to all periodic fevers, including the imperfect, and even to the subintrants and remittents of the older authors. . . . Completely practical and based on experience.[10]

Haller's own successful experience with Peruvian bark administered to him by Jesuits was recounted by Morgagni.[11]

An excellent example of early nineteenth-century opinion has been bequeathed by Kurt Sprengel, who wrote that Torti earned great fame by his masterly depiction of the manifold variants of the intermittent fevers, arranging them according to type, epidemic constitution, and benign or malign behavior. None of his predecessors, says Sprengel, had observed with such accuracy or recognized and taught with such clarity the diagnosis of various forms, such as the subintrant, the complicated, and the larval varieties. And no one had presented so well the proper use of the bark as the only drug that can overcome intermittent fever.[12]

In his detailed analysis of the pernicious intermittents that occurred in Rome in 1819–21, Francesco Puccinotti built directly on Torti's taxonomy, elaborating it to the fullest extent. That Torti had been receptive to the possibility of various later developments is shown in a passage that Puccinotti quoted from the third book of the *Therapeutice*.[13]

Salvatore de Renzi, in an appropriately ample analysis, referred to Torti's exact determination of the indications for using the bark in pernicious fevers, in which the drug had been either avoided or given in inadequate amounts, or late, or at the wrong times. Moreover Torti's statements were based on experience and not on theory. "His merit consisted in his having clearly separated one family of fevers from all the others with which they had been confused, and in his having found the true connective link among these sicknesses that are of varied appearance, and in having reduced them all to a single basis, indicating that the bark is the only and certain means of overcoming them."[14]

More clearly than other historical analysts, De Renzi recalled details demonstrating Torti's additions to clinical knowledge. For example, Torti had pointed out the dangers of the delays that were caused by preparatory treatments; he established the fact that recurrences are inherent in the nature of intermittent fevers; and he recognized that dropsy and visceral [i.e., hepatosplenic] enlargements are not caused by the bark but are relieved by it. De Renzi's conscientious analysis thus did justice to elements of original observation that had received less than adequate emphasis from earlier encomiasts.

With the accurate appreciativeness that is not rarely attributed to the French, P. V. Renouard wrote of Torti that "no one had before demonstrated with so much force and reason, the superiority of cinchona over all other remedies, in that class of diseases, and no one had refuted in so victorious a manner, the objections of its adversaries. He wrote at the beginning of the eighteenth century, from which period we may regard the cause of cinchona as won."[15]

Armand Trousseau, a masterly physician and teacher deeply interested in therapeutics, distinguished three principal methods of administering cinchona: Torti's (also called the Roman method), Sydenham's English method, and a French method based on the work of Bretonneau. This arrangement obviously accords high rank to Torti. The repeatedly reissued treatise on pharmacology which Trousseau wrote with Pidoux repeatedly recognized Torti's contribution.[16]

The Spanish historiographer Hernández Morejon wrote, briefly and mistakenly, that "Francesco Torti, although he determined the methods of administering *la quina* in all kinds of intermittents . . . was undoubtedly the cause delaying the advance of the drug, since he established as an incontrovertible principle and undeniable maxim that the drug *is effective against no ferment other than the intermittent*" (italics in the original).[17]

The magisterial William H. Welch of Baltimore appropriately ends our procession of cognoscenti. After mentioning very briefly the great classic works of Sydenham, Morton, Ramazzini, and Lancisi, Welch adds:

Especially complete and keen in analysis is the nosography of Torti, whose classification of malarial fevers, particularly of the pernicious and mixed forms, has been followed by most subsequent authors. The diagnostic as well as the therapeutic value of the preparations of Peruvian bark was recognized, and assisted materially in the discrimination of the malarial fevers from the other so-called essential fevers. It is interesting to note the relative accuracy of diagnosis and of description of the group of malarial fevers from the latter half of the seventeenth century onward, in contrast to the confusion which existed regarding the other essential fevers until the discrimination of the latter by the pathological-anatomical studies of the present [nineteenth] century.[18]

Since Welch's paragraph combines exact judgment of Torti's contribution with correct appraisal of its replacement by later discoveries, his comment leads us to the present era.

The total roster of verdicts shows early and deserved appreciation, a single episode of painful hostility with long aftereffects, and permanent establishment in the ranks of the classics. Torti's enduring fame rests on the *Therapeutice specialis*. This work affords only a few glimpses into his ability in the diagnosis and treatment of diseases other than intermittent fever. What treasures of knowledge or insight may be hidden in his unpublished consultation reports we cannot judge until they have been subjected to careful study.

Important Later Editions of the *Therapeutice Specialis*

The *Therapeutice specialis* of 1712 is known or believed to have been followed by eleven versions, not all of which are adequately documented. Since information about these publications is given in Appendix D, only the most significant or interesting are considered in this chapter. Their value lies in the extent to which they reveal the extension of Torti's experience, the advance of his ideas, and the continuation of his defenses.

The careful reader observes that almost all of Torti's new insertions consist of complete paragraphs or series of complete paragraphs; rarely has the wording elsewhere been emended. Hence most of what appeared during 1730–1821 under the title *Therapeutice specialis* consists of reissues that hardly deserve to be considered new editions. With this body of material successive editors and publishers included selections from Torti's other writings, as well as introductions, dedications, and supplements by other hands, and Muratori's biography of Torti.

In 1730, eighteen years after printing the *editio princeps*, Soliani of Modena issued a second edition, designated as *editio altera auctior*. Professor Di Pietro, a leading authority, has distinguished it as fundamental, since its text—mostly the version of 1712 plus several intercalations—is reprinted in the later editions.

The 1730 version is dedicated to Sir Hans Sloane, Bart., a fact that may reflect Torti's connection with the Royal Society of London. The engraved frontispiece includes a portrait of Torti by Francesco Maria Francia (1657–1735), a Bolognese who had worked at times in Modena and Parma. He is known to have produced more than fifteen hundred pages of work, which a German encyclopedist has declared to be of very variable merit.[19]

In introducing his second edition Torti says, attractively, that, on being asked by the publisher whether there were new materials to be inserted, he had replied that he had more to delete than to add. He thinks that his text contained much that future readers would find superfluous, since he had been obliged to counter the now obsolete contentions of humoralists (*humoristarum*) and to establish the harmlessness and the value of the bark. He surmises, further, that ultimately his own theories might prove unacceptable in turn. He suggests, also, that the reader examine his *Responsiones*, into which he had inserted, piecemeal, the dissertation of Ramazzini, who had judged too narrowly the correct use of the bark and had described its abuses too broadly.

Torti then tells of the untrained persons who had used the drug excessively, to the detriment of its reputation. "Indeed, I never thought

that what I had predicted . . . would come true even in the days of my
youngest grandchildren, namely that the drug which once was rejected
and forbidden would gradually come to be desired by everyone and
would become an obstacle to its own acceptance. . . . It is often used
needlessly and harmfully, and the entire supply from the realm of
Quito will prove insufficient."

In order to resist this unwise prodigality Torti advises the reader that
after he has studied carefully the treatment of pernicious intermittents
with large doses of the bark and has learned the treatment needed in
urgent cases, he should also study the administration of the drug in
other fevers and the precautions to be observed in various circumstances. Torti's emphatic excursus on abuse of the bark suggests that
the influence of Ramazzini's attack, launched sixteen years previously,
had not lost its force. The statements of the two opponents can be taken
conjointly as advances in the historical process by which the properties
of the bark came to be defined.

The first of the noteworthy additions made in 1730 in the text proper
appears in the fifth chapter of book 1, which deals with the failure of
the Peruvian bark to produce perceptible evacuations (56–57). Torti
took occasion to attack the hypotheses and procedure of Johannes Do-
laeus (1651–1707), who had attributed intermittent fevers to obstruction of chyliferous ducts and stagnation of chyle and therefore had
treated such fevers by adding laxatives to the bark. In disapproving
both the theory and the practice, Torti also attacked the opinion of Bellini (see Appendix A), who had asserted that the fevers were caused by
sluggishness or *lentor* of viscid materials, either innate or acquired.
Torti's verdict adds to the evidence that Bellinian lentor was a short-
lived guess.

In book 1, chapter 10, Torti updated his text by the insertion of three
additional case reports (126–30) containing observations gathered at
the bedside in 1709 and 1728. These were intended to illustrate un-
satisfying results of treatment given either in the beginning or during
the course of intermittents, especially of the depurative type.

Much more extensive is a new inclusion that appears in book 5
under the medieval subtitle, *Quaeritur tertio* ("It is asked, thirdly")
(530–42). This query is in part an echo and in part an elaboration of
comments that Torti inserted into the preface of the same edition (see
above). Torti's subtitle translates as follows: "It is asked . . . whether
because of the fact that the Peruvian bark is naturally harmless, it may
be used indiscriminately as a trial (*tentandi gratia*) in fevers and diseases of all kinds, including those in which it is commonly understood
to be useless. The answer is in the negative." We may observe at the
outset that the word "indiscriminately" begs the question.

Torti says that the bark should not be used unless there is a rational
conjecture that it can be helpful and such conjecture is not counter to
the common experience and the common statement of established
writers accustomed to its use. These two conditions can be present simultaneously only in diseases and cases in which no trial has been
made by the better practitioners and in which there exists a theoretical
reason, founded either on sound hypotheses or on several observations
based on analogy (530).[20] When these conditions are present simultaneously, natural harmlessness of the drug can excuse even a harmless
trial, but when these conditions are absent or their opposites are present, the same trial must be considered not only irrational, but is either
ridiculous and unwise or rash, or perhaps harmful.

Here Torti has presented not merely a rationale for the use of the
bark but a rationale for the trial of any and all new drugs. In his reasoning he relies on the experience of respected authors and on analogy.
Where he requires that the drug be harmless he has begged the question once again.

Later he says, wisely, that the rationale for using a drug should depend not on harmlessness but on usefulness. He had always asserted
that the bark is harmless as far as its substance is concerned, and he
had proved this by observing the obsolete principles of its opponents. "I
have said a thousand times in this treatise," he adds, "that harm can
come, not from its substance but from premature and ill-timed administration, even though the drug itself is harmless. Indeed, it is harmful
only when it halts a fever that should not be halted, that is, a depuratory fever" (531).

The drug, Torti remarked, is the dry bark of a foreign tree unknown
to us. This statement is dated 1730, seven years before La Condamine,
traveling in Loja (now Ecuador), first caught sight of the wonderful
tree;[21] it was never corrected in the subsequent editions, when the origin of the bark was well known.

Torti concluded that the bark should always be avoided in diseases
in which it is not really indicated. He also avoided *prophylactic use.*
Because of the large importance of quinine prophylaxis to the human
race, a generous sample of Torti's little-known statement is given here-
with.

Neither for healthy people, for preventive purposes (*ad praecautionem*), for example, at a time when the fierce constitutions and weathers of periodic fevers
prevail, have I dared up to now, nor would I at present dare to propose [it]. This
is not because I disapprove it but because I am uncertain, although about this
kind of procedure, which is inherently not irrational, there is no contradicting
experience and what is available is favorable. It has been given to persons convalescent from these fevers and, for precautionary reasons it has been given,

with benefit, to persons prone to have relapses, and indeed, necessarily. We know that it has been given under this designation, to completely healthy people, and usually was given annually to the late unconquerable King Louis XIV of France. And yet since an experiment of this kind with regard to healthy people will always be uncertain (*experientia hujusmodi respectu sanorum semper incerta futura sit*) when it has turned out favorably—for we do not know whether a person who has taken the drug preventively and has remained unharmed would or would not become sick if it were omitted. It only can be a test by contrasts (*experientia de opposito*), to show whether someone who has taken the drug for prophylaxis nevertheless becomes sick equally with those who have not taken it. Hence up to the present I have thought it best to keep away from an experiment of this kind, and to leave it to others. As I have said, I do not know what it might do in the different tendencies of different bodies. (538)

In these statements we can see that the notion of prophylaxis was fully formed in Torti's mind and that he did not regard the procedure as new or very strange. The element of experimental control is not excluded. But the seventy-two-year-old veteran was not the bold infantryman of earlier decades, and the traditional conservatism of the practitioner inhibited a demarche into the unknown. It is significant that in 1914, Henry C. Carter, a man widely experienced in preventive medicine, wrote that he had not heard of quinine being used prophylactically before 1847.

These important comments, together with the other addenda mentioned on previous pages, fully justify Professor Di Pietro's high opinion of the edition of 1730.

The third edition, published by Basilius of Venice in 1732, bears official permissions dated 1730 and 1731. In addition to the text of the *Therapeutice specialis* it contains reprints of the earlier dedications to the Duke of Modena and Sir Hans Sloane and the text of the *Responsiones jatro-apologeticae*, reprinted completely.

In 1743, two years after Torti's death, the fourth edition of the *Therapeutice specialis* was published in Venice by Basilius. This well-stocked version contains: reissues of earlier dedicatory epistles; a biography of Torti by his intimate friend and correspondent the Abbot Lodovico Antonio Muratori (1672–1750); three letters from Torti to Muratori; a reissue of Torti's *Responsiones jatro-apologeticae;* and reissues of Torti's two epistolary dissertations, originally dedicated to Ramazzini, on the movement of mercury in barometers (1695, 1698). Clearly it is a major edition.

In his biographical essay Muratori mentions the medical and scientific benefactions of the Este family, which included assistance given to physicians such as Sancassani and Pacchioni, as well as support of the medical school at Modena. With these remarks Muratori included a few personal observations, namely that Torti had a fine and lively intelligence, a retentive memory, and exceptionally keen judgment.

Torti's missives to Muratori are labeled *Tre lettere* (three letters). They are marked in the text as first, third, and fourth letters, with the intercalated explanation that the second is missing.

Editions issued between 1755 and 1781 are not described in this chapter; ample details appear in Appendix D. Under the year 1821 Di Pietro records an edition published in Louvain. I have been unable to corroborate the existence of this version.

In their introductory note to the two-volume version of the *Therapeutice specialis,* which was published by Bassompierre of Liège in 1821, C. C. J. Tombeur and O. Brexhe of that city mention the difficulty of obtaining Torti's book, which had become scarce and very expensive. This statement implies that as late as 1821 the *Therapeutice specialis* was still considered useful or even necessary.

In their excessively concise introductory statement the young Belgian editors[22] underestimated the ratiocinations of earlier centuries and referred to the difficulties that Torti experienced in applying the Peruvian bark to the treatment of intermittent fevers. Learning the need for a remedy, he had tried in every way to disentangle the chaos of the intermittent fevers. Although he trusted experience more than hypotheses, he judged that mere observation was ineffective without the support of reasoning.

The Term Mal' Aria

In literary and scholarly discussions it is customary to use the word *ghost* to signify a persistently cited nonexistent work or a persistent erroneous allusion. The latter meaning, unrecorded in the reliable second edition of *Webster's New International Dictionary,* is approached in the *American Heritage Dictionary* (1981), which declares a ghost to be, *inter alia,* a nonexistent publication listed in bibliographies. On this reckoning, quasispectral status, at the very least, must be accorded to the belief, widely and confidently stated but never properly documented, that Torti introduced the word *malaria* into the medical literature.[23]

As I have reported elsewhere,[24] investigations made by H. H. Scott, by H. B. van Wesep, and by Paul Russell and amplified by me failed to discover the term *malaria* in Torti's *Therapeutice specialis* of 1712 or in his *Synopsis* of 1709, or in four manuscript consultations composed by Torti.

Two specialized Italian dictionaries yielded a modicum of encouragement in that the word *malaria* appears in both. The *Dizionario eti-*

mologico by Cortelazzo and Zolli (1983) presents the word *malaria* (not divided into two parts) as one of numerous subentries under the word *malo* and indicates that the term *malaria* was used by one B. Guarini in 1572. This notation is not elaborated. Information obtained directly from Professor Cortelazzo by correspondence cites *La Idropica* ("The Dropsical Woman"), a play by Battista Guarini (1538–1612) of Ferrara. This work is believed to have been written about 1572 and was first published in 1613 in Venice. A standard modern edition was issued in 1950. The critical passage, in Act 1, Scene 1 of the play, as given in the edition of 1950, reads "feci credere al padre, che fosse inferma di malaria poco men che incurabile (I made the father believe that she had an almost incurable case of malaria)" (296). However, when the word in question is examined in the original edition of 1613, and especially when the text is magnified, it is seen to be not *malaria* but *malatia* (see Fig. 7). Hence the Guarini text cannot be accepted in evidence.

The standard *Dizionario etimologico italiano* of Battisti and Alessio makes the following statement: "malaria f[emminile] (a[nno] 1571, Tatti), -*ico* (a[nno] 1902); 'aria' insalubre ('mala') di luoghi paludosi; med[icina] (XIX sec[olo]), forma febbrile infettiva . . ."[25] This signifies that the Italian word *malaria* was used by one "Tatti" in 1571 to refer to bad air emanating from swampy places and that the term was used in medicine in the nineteenth century. It is known that Giovanni Tatti is the pseudonym of Francesco Sansovino (1521–86), who wrote a treatise on agriculture, published in 1560, which uses the expression *corrotta & mal' aria* (corrupt and bad air).[26]

Angelo Celli found the term *male d'aria* in seventeenth-century Italian documents held by the Archivio di Stato of Florence.[27] Additional information is given in an essay by Anna Celli-Fraentzel.[28] In discussing malaria in Rome and its environs in the seventeenth century, she wrote that at this time the names "tertian" and "quartan" and the general expression "malignant fever" dwindled steadily and gave place to the terms "air sickness" and "sickness from the air" (*male d'aria*). She referred to a document dated August 30, 1648, in the Archivio di Stato at Florence,[29] and added that "from now on, through this typical designation it is possible to distinguish the various epidemics of malaria much more certainly from other epidemics."

These facts show that the term *male d'aria* was in use for almost a century before Torti was born, but the question of who introduced the term *malaria* into medical usage remains unanswered. Nothing has been found thus far that points to Torti as the source.

So far as I have been able to ascertain, the attribution of the word *mal aria* to Torti appeared for the first time in the second edition (1917) of Fielding H. Garrison's *An introduction to the history of medicine:*

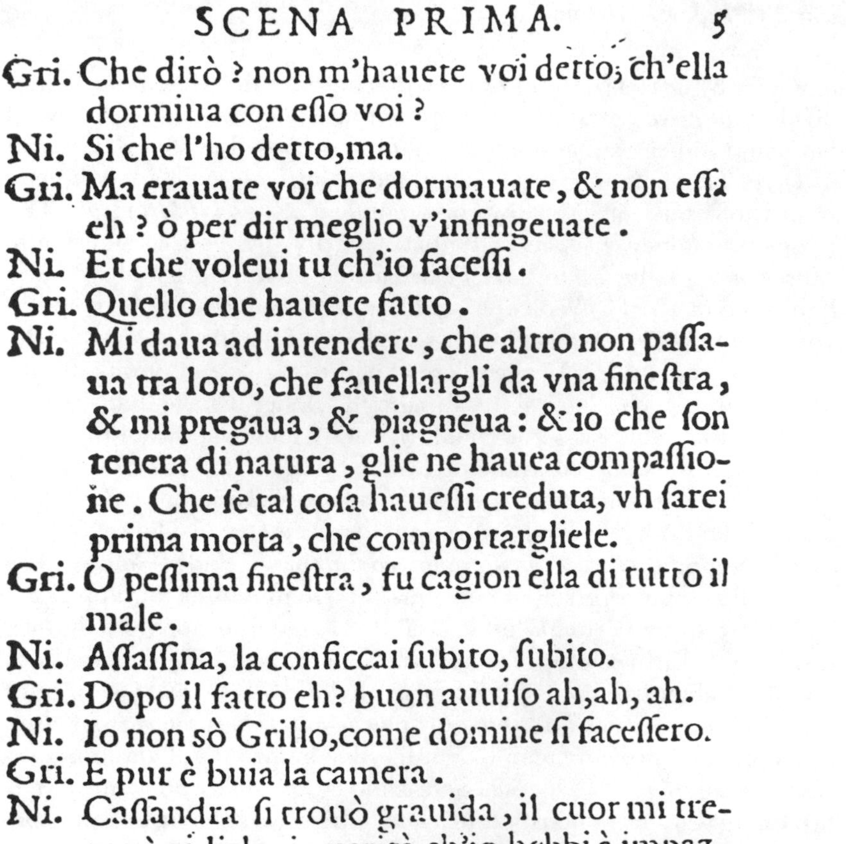

Gri. Che dirò ? non m'hauete voi detto, ch'ella dormiua con esso voi ?

Ni. Si che l'ho detto, ma.

Gri. Ma erauate voi che dormauate, & non essa eh ? ò per dir meglio v'infingeuate.

Ni. Et che voleui tu ch'io facessi.

Gri. Quello che hauete fatto.

Ni. Mi daua ad intendere, che altro non passaua tra loro, che fauellargli da vna finestra, & mi pregaua, & piagneua : & io che son tenera di natura, glie ne hauea compassione. Che se tal cosa hauessi creduta, vh sarei prima morta, che comportargliele.

Gri. O pessima finestra, fu cagion ella di tutto il male.

Ni. Assassina, la conficcai subito, subito.

Gri. Dopo il fatto eh? buon auuiso ah, ah, ah.

Ni. Io non sò Grillo, come domine si facessero.

Gri. E pur è buia la camera.

Ni. Cassandra si trouò grauida, il cuor mi trema à ridirlo. in verità ch'io hebbi à impazzare: ma che? il fatto, era fatto, e frastornare non si poteua.

Gri. Troppo è vero.

Ni. Io me n'auidi prima di lei, & hauendola confortata à starsi nel letto, feci credere al padre, che fosse inferma di malatia, poco men che incurabile. Onde fu ageuol cosa, che per guarirla, egli si risoluesse à conforti del nostro Medico, che era (vedi ventura) parente stretto di Flauio, di mādarla quì in casa di madonna Gineura, che fu nostra padrona,

B 3   drona,

FIG. 7. Guarini, *La idropica*, 1613, page 5. Courtesy of Library of Congress. The page has been enlarged from 91 × 131 mm. Line 27 (*arrow*) reads *malatia*, not *malaria*. The double *t* in *letto*, in preceding line, also shows the form of the letter *t* clearly.

"Torti . . . wrote an important treatise on the pernicious malarial fevers (1712), which practically introduced the employment of cinchona bark into Italian practice and introduced the term *mal aria.*" The same statement appears in Garrison's third edition (1924, 381) and, with minimal modification, in the fourth edition (1929, 367). It is not found in the first edition (1913). The great popularity of Garrison's book could explain the wide dissemination of the unsupported statement.

12 The Bark: Botanical, Geographical, and Commercial Factors

Botany

The preceding chapters have described the discovery of the Peruvian bark by Europeans and the spread of the drug to Europe and other continents. The narrative has referred only to the bark, since the identity of the tree, as has been stated above, was not revealed until the travels of Joseph de Jussieu (1735),[1] the report by Charles Marie de la Condamine (1740),[2] and the somewhat earlier travels of the obscure Scottish surgeon, William Arrot (see Fig. 8). The probable earliness of Arrot's observations in Peru suggests that this Caledonian may have been of greater importance than historians have recognized, but he published nothing and the facts of his life have resisted detection.[3] These events occurred, or are thought to have occurred, during the final lustrum of Torti's lifetime, a century after the discovery in Peru.

We have already noted Torti's remark of 1730 that the Peruvian febrifuge is the dry bark of an unknown foreign tree, *aridusque cortex arboris exotici nobis ignoti* (532).[4] This comment signifies that physicians, pharmacists, and patients had been dependent on a drug, possibly the most important and certainly one of the most significant historically in the entire pharmacopoeia, whose identity was unknown. It is therefore necessary for the historian to review the meager correct information and the much more extensive misinformation that appears in available records. Data of this kind are apt to be fortuitous, sporadic, noncumulative, and unreliable. The botanical part of the difficulty is attributable mainly to the fact that a valid and dependable distinction had not yet been established between the tree later known as cinchona, source of the great febrifuge, and trees of the genus *Myroxylon*, the

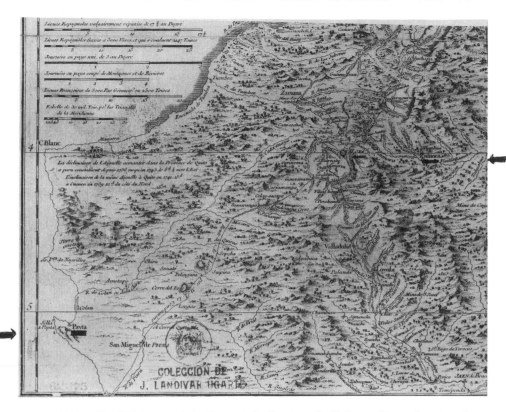

FIG. 8. D'Anville, J. (1697–1782): *Carte de la Province de Quito au Perou dressé sur les observations astronomiques . . . de Mr de la Condamine*, 1751. Courtesy Map Division, New York Public Library, Astor, Lenox, and Tilden Foundations. The area reproduced here represents approximately one fourth of D'Anville's chart. It includes part of the Pacific Coast. At 4°S is *Loxa* (Loja), the most important inhabited place in the region in which the Peruvian bark was found by Europeans (ca. 1630?). Also shown are *Piura*, a primary collecting station; the Pacific port of *Payta*, used for obligatory shipment to Panama; the town of *Zamora*, east of Loxa; and the Rio de Zamora, a tributary of the eastward-flowing Marañon-Amazon system. The contributions of Condamine's expedition, and of Jussieu, are discussed in Chapter 12.

balsam tree. An additional aliquot of confusion stemmed from *Smilax china*, commonly mentioned in the Renaissance literature as chinaroot and honored by the comments of Vesalius.[5]

Fortunately, much of the early literature was reviewed by a skilled investigator, Alec W. Haggis (1889–1946) of the Wellcome Historical Medical Museum, who had within his reach the scientific and literary resources of London.[6] His work has been used repeatedly in preceding chapters, and in the present chapter we can scarcely do better than to start by following his lead.

An example of the early difficulties, botanical and also linguistic, is provided by Pietro Castelli (1570?–1661), professor of botany in Rome. Of his *Responsio chymica* Haggis (1941) says:

There is no evidence whatsoever that, at the time of writing, Castelli had examined as much as a fragment of the bark, nor had he used a single dose of the powder. . . . The explanation of Castelli's sequence of error seems to be that about 1623 he had in his possession *Quina-Quina* seeds, i.e., the *Pepitas de Quina* (of Peruvian balsam) known in Italian as *China China.* When in 1653 he was questioned by Hieronymus Badus regarding Cinchona, which had become known in Italy as *China China,* he concluded that Cinchona was the remedy of which he had possessed the seeds thirty years before. (446–48).

So says Haggis about Castelli. Of Sebastianus Badus he observed: "Not one true physiological characteristic of Cinchona does he give, although his work stands accepted as the greatest of the early authorities on the remedy" (450–51).

A startling result of Haggis's work is the demonstration already cited (Chapter 4) that Richard Morton had described the Peruvian tree incorrectly but had given an exact account of the bark, showing that he had seen, and presumably used, genuine samples of bark at least occasionally if not invariably.[7]

If we jump from the confused early efforts to a modern presentation well beyond the temporal limits of this history, we find that several principal species of cinchona are now accepted. These, exclusive of hybrid forms, are:[8]

Cinchona succirubra Pavon and Klotsch
C. ledgeriana Howard (Moens and Trimen)
C. calisaya Weddell
C. officinalis Hooker

In contrast, the *Gray Herbarium Index* (1968), which is oriented toward botanists and bibliographers, not toward pharmacists or physicians, lists forty-three specific names under the genus *Cinchona.* In this series the term *Cinchona officinalis* is followed by the names of three varieties.

In 1704, the widely traveled Dr. William Oliver, F. R. S., wrote:

Peru Bark, comes from a Tree about the bigness of a plumb Tree. . . .'Tis gathered in Autumn, and the Rind taken off all round. . . . This account I received from an Ingenious Apothecary at Cadiz in Spain, A.D. 1694 who had lived in Peru, and seen it growing, and gathered it several times: From this History I made this Observation, that probably China China, or the Rind of the Fruit, was first only in Use, and the more powerful Medicine, used in smaller quantities, and that the Bark of the Tree came not into play till some time after; when the Vertues of it, known in Europe, occasioned a greater demand for it.[9]

As an authoritative twentieth-century teacher remarked, "The constituents of cinchona vary, especially quantitatively, in the numerous species and hybrids, and indeed in individual trees and in different parts of the same tree."[10] With respect to this problem the state of knowledge a century earlier, in 1855, is shown by Trousseau and Pidoux, who complained that the samples sold under the name of *Calisaya* "nowadays" contained very little quinine (2:327).

Still earlier, in the eighteenth century, the suspicion was voiced "that the Peruvian bark in common use [in England], was very inferior in power and efficacy to that recommended by the early writers on the subject." It was surmised, further, that the Spaniards in South America might have given more careful attention to samples that were intended for Spain than to samples intended for foreigners. In 1779 a Spanish ship en route to Cadiz was captured and taken to Lisbon. Her cargo consisted chiefly of Peruvian bark, part of which was later sold in London. The samples, being large and coarse, were accepted reluctantly, but when they were tested in hospitals they proved to be highly efficacious.[11] These facts show that, in addition to the well-known problems of adulteration and deterioration, botanical variation and diversity of chemical content must have played a large role in the production of clinical misunderstanding and failure when the Peruvian bark was used.

As one leading treatise tells us, the cinchona contains some twenty-five closely related alkaloids.[12] The alkaloids are contained in parenchymal cells in all parts of the tree; the bark is the richest, especially that of the roots. Connected with this, an unexpected fact, not properly within the scope of the present history, is the observation by Jean Baptiste Senac (1693–1770) that the bark can be used to control cardiac palpitation: "Relief has often been found in various remedies having very different properties; these are stomachics, cordials, and sedatives. . . . Of all the stomachics, the one whose effects have seemed to me to be the most constant and rapid in many cases is quinquina mixed with a little rhubarb."[13] The physician reader will at once recognize that this effect is due to quinidine.

Also outside our scope is the use of the Peruvian bark in infectious diseases of domestic animals. This use is mentioned sporadically in the literature, for example in Ramazzini's description of a bovine outbreak.[14] It is mentioned also in a broadside issued in Bologna and Parma in 1746 and in one issued in Bologna on the twenty-second of Thermidor (August 10), 1800.[15]

Geography

The Peruvian bark that first became known to Europeans was obtained from trees in the Andes Mountains at altitudes of 2,500 m, especially in an area about 14 km south of the town of Loxa (also written Loja), situated at 3°59'S, 79°16'W, and near Malacatos (see Fig. 9). The district, formerly part of the Audiencia of Quito in Peru, now belongs to Ecuador. In 1767–68, more than a century after the discovery of the Peruvian bark, the Spanish government established in this area a cinchona reservation that had the special purpose of supplying febrifugal bark to the royal pharmacy (Real Botica) in Madrid.[16]

One of the earliest geographical statements, written at an unknown date by Arrot, was published in 1737: "But the true and genuine fine Jesuits Bark . . . is only found from about five to fourteen Leagues round the City of Loxa. . . . This city is situated between two Rivers, that run into the great River Marannon, or of the Amazons, and lies about 100 Leagues from Payta. . . . The Places about Loxa, where this fine sort are found, are, La Sierra de Caxanuma, Malacatos, Yrutasinga, Yangana."[17] The bark was collected during most of the year except for the rainy season, activity tending to be greatest in autumn. The harvested material was carried 240 km southwestward to the town of Piura in the coastal plains. It was then conveyed about 90 km to the port of Paita for transfer to ships. Paita served as the principal entrepôt of the Pacific until 1741, when it was sacked and burned by pirates. Alternative routes used in transfer of the bark passed through Malacatos to Guayaquil and Callao.

The trade in Peruvian bark was not long in existence when Spanish authorities became aware that noteworthy amounts of the product were being abducted by smugglers. Almost incredibly, these evildoers were able to take the bark *eastward* to the great Marañon River, a tributary of the Amazon, and thence, after a total trajectory of 3,200 km, to the coast of the Atlantic (see Fig. 10).

Although Loxa is no more than 200 km from the Pacific Ocean (by measurement made along the fourth parallel of south latitude), the drainage of the area is *eastward*. Near the cinchona trees of that district there is the Rio Zamora, which flows northeastward and then southward, to join the river Paute and form the Rio Santiago.[18] After a further east-southeastward course of approximately 200 km it enters the Marañon. At present the lower Rio Zamora is navigable by small motorboats.[19] This river is cited here merely to exemplify the direction of drainage. I have found no evidence identifying the smallest of the streams that were actually used in the illicit transport, nor is it known

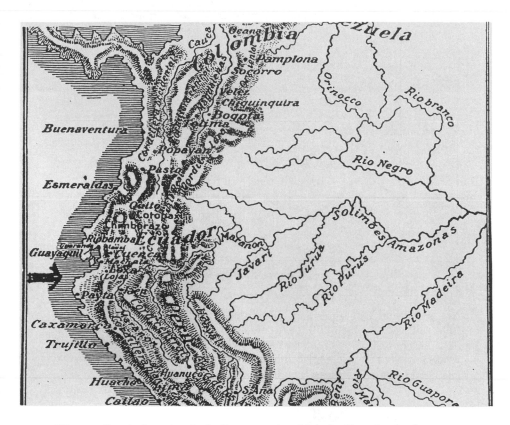

FIG. 9. Western South America, including areas in which the Peruvian bark was obtained. The arrow points to Loxa (Loja). Payta, the principal port of shipment, is on the Pacific coast, southwest of Loja. See also Chapter 12. From Tschirch, 1923. New York Academy of Medicine.

exactly which parts of the transmission across South America were performed overland during the earliest period.

The eastward route across South America became known comparatively soon after the arrival of the Spaniards. In his *General and Natural History of the Indies*, written in 1535–57, Gonzalo Fernando de Oviedo y Valdes (1478–1557), historiographer of the Indies and governor of Santo Domingo, tells of Captain Francisco Orellana, who in 1542 discovered the River Marañon, which crosses the continent from west to east and empties into the Atlantic Ocean.[20] Orellana is believed to have reached the Marañon via what is now called the Napo River, which originates in northern Ecuador. It should be noted in addition that the crossing from east to west, also accomplished by way of the Napo, did not occur until almost a century later, in 1638.[21]

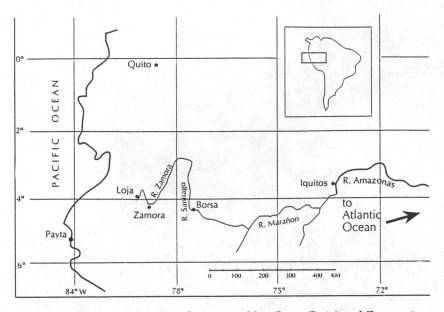

FIG. 10. Prototype of the smuggler's route. Near Loxa (Loja) and Zamora is
the Rio Zamora, which ultimately connects with the Amazon and leads to the
Atlantic coast. Tracing based on *The Times Comprehensive Atlas of the World*,
plate 119. Scale, 1:500,000. © John Bartholomew and Son, Ltd. Lambert
Zenithal Equal-Area Projection. Derived by permission.

A colored engraved map of North and South America, made by the
Dutch cartographer Jan Mathijsz[oon] (1627–87) and thought to have
been issued after 1650, shows rivers in Peru going *eastward* into the
Rio de Orellana [?], which enters the Amazon.[22] And before that, Paita,
Loxa (Loja), Piura, and the eastward drainage into the Marañon-
Amazon system appeared in the earliest of the famous atlases of Abra-
ham Ortelius (1527–98), the *Theatrum orbis terrarum*, published in
Antwerp in 1570, 1579, and 1584.

Two facts greatly increase the historical interest of the west-to-east
smugglers' route. The first is the anthropologists' discovery of evidence
probably at least five thousand years old that cultural relations existed
between peoples of the Peruvian coastal highlands and those of the
Amazonian rain forest and that a tributary of the Marañon was important to the contact.[23]

The second is that the use of the west-to-east route across South
America, initiated or anticipated in prehistoric times, did not cease
with seventeenth-century smugglers of Peruvian bark. On August 28,

1988, the *New York Times* described similar west-to-east travel for the surreptitious transfer of coca from Peru to the Atlantic Coast.[24]

Contraband was also conveyed, on a large scale, from east to west. For example, Portuguese are known to have moved goods from Portugal to Brazil and the Rio de la Plata, then by land across Paraguay and the realm of Tucuman to Potosí and Lima, at which point the shipments entered the domain of respectable commerce. The deviation is relevant to the transfer of Peruvian bark in that it was based on extensive bribery of officials, who usually obtained their positions by purchase.[25] Other interesting information about the route from the Atlantic Ocean to the Pacific by way of the Rio Plata has been presented in an important volume by Spate.[26]

From Paita and a few other Pacific ports the Peruvian bark traveled by ship approximately 1,200 km to the city of Panama, on the southern coast of the isthmus (Fig. 11). This journey usually took about three weeks. On approaching Panama the ships anchored off the island of Perico, about 12 km away; the cargoes were then taken ashore in lighters. This procedure was necessitated in part by the tides at Panama.

Like the other treasures of Spanish kings, the bark was then carried northward, on the backs of men (including slaves) and animals, to Portobelo on the Atlantic coast, Nombre de Dios having been abandoned in 1597 because of intermittent fever and other diseases. In the eighteenth century a paved transisthmian causeway replaced the more difficult mule track.

Incredibly, the immense traffic included not only the silver taken from Peru; almost everything from Buenos Aires was transported overland across the Andes to Lima. It was then transferred to ships, taken to Panama, carried across the isthmus, and conveyed by galleons to Spain.[27] By the beginning of the seventeenth century the use of galleons had declined greatly, an alteration that was part of the general decline of Spanish foreign trade in consequence of increased local manufacturing and simultaneous increase in foreign competition and contraband.

As for the city of Panama, Thomas Jefferys, royal geographer (d. 1771), described the intricate procedure as follows:

The ships from Guayaquil bring cacao, and jesuit's bark, which always meet with a quick exportation here, especially in times of peace. . . . As soon as ever the galleons enter the port of Carthagena, an express is dispatched over land to Panama, from whence he proceeds by sea to Lima. In the mean time all the necessary preparations are made for conveying the treasure from Panama to Porto Velo. The viceroy of Peru, on the other hand, makes all imaginable dispatch in sending the Lima fleet, escorted by an armadilla, or small squadron of

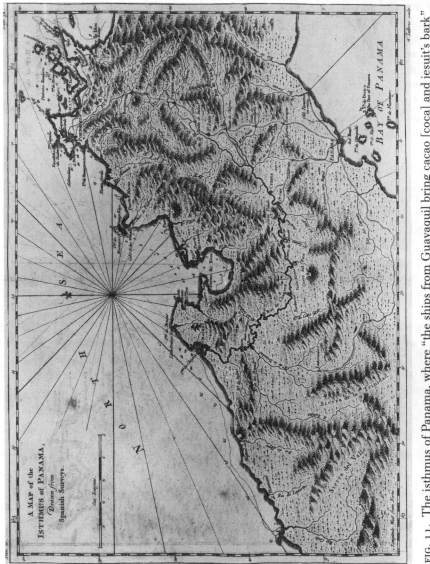

FIG. 11. The isthmus of Panama, where "the ships from Guayaquil bring cacao [coca] and jesuit's bark" (Jefferys, 1762, 32–33). The chart shows the land route from the city of Panama to Portobelo, also the Chagres River, way stations, and the ruined cities of Old Panama and Nombre de Dios. Courtesy Rare Books and Manuscript Division, New York Public Library, Astor, Lenox, and Tilden Foundations.

men of war, to Panama, where, as soon as they arrive, they are unladen and the goods forwarded for Porto Velo. The Lima fleet then sails to Perico, which is the port of Panama . . . and there waits the return of the European goods from Porto Velo.[28]

Jeffreys added that in 1740 the town of Venta de Cruzes, a place of storage, surrendered to the English, who found in the customhouse 4,300 packages and bags of "Guayaquil cocoa, jesuits bark, and Spanish wool, ready to be shipped."[29]

The land route across the isthmus was about 80 km long, and the crossing usually took four days. It was available only during the dryness of summer. In the winter, when rains and floods precluded its use, the longer and less expensive Chagres River route was used instead.[30] Facilities for storage and trading existed at Venta Cruz (or Cruces), 30 km from Panama and situated at the head of navigation on the Chagres (Fig. 12). This place was the main transisthmian station.[31] The river route required three to twelve days; it was faster when the water was high. Charles Boxer has referred to the entire procedure as "one of the more patent absurdities of the Spanish colonial administrative system."[32]

From the isthmus the goods went on to Havana and then to Cadiz or Seville, the Casa de Contratación having been transferred to the latter city in 1717–18. Under favorable conditions, ships departed from Panama in January, proceeded to Havana, and started across the Atlantic, under convoy, in or after the middle of March. Delayed departures were usual. A. P. Newton has given a slightly later schedule: "the treasures of gold and silver coming from Peru by the South Sea were all collected at Nombre de Dios in May."[33] The route to Europe led through the Bahama channel, continued between the Virginia capes and the Bermudas, passed due east to the Azores, and then proceeded to Spain. In and after the late sixteenth century Spanish maritime commerce, like the political and military fortunes of Spain, suffered a decline, which was accelerated by the activities of the Dutch West India Company.[34]

Almost certainly there were incidents in which shipments of bark were stolen from warehouses and in ports. But they appear unlikely to have been as dramatic as the instances of capture at sea. Piracy was at its height in most of the seventeenth century. In 1709 Sir George Rooke (1650–1709), admiral of the fleet, captured a number of French and Spanish galleons in the harbor of Vigo. Red Peruvian bark was part of the plunder; its decoction proved to be much stronger than the bark commonly used in England, and much more efficacious.

In transportation from one European port to another, part of the

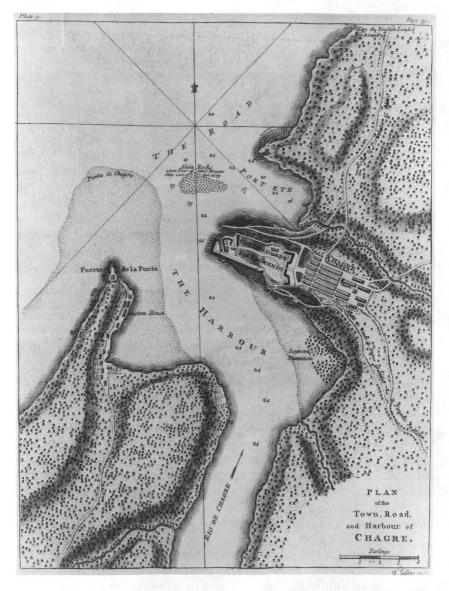

FIG. 12. Plan of the town road and harbour of Chagres (Jefferys, 1762, 30–31). Note the customhouse on the western shore of the harbor. Raided by Admiral Vernon in 1740, it yielded a large amount of Jesuits' bark. Courtesy, Rare Books and Manuscript Division, New York Public Library, Astor, Lenox, and Tilden Foundations.

traffic was conducted by ships from Marseilles and other Mediterranean ports. Before the beginning of the eighteenth century the shipping came to be dominated by the Dutch; the cargoes are known to have included Peruvian bark.[35]

Transatlantic traffic included not only the officially authorized shipping of Spain but also the rival shipping of other European countries and the heterogeneous shipping conducted by pirates. The latter at times enjoyed somewhat elaborate organization.[36] Since the war between Spain and the Netherlands was resumed in 1619 and resulted in the destruction of Spanish fleets, such quantities of Peruvian bark as later came to be sent to Venice by water were limited to Venetian, English, and Dutch ships, the last named being dominant.[37] Conveyance to Venice is especially important in the present history because it is probable that a large portion of the imported drugs used by Francesco Torti and his north Italian colleagues had arrived by way of that city.

Over the terrestrial and maritime routes four methods of distribution existed. The earliest was that by priests, officials, soldiers and their families, and miscellaneous travelers such as the numerous servants who are listed, sometimes anonymously, in the archives of the Indies. The second group of distributors were merchants. A third class consisted of nobility and royalty who, in the tradition of the Queen of Sheba, made gifts of the wondrous drug to foreign dignitaries. This was important because, in the case of the Peruvian bark, it amounted to an increase in geographical distribution and also because the transfer was conducted at highly influential levels. Still another class of distributors consisted of pirates. The third group, the royal donors, left occasional or incidental records. The pirates left accidental records, which were sometimes the result of unsuccessful encounters at sea.

As to eminent persons Sturmius remarked that the bark of the Peruvian tree is esteemed so highly that it is even given to the great as a gift, *ut etiam magnatibus dono mittantur.* Indeed, Sturmius wrote that in 1654 the Spanish ambassador in the Hague had asked him to give an opinion on a batch of bark that the ambassador had received as a gift from Archduke Leopold.[38]

Documents in the Archivo General de Simancas record gifts of Peruvian bark sent in 1772–86 to the empress of Hungary, Pope Clement XIV, the duke of Parma, the electress of Bavaria, and the general commissioner of holy places in Jerusalem. In addition an *arroba* (11.5 kg) was regularly given to ambassadors on their return from foreign duty.[39]

It is easy to assume that the long delays of shipment, transshipment, and storage, the changes in altitude, temperature, and humidity, and the exposure to other cargoes would exert a harmful effect on packages of Peruvian bark. Indeed, even in the latter part of the eighteenth century, after the Spaniards had been shipping the bark for a century and a half, the official records contain numerous reports of spoilage. For example, a collection of documents limited to the years 1764 to 1798 tells us that in 1767 all the *quina* that came from the royal properties arrived rotten because it had been packed in damp bags and had not been handled carefully at the time of collection. Some of the bark had been shipped with other plants; some was totally useless and had to be incinerated.[40] At about the same period Hipólito Ruiz López, a respected botanist, wrote that the bark was often harvested improperly and transported badly.[41]

Lest it be thought that deteriorated bark was invariably inert or harmful, at least one piece of countervailing evidence must be considered. On May 6, 1776, Dr. Eugenio Escolano and five of his colleagues at the General Hospital of Aranjuez tested samples of allegedly useless bark (*la quina llamada inutil*) on sufferers from tertian fever and found it to be effective.[42] This report signifies that it is especially difficult to judge what quantities of active drug were actually used by physicians and apothecaries before the nineteenth century.

We lack satisfactory reports of the time—or the range of times— required for each stage in the long odyssey of the Peruvian bark, nor do we know the customary length of the delays in warehouses.[43] Yet it is clear that if, as usual, the bark was gathered in the Andes in autumn, it could hardly reach a European apothecary before the subsequent autumn, even if the moving accidents of flood and field were at a minimum. In the turbulence of war, piracy, shipwreck, and weather, a longer course would be inevitable.[44]

Price

Information about the price of Peruvian bark is apt to be fragmented, elusive, poorly documented, and otherwise incomplete. Much of what is available falls outside the temporal limits of this history.

According to a familiar story, Juan de Vega—whose name is printed incorrectly as often as not—after having served as physician to the count of Chinchon returned to Spain and, about 1640, sold the bark in Seville at 100 *reales* a pound. This story is not improbable; it has parallels in the history of ipecacuanha and kousso, but it lacks satisfactory documentation. Its survival may have been caused by the prestige of Condamine, who added that samples of the bark were later adulterated, lost repute, and were sold in Panama for half a piastre per pound.[45] No comment from de Vega is known to be extant; we do not know his side of the story. Another well-known anecdote has been be-

queathed to us by Sturmius, who wrote that in 1658 the bark was rated
in Brussels at 60 florins for twenty doses but was unobtainable even at
that price.[46]

Still more famous is the story of the high prices charged in England
and France by Talbor in 1678–79 and his attempt to establish a monopoly. In 1678, says Cabanès, referring to de Blegny, the bark, which
had been sold at a golden *écu* for two drachms, declined to twenty-five
or even twelve francs a pound.[47] Dewhurst adds that at one time the
price was £15 per pound, whereupon Louis XIV bought large amounts
in Cadiz and the rate then fell to £5.[48]

In 1653 Guy Patin mentioned a charge of 40 francs for "une prise,"
which could be either a single dose or a single course of treatment.[49]
An anonymous book printed in 1689 says that Peruvian bark of the best
quality was selling in Paris at 12 to 20 sols per ounce.[50]

A student of Spanish archives has found evidence of severe fluctua-
tion in the value of the bark in Peru during the final decades of the
seventeenth century. The apparent effectiveness of the product had led
to great demand and exalted prices in the European market. By 1690,
probably because of adulteration, esteem faded and thousands of
pounds lay unsold in Piura and Payta.[51]

It is not unusual to encounter the accusation that the Jesuits in Europe sold the bark at excessively high prices and gained great profits.
The generosity of Cardinal de Lugo is established by repeated testimony, and any remark by Guy Patin was almost certain to be bilious.
Statements by others could be true, or deeply dyed by anti-Catholic or
anti-Jesuit emotion. The seventeenth century glowed with the fires of
early modern science but also seethed with religious hatred. It would
not be utterly repellent to our present views if the Jesuits overcharged
the rich in order to protect the poor.

A group of facts approaching coherence was given by Marret, editor
of Chomel's dictionary of economics. According to this compilation,
which appeared in 1732, *quinquina* was not being taxed anywhere in
France, except Lyon, where the imposition was 3 sols per pound; and
in Amsterdam the price was 36 to 54 sols per pound (214).

Those who undertake to study the prices of Peruvian bark look especially to Amsterdam for information, since that city speedily became
the world center of the cinchona trade. The holdings of the hospitable
Economisch Historische Bibliotheek in Amsterdam contain weekly
and biweekly quotations (the so-called *Cours van negotie*) of the Amsterdam exchange from 1650 to 1712. These regularly include the
prices of approximately twenty-five drugs, such as Roman alum and
Radix china. It was therefore a disappointment that listings for *cortex
chinae* do not appear until March 17, 1777 (Fig. 13), especially since

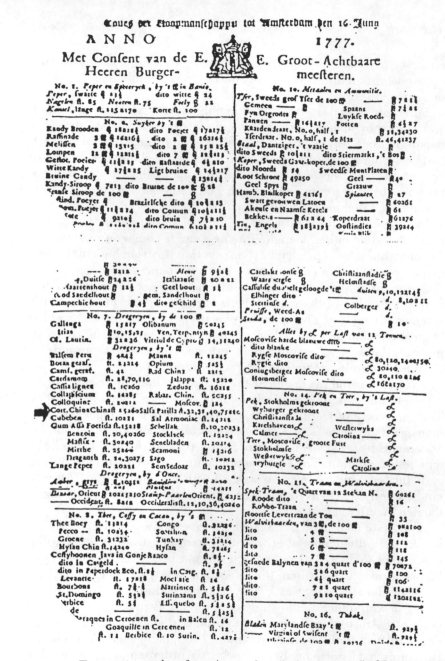

FIG. 13. Two sections taken from Amsterdam "price-currents" of June 16, 1777. In the upper section, list no. 1 reports the prices of pepper and spices. In the lower section, no. 7 is a list of drugs; the arrow points to Cort[ex] China China at 15 to 60 stuivers for 100 pounds. The entire document is reproduced in Posthumus, 1943, 1:xxxvi. Courtesy of Economisch-Historiche Bibliotheek, Amsterdam.

occidental bezoar, an Andean product, appears as early as 1650 and the lists also include other drugs from the Western Hemisphere, such as ginger from Puerto Rico, and mechoacan, a Mexican purgative. It is difficult to explain the absence of Peruvian bark for a century after the Dutch had established dominance in its transportation and sale. The listing ends on December 23, 1782. New and valuable information is expected from research being conducted by an American scholar. This work is more than likely to amplify and supersede, for Holland and also for other European countries, the fundamental contribution of N. W. Posthumus (1946–64).

During the available six years of record, the price was quoted in Amsterdam almost always at 12 to 60 florins per 100 pounds, but during 1779 the range usually was a little narrower, namely 25 to 60 florins.

Spanish records, rich in information on the prices of drugs, will reward extensive exploration. For example, the manuscript records of the royal hospital of Nuestra Señora de Esqueba in the city of Valladolid, preserved in the *ayuntamiento* (city hall) of that Cervantean municipality, contain copies of numerous prescriptions for *Puluis quarangi*—*quarango* being the Quechua name for Peruvian bark[52]—usually in amounts of one and a half drachms and priced most often at 58 maravedis, the extremes being 51 and 64.[53] During 1703 the price of the pharmacist's prescription (not the price of the merchant's drug) rose from 51 maravedis to 58. In 1704 it declined to 51 and in 1712 to 48. Throughout 1713 it was constant at 48. On two occasions in 1713 smaller amounts, namely one drachm, were issued at the smaller price of 34 maravedis. The drug was dispensed invariably as a powder, without admixture.

Abundant information about the price of the Peruvian bark comes to us from German sources (see Table 1 and Fig. 14). In the study of this material, and also for the list of equivalents that follows, I have been fortunate to have the guidance of Professor Dr. Erika Hickel of the Abteilung für Geschichte der Pharmazie und der Naturwissenschaften, Technische Universität Braunschweig.[54]

1 thaler	= 36 mariengroschen
1 mariengroschen	= 8 pfennig
1 libra [ca. 360 g]	= 12 ounces
1 ounce [ca. 30 g]	= 8 drachms
1 lot	= 1/2 ounce
1 quent or quintlein	= 1 drachm

With these scattered fragments of information inference must be cautious and limited, doubts being at least as numerous as certainties. It is observable, for example, that in the foregoing list prices are quoted

TABLE 1   Prices of Peruvian Bark in Germany, 1663–1746

	City	Price
1663	Regensburg	
1668	Frankfurt am Main	
1669	Leipzig	
1669	Frankfurt am Main	1 drachma = 50 kreuzer
1677	Straubing	1 drachma = 30 kreuzer
1680	Freiburg	1 lot (½ oz) = 2 reichstaler
1680	Frankfurt am Main	1 drachma = 50 kreuzer
1681	Jena	
1682	Celle	
1687	Ulm	1 drachma = 12 kreuzer
1696	Jena	
1697	Hof	1 loth = 12 kronen
1700	Halle	
1710	Frankfurt am Main	1 loth = 10 kronen
1710	Rotenburg	1 loth = 10 kronen
1711	Bremen	1 loth = 8 schilling
1713	Berlin	
1714	Frankfurt and Leipzig	1 loth, 4 groschen
1715	Berlin	
1715	Mühlhausen	
1718	Frankfurt am Main	1 loth, 12 kronen
1726	Anhalt-Zerbst	1 loth, 3 groschen
1726	Brandenburg	3 groschen
1735	Wirtemberg	
1737	Ulm	
1739	Münster	
1745	Lübeck	
1746	Schweinfurth	1 loth, 5 schilling

Source: Based on Tunmann, O., 1910, in Tschirch, *Handbuch der Pharmaco-gnosie,* 1 (pt. 2): 810–35. Leipzig: Tauschnitz.
Note: Where no entry appears in the last column, the original is blank.

in only about half of the reports. It will be noted that at Frankfurt am Main a drachm of Peruvian bark was priced at 50 kreuzer in 1669 and also in 1680—that is, there was virtual constancy over the short span of a decade. In the same city in 1710 the drug was priced at 10 kronen for 1 loth (4 drachms) and in 1718 at 12 kronen for the same amount.

The German data present a special pitfall for those who attempt to study the taxation of drugs. Apart from the fact that drugs were not taxed in Germany during this era, the German language uses the fem-

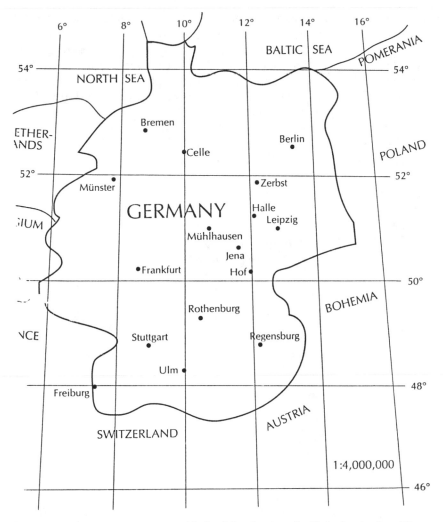

FIG. 14. German cities that established fixed prices for Peruvian bark, 1663–1746. Based on data from Tunmann in Tschirch, *Handbuch der Pharmacognosie*, 1910.

inine noun *Taxe* to mean *both valuation and taxation;* rarely it is used to mean *tax, impost,* or *rate.*[55]

Apart from the Dutch, Spanish, and German sources a large body of English material is extant in the inspector general's ledgers of imports and exports for the years 1696 to 1780.[56] In this series, which I have sampled extensively but have not read *in toto,* usable information about the Peruvian bark is scarce. In one folio, no. 103, dated 1696–97, we read that "Cortex Peru" had come from Spain in "English shipps." The very next line contains an entry in which the drug is labeled "Jesuits Bark." A later folio (no. 112) in the same series states that Cortex Peru worth £460 had arrived from Jamaica; obviously this must represent an instance of transshipment. A list of drugs sent from London to East India is designated "Medicines, 2 chests. At 10£ per chest." Other entries state, cryptically, "Druggs"; obviously there is no hint as to whether or not such shipments included Peruvian bark, nor can such entries be used as a basis for statements about prices of this drug. The scarcity of entries that mention the bark suggests, but does not prove, that the drug was relatively unimportant in English commerce at this time. As Edward Gibbon wrote, in the penultimate sentence of his immortal history, "The historian may applaud the importance and variety of his subject; but, while he is conscious of his own imperfections, he must often accuse the deficiency of his materials."

13 Epilogue

Some Historical Parallels to Peruvian Bark

During most of this book attention necessarily has been limited to the history of a single drug—cinchona. This procedural method, if it has brought to reader and author the benefits of clarity and continuity, may have risked falsification of perspective, since it may produce the incorrect impression that the events described are unique, whereas wider study reveals many of them to have had precedents or parallels. The history of another drug—ipecacuanha—reveals a surprising parallel to what has been said of cinchona.[1]

These resemblances include the following: (a) derivation from a tropical plant used by American Indians; (b) discovery during the era of exploration and colonization; (c) discovery by missionaries (Jesuit or other)[2]; (d) early botanical and nomenclatorial confusion, which was almost inevitable during the two and a half centuries that elapsed between Columbus and Linnaeus; (e) resultant mistaken use of inert or unsuitable plants, with failure and consequent mistrust by apothecaries and physicians; (f) transmission to Europe via the Iberian peninsula; (g) early clinical trials in European hospitals; (h) early resistance to adoption in Europe; (i) secrecy of some early formulations; (j) early treatment of royalty (French, especially)[3] and other highly placed personages, and early approval by them; (k) bestowal of monopolies; (l) wealth and fame of physicians or others who received monopolies; (m) different degrees of approval in different European countries; (n) early reputation as a specific; (o) special publication of instructions for use; (p) discovery of active principle in France in the early nineteenth century.

This list does not pretend to be complete. Moreover, a study going beyond the limits of the present investigation would probably yield additional parallels and would issue in an instructive generalized depiction of drugs introduced from the New World.

The history of cinchona differs from that of ipecacuanha in at least one important respect. Before the era of artificial cultivation in Java, cinchona had extremely small areal distribution and hence small production. The marked effectiveness of the drug led to early scarcity and early adulteration. I have not found reports of adulteration of ipecacuanha.

A curious parallel, interesting but imperfect, is supplied by the so-called Goan stone (*pedra de Goa*), a secret drug, not botanical, produced by the Jesuit secular brother Gaspar Antonio.[4] Widely disseminated by Jesuits, it even reached the Chinese emperor in Peking. Its large commercial success led to the manufacture and circulation of imitations, until the Jesuit procurator in Goa secured a monopoly from the metropolitan government in Portugal.

Another interesting but imperfect parallel comes from Ethiopia. Pankhurst has shown that an Abyssinian plant called *kosso*, whose flowers and seeds contain an anthelmintic, was reported by at least three seventeenth-century Jesuit missionaries.[5] In the nineteenth century a French diplomat brought back from Ethiopia thirty thousand doses, which he attempted to sell for 22,000 guineas.

Summary

It is obvious to the reader that this history, like most others, is based in large part on written records. It has often been necessary to interpret these materials as they would have been understood in their own time and also as they are regarded in the light of modern knowledge.

With respect to the discovery of Peruvian bark by Europeans and with respect to the European and extra-European dissemination of the drug, the exposition has relied heavily on Jesuit achievements, many of which were reported by non-Jesuits, especially physicians. Other possible sources, commercial and governmental, have been found to be scantier and less accessible. In addition, some deposits and some repositories have not been surveyed with adequate thoroughness. While the history of commerce has existed for well over two hundred years, the special history of prices is relatively new.

At present, however, there is no reason to suspect that even a thorough search of commercial and governmental records would yield evidence that would nullify any important part of the account that has been presented. For the limited period that has been examined in this book, the Jesuits' bark is unlikely to emerge as a merchants' marvel or a buccaneers' bonanza.

It now appears probable that the methods of paleopathology and paleoserology will become applicable to at least a few of the historical problems that have claimed our attention. It may become possible to obtain important information from the cadavers of persons who lived in the seventeenth or eighteenth centuries and whose clinical histories describe sickness or death caused by intermittent fever. Some of these histories mention also the use of Jesuits' bark. For example, Francesco Torti stated that in 1696 he saved himself from death by taking six drachms of the powder in a single drink.[6] He lived forty-five years longer (until 1741), and his body is buried in Modena in the parish church of Sant' Agostino.[7]

If the entire process of production and consumption of Peruvian bark is viewed as a system of primary causes, subsequent intermediate causes, and ultimate results, it is recognizable that extant knowledge of the subject has many gaps. We possess detailed information about primary events, such as collection and transportation. Of intermediate phenomena such as prices, taxes, and vagaries of supply, our knowledge is fragmentary. We have abundant information about the end of the process, that is, the variable effectiveness of the drug, consequent variations in dosage, and the predominantly successful therapeutic results that were obtained even in very severe cases. The total of difficulties and obstacles was incapable, except temporarily and intermittently, of destroying the reputation of the bark, and it does not appear probable that this overview of the process will be altered by accessions of new historical information.

Torti's contribution consisted of clarifying the worst part of the problem—the dangerous pernicious cases. It is wonderful that this could be done entirely by means of clinical knowledge, without important cooperation from morbid anatomy, before the advent of useful laboratory examination, before the discovery of the plasmodium, and before the recognition of the most dangerous plasmodial species.

The history of the Peruvian bark from the time of de Lugo to that of Torti can be regarded also as a problem in the acceptance of innovation. Examined in this way, the bark had several features in common with other novelties, and several differences.

Five facts were of major importance at the outset: the active principle in the bark resisted destruction during transportation; the bark arrived in Europe when the incidence of intermittent fever was high; the disease was easily recognized in a great many cases; the drug was promptly effective; and toxic effects were few. The stage was therefore set for a convincing demonstration, as judged by the simple criterion of *post hoc ergo propter hoc.* Such demonstration was given promptly by Fonseca, de Lugo, and Puccerini in Rome and by Badus in Genoa.

Other favorable elements were the presence of educated, widely traveled, and influential clergy, the existence of a well-organized hierarchy, the skillful organization of the Jesuit order, and the absence in Italy of strong anti-Catholicism such as was to resist acceptance of the bark in England.

There is no evidence that while the first large-scale experience with the Peruvian bark was being gained in Rome and Genoa, the strangeness that so often obstructs innovation played a large role, but difficulties ensued elsewhere and were followed by acceptance. Once established, the bark fluctuated in esteem but was not discarded. And, unlike many new inventions and ideas, it was not an example of multiple simultaneous discovery. Being relatively simple, it underwent no important modification for almost two hundred years.

Competing contenders, such as have troubled the progress of other innovations, are not absent from the history of cinchona. Antimony, the most noteworthy rival, has been considered in detail in the addendum to Chapter 5. As the decades unrolled, neither drug expelled the other; both are in use today, for different therapeutic purposes, more precisely defined.

Especially conspicuous in the history of the bark is the role of the highest social strata, exemplified by the decisive participation of Louis XIV. In an exactly analogous way, codes of dress and manners followed royal or noble leadership. That the prestige of the influential might have complicating effects has been shown by the cases of the viceroy Ferdinand and the archduke Leopold.

The chief obstacles to acceptance of the bark were doctrinal: the Greek beliefs, widely held, that perceptible evacuation was essential to cure and that a drug alleged to be hot was counterindicated in a fever. The opinions that the learned had obtained from books could not prevail against the relief that the sick received from the drug. Moreover, the prestige of antiquity was losing its strength.

Other obstacles were inherent in the practice of medicine, for example, uncertainties of clinical diagnosis, especially in the absence of the necessary fundamental knowledge. In this category belonged the chaos of nosologic taxonomy and an inadequate recognition of pernicious intermittents. Here the contribution of Torti proved to be of great importance.

The discovery of the Peruvian bark by Europeans and its transmission to Europe and other continents is merely a single case. Historians should now proceed to consider other cases concomitantly, such as that of ipecacuanha, in order to form an accurate general understanding of the process of discovery and spread of drugs from America. Nor need the research stop there, since analogous studies of Asian drugs, a process that began in antiquity, would produce a somewhat different portrait as well as an instructive contrast. Histories of individual drugs and groups of drugs exist, but the general principles of their discovery deserve much additional study.

That similar considerations apply to plants used for food and for other purposes has long been evident from the research of Alphonse de Candolle. That the same train of observation and reasoning can also be extended to cultural traits has been brought to our consciousness by the work of travelers and the analyses that have been made by cultural anthropologists. Thus our observation expands the world that we see, while our thinking enlarges and complicates the cosmos to which it is directed.

The Intermittent Fevers as
Understood in the Seventeenth and
Early Eighteenth Centuries

IN EXPLORING the early history of the Peruvian bark it is
desirable to examine the concepts of intermittent fever (with necessary
reference to the concepts of fever in general) that were entertained in
the seventeenth and early eighteenth centuries. Because these concepts
drew heavily upon Galen, we cannot avoid starting with a discussion of
this famous and difficult source.

The Galenic Foundations

The extant writings of Galen include one major treatise
devoted specially to fever, his *De differentiis febrium* (On the kinds of
fever, K7. 273–405). This essay is supplemented by a host of incidental
and miscellaneous comments distributed through other parts of the
Galenic corpus.[1] From these we must isolate the statements that have
to do with definitions, categories, and causes.

Fever, says Galen, is abnormal heat in which the heart is involved;
unless the heart is heated, fever is not present (K7. 283). Like fire, fever
has many kinds and many causes (K7. 282).

Ephemeral fever (*febris diaria, febris ephemera*, K10. 666, K9. 695)
is an affection of spirit in which the blood is heated but not putrefied
(K7. 295). It must be distinguished from quotidian fever, which is mentioned later.

Putrid fevers occur in the humors;[2] accordingly there are four kinds.
The first of these, the synochal or continued fever, exists in the blood.
For example, if menstrual products are retained, the patient becomes
overfilled with blood. If the blood putrefies and a fever develops, it is
synochal (K17A. 807).

Galen also regarded as humoral the three major intermittent fevers—the quotidian, which comes from rotting phlegm; the tertian, from yellow bile; and the quartan, from black bile (K7. 336).[3] To complicate the subject, he stated that yellow bile can also produce synochal or continued fevers, of which he recognized three varieties (K7. 336–37). A special problem is semitertian fever, a composite of continuous quotidian and intermittent tertian (K7. 385; 9. 673; 9. 680). It was very common in Rome (K17A. 121), and was dangerous (K17A. 945).[4]

One important category remains to be considered. This is hectic fever; unlike ephemeral and putrid fever, it is located in solid structures (K7. 313–14; 10. 699). The term *hectic*, used in this manner by Galen, is sometimes confusing to modern readers, since today's physician limits it to high, "swinging" fevers, especially those that occur in sepsis and acute miliary tuberculosis.

Until recent times tertian and quartan fevers were regarded as different diseases, as is shown by the fact that they were attributed to different humors.[5] Nowadays, in contrast, we think of human malaria as a single disease of which the tertian and quartan fevers are varieties. For reasons that appear mysterious, almost every premodern writer discusses or mentions quartan fever before tertian. Perhaps the relative mildness or benignity of the tertian caused it to take second place, or the greater chronicity of the quartan and the more conspicuous character of its complications earned prior mention.

According to ancient doctrine a fever might change from one kind to another (K7. 310; 7. 466; 18B. 279; 10. 665); the concept of specificity was virtually nonexistent. Variant forms, however, were recognized; thus, an exquisite or exact tertian (K7. 371; 17A. 233) was distinguished from an inexquisite, mixed, or spurious tertian (K11. 26–27). Analogous considerations applied to quartans (K11. 30).

Galen believed that fever had numerous causes, such as anger, sadness, burns, insomnia, drunkenness, indigestion, and satiety (K7. 279). He recognized that fevers might arise from the hypochondria (K16. 245), an opinion that doubtless contributed to later confusion about the vaguely defined afflictions designated as hypochondriasis. He discussed a cryptic statement of Hippocrates that chills came from the upper abdomen, fever from the lower (K17B. 299). In Galen's opinion, just as quotidian fever rarely occurred unless there was disease at the mouth of the stomach, quartan fever did not occur without disease of the spleen, or tertian without disease of the liver (K11. 18).[6] The discovery of the preerythrocytic and exoerythrocytic lesions of malaria, situated in the liver, must be reckoned an astounding historical coincidence.[7]

Another coincidence, equally astounding, concerns a disease that occurred in Rome in the late seventeenth century and was treated unsuccessfully with the Jesuits' bark. This condition, discussed by Giorgio Baglivi (1668–1707) under the designation of *mesenteric fever*,[8] was almost certainly typhoid fever, plus occasional cases of salmonellosis and amebiasis. The recognition that mesenteric fever was abdominal, was—by coincidence—highly compatible with the Hippocratic and Galenic opinions that have just been discussed.

Toward the end of this appendix I will suggest that ancient theories of fever—especially ancient incrimination of the hypochondria, the liver, and the spleen as participants—would later favor the development of abdominal palpation.[9] The evidence is fragmentary but not negligible.

In his remarks on fevers, as in his discussion of many other subjects, Galen occasionally contradicted himself; sometimes he did this in a perplexingly intricate manner. To those who enjoy dialectic acrobatics I recommend several Galenic dicta that describe the pulse in putrid and other fevers.[10]

That Galenic concepts of the fevers were dominant for many centuries is well known. Striking evidence of their persistence in medical opinion had been recorded in the early nineteenth century. In Philadelphia in the year 1807 Charles Caldwell included the following statement in his translation of a treatise by Jean-Louis Alibert:

Here [in the United States] the practitioner, when called to a case of malignant intermittent, must reduce the tumultuous and excessive action, and remove the inflammatory diathesis of the system, before he can venture to exhibit the bark. These ends he can attain only by bloodletting, purging, and perhaps vomiting and sweating. If he venture on the use of the bark in any form, previously to this evacuating process, he never fails to injure his patient. For, to exhibit that remedy during the continuance of an inflammatory state of the system, is, emphatically, adding fuel to fire. Should such practice even succeed in removing the disease, it almost inevitably produces visceral obstructions in its stead. (v)

Mercatus

Galenic doctrine having been dominant in the Western world from ancient times at least until the middle of the eighteenth century, it would be supererogatory for us to consider each medical author, or even each important medical author, whose writings were composed during this period of almost two millennia. Instead, we can bridge the interval and compress the narrative by taking as a single sample of that entire period the *Praxis Medica*[11] of Ludovicus Mercatus

(1520–1606), professor of medicine at Valladolid, personal physician and protomedicus of Kings Philip II and III of Spain, and as conservative as these honors would suggest. His impressive systematic treatise combines the large experience and learning of its author with the doctrines of Galen, which he elaborated more than he clarified. Its tenor is demonstrated adequately by the following excerpts from his discussion "On the exact tertian," which is part of the section on the nature and cure of putrid fever.

Without doubt physicians usually understand many different things by the term *tertian*. First is the simple tertian, that which Galen acknowledges in book 2, chapter 3 of *The kinds of fevers* [K7. 339–41], namely the illegitimate tertian, which the same author in chapter 5 of his third commentary on Hippocrates' *Epidemics* I [K17(1). 233] calls an extended tertian.[12] Indeed, physicians sometimes use the term *tertian* with an addition, for example *semitertian* or *hemitritean*. . . . A tertian is designated in another way when we call it double, because in the time of quiescence, that is, on the day between two paroxysms, another attack supervenes, and this constitutes a double tertian. Finally, the term *exquisite tertian* is customarily applied to the fever that is true and legitimate and comes from yellow bile putrefying in the ends of vessels. . . . The exquisite tertian is one of the burning fevers; both kinds come from ignition of the same humor, namely yellow bile, although the tertian differs from burning fever because of its intermittence and in the kind of heat, as Galen says. (526)

These excerpts have been selected as demonstrations of Mercatus's Galenism. That, like many another confirmed Galenist, he was capable of independent thought and observation[13] is shown by the following remarks:

On the pernicious tertian. Included in the class of fevers that produce paroxysms on the third day is this pernicious species, not adequately reported or known, and accompanied by high mortality among patients and astonishment among physicians. It occurs more infrequently and hence is harder to recognize; its attack is more serious and because of ignorance it produces greater terror and bewilderment. Who would ever believe that a tertian fever could become deadly? (539)

Whereas previous physicians, ancient, medieval, and modern, had observed that tertian fever, usually a mild ailment, sometimes produced overpowering psychic disturbances and death,[14] Mercatus recognized these cases as representing a distinct form of intermittent fever. His discussion describes six ways—all of them chiefly theoretical and not readily understood by the modern reader—in which a tertian fever may become pernicious. The merits of his contribution have been obscured by latinity, verbosity, and the passage of time.

Spigelius

In 1624, Adrianus Spigelius (Adriaan van den Spieghel, 1578–1625), an eminent surgeon, anatomist, and botanist, issued his *De semitertiana libri quatuor.*[15] This treatise attempted to define and describe a difficult concept or syndrome inherited from Greco-Roman antiquity,[16] and especially to distinguish it from double tertian fever. In his exposition Spigelius drew upon extensive clinical, anatomical, epidemiological, and pedagogical experience gained in the Low Countries, in northern Italy, and in central Europe. Several of the fevers that he described in his book were quite probably malaria; one was possibly typhus.[17]

His anatomical writings, overlooked by historians of malaria, contain additional hints of his clinical knowledge and alertness. For example, in his *De humani corporis fabrica* he says he had noticed that inhabitants of dry districts have smaller spleens than denizens of swamps (1: 240) and that in cases of splenic "inflammation" a hand placed over the left hypochondrium might detect that the spleen seems to be palpitating (1: 179).

These Spigelian passages have at least one additional merit for the modern reader, since they put him on notice that, in books written in earlier times, discussions of what we can now recognize as malaria or some special aspect of malaria, do not necessarily occur in chapters devoted to intermittent fever but may be found instead in paragraphs or chapters devoted to the spleen. An interesting example is to be found in the *Affections (Peri pathōn)* of Hippocrates. In this treatise section 18 deals with tertian and quartan fevers, and section 20 is devoted to enlargement of the spleen.[18]

In the introduction to his treatise on semitertian fever Spigelius asserts that even skilled physicians confound this ailment with the double tertian.[19] In the former disease the attack lasts eighteen hours, whereas in tertians the duration is twelve hours (2: 2, 5). It is established, he says, that the proximate cause of genuine semitertian is a double humor that possesses putridity and consists of excrementitious bile and phlegm. Elsewhere he adds:

All semitertians have their putridity not within blood vessels but outside them. For as often as I think about what I have seen in the treatment of putrid fevers, *whether intermittent or continued* [italics added] and what I have seen in the dissection of those who have died of these fevers—and especially from semitertians—I can acknowledge nothing else than that the putridities of intermittent and continuous fevers have always been within the vessels and rarely outside them; on that account I have always found the tinder (*fomitem*) of the semiter-

tian in the vessels, mainly in the smaller ones. For in dissected cadavers inflammations produced from bilious and pituitous blood had formed around the hepatic concavity, in the stomach, intestines, . . . omentum, and spleen, and were
rapidly fatal. (2: 8–9)

While this statement suggests extensive anatomical experience, the location of the observed changes arouses suspicion of peritonitis or postmortem autolysis.

After these comments Spigelius goes on to recount the histories of
two fever patients whom he had observed. Apparently he often used
abdominal palpation. In his first case he specified: "I palpated both
hypochondria but by touch I could detect no swelling worthy of mention" (2: 9).

In the second of the two cases he performed an autopsy, and the
findings are reported with the clinical discussion (2: 9). In this instance
the relatively abundant detail includes *no* convincing evidence of malaria, but the text exhibits the dominant Galenic concept of semitertian
fever and shows that this was supported—rather than being refuted or
even threatened—by detailed dissection. The patient was the manser-
vant of a Swiss nobleman. He had had fourteen days of dysentery, and
a fever that lasted about two months. Death occurred soon afterward.
A painful swelling in the liver had been detected by palpation.

Spigelius states that he dissected the cadaver not merely in order to
view the tinder of the fever, which he had always believed to be situated
in the veins of the liver and mesentery, but also in order to examine
carefully the reason why, as far as he could tell, the patient had been
afebrile for five days before death.

He found the stomach to show mild inflammation of its innermost
coat. The liver was greatly enlarged, and Spigelius either sectioned it
or broke it apart.[20] The spleen is not mentioned. Spigelius concluded:
from this history it is manifest to anyone that this double fever—tertian
and simple—had its main source in the portal veins, which are spread
out through the hepatic substance, the mesentery, and omentum, and
the stomach, since there was no other structure, no other place, no cav-
ity, outside the veins, which contained biliary and pituitous humor. In
other words, Galen was awarded full marks.

In his discussion of quartan fever Spigelius says that when the
spleen is swollen, the swelling does not come from the flesh or parenchyma (*non caro lienis, quae parenchyma dicitur*) but from filling and
distention of the numerous venous and arterial branches that are scattered throughout the organ. The same occurs in other soft structures
such as the testes which have very many veins and arteries (2: 10). This

statement implies, somewhat indistinctly, that the anatomist regularly incised these organs when he performed an autopsy.

In two cases of continued fever (2: 10–12), one of which was considered to be a semitertian, the other a double tertian, autopsies revealed that the cause was not putrefaction of blood or bile in the great vessels but inflammation in the intestines and the hepatic concavity. Since the causative humor was bilious and pituitous blood, its putrefaction gave the impetus for fever on single and alternating days. An accessory cause was constriction and obstruction of channels, including vascular channels, in the skin and the abdominal viscera.

Spigelius says that while semitertian fever has no distinct pathognomonic signs, it is differentiated from the continuous tertian, which is characterized by chilliness and shivering (2: 17). It is set apart from the double tertian by the length of the attacks and the form of the daily recurrence.[21] These and other differentials he illustrated by case histories and supplemented by discussion of subtypes, prognosis, and treatment.

Another treatise by Spigelius deals with plants. This work first appeared in 1606. The latest recorded edition, dated 1633, contains no mention of Peruvian bark and hence offers what can be taken as an uncertain *terminus a quo* for the introduction of the drug into northern Europe.

In his effort to understand the ancient nosologic concept of semitertian fever, Spigelius was confronted by an ill-defined congeries, which quite probably included some cases of malaria, even more probably included typhus, and almost certainly embraced also a miscellany of other febrile conditions such as typhoid fever, cholangitis, and sepsis. The not infrequent use of autopsy, added to the use of bedside methods (which included abdominal palpation), served merely to confirm Spigelius's Galenic beliefs and did nothing to alter them. He dissected in order to find where morbid humors had been deposited.

Harvey and Willis

Spigelius's book on semitertian fever appeared in 1624. At this time his exact coeval William Harvey had been working on the circulation of the blood for at least eight years.[22] Hieronymus Fabricius ab Aquapendente, a Galenist, had been the teacher of both Harvey and Spigelius. The latter followed his teacher's Galenism, whereas the former was more inclined toward Aristotle. Harvey's great influence on concepts of intermittent fever was soon to emerge in the ideas of Willis.

The importance of Thomas Willis (1621–75) in European medicine has never been seriously contested and is not reduced by recent research.[23] Dewhurst has shown that Willis went through a long preliminary period of transition from Galenism toward iatrochemistry. His concepts of fever appeared first in 1659 in his *Diatribae duae medicophilosophicae: quarum prior agit de fermentatione . . . altera de febribus.*[24] As this title shows, the two essays were prepared and issued together. Indeed, the first points toward the second: "On fermentation of the blood, both natural and febrile, more would be said here, were it not that I reserve consideration of this for a special treatise in which fevers will be discussed" (16).

The essay on fermentation bears a significant subtitle, which can be rendered, "On the inorganic movement in natural bodies." In all fermenting bodies, says Willis, heterogeneity[25] of parts or particles is found (*reperitur partium aut particularum heterogeneitas*); the movement in fermentation is caused especially by the struggling and straining of these against one another. He favored the Paracelsian doctrine, which classifies them as spirit, sulfur, salt, water, and earth. He referred to this system not as established fact but as *haec hypothesis* (2).

The earliest beginnings of life come from spirit in the [embryonal] heart, recognizable as a little fermenting speck; the speck is reminiscent of Harvey's embryological observations. Fermentation in the fireplace of the heart (*in cordis foco*) (16) is an important cause of the blood's circulation and effervescence.

Fermentation, says Willis, has a role in many diseases. Indeed, the sulfurous and spirituous part of the blood, activated excessively, boils immoderately in the vessels, like bubbling wine. By this process fevers of various kinds are kindled (19). Likewise, the cure of many diseases is accomplished by regulating fermentation (19).

All things are filled with fermentation. Fermentative movement is observable in the death, putrefaction, and corruption of bodies (31), and the corruption of any object is merely the separation of parts that were previously joined (34).

The essay on fevers, as already stated, is a direct sequel to the essay on fermentation. The ancients erred, says Willis, because they held false doctrines concerning the movement of the blood. Lacking a firm and stable basis, their pyretology was speculative, specious, and deceitful.

The preface to the "De febribus," published in the edition of 1659 and reprinted without alteration in the *Opera Omnia* of 1681, contains historically important statements, from which a historically important inference can be drawn. It portrays the destruction of old medical beliefs as a consequence of Harvey's discovery, and it describes the present task as consisting of the removal of the ruins. The preface contains not one word about the Jesuits' bark. Indeed, the 1659 text of the "De febribus," as Chapter 4 of this history has shown, mentions the drug not at all in the discussion of tertians and with noticeable brevity in the discussion of quartans. Hence the preface to the "De febribus" allows us to observe that *in the view of Willis the bark could have played no more than a secondary role in the downfall of Galenic doctrine.* This interpretation differs from that of the eminent Max Neuburger, who stated: "No other event contributed to such a high degree of exposure of the deficiencies of Galenism but also of iatrochemistry and iatro-mechanics as the introduction of the [Jesuits'] bark."[26]

Willis's opinion is supported by a remark of Jean Riolan (1580–1657), son of the famous anti-Harveian. In his *Encheiridium anatomicum* published in 1649, an early time in the (European) history of the Jesuits' bark, he wrote: "You see how great is the need of circulation of the blood in the movement of the heart, and how the circulation is conducted, without regard to confusion and disturbance of the humors and the destruction of ancient medicine (*citra confusionem et perturbationem humorum, et veteris Medicinae destructionem*)" (222).

A fever, Willis continued, is only a fermentation or immoderate heat introduced into the blood or humors (1: 63, SP 57).[27] The blood becomes hot and by its fervor must be purged of its filthiness. In addition, "it may lawfully be suspected" that the fluid which waters the brain and nervous structures is often affected; this may cause rigor, convulsion, delirium, and frenzy.[28]

Chyme, a nutritious juice, enters the blood continually, and a serous latex perpetually departs from it. In addition, the blood contains five kinds of particles, which have been mentioned: watery, spirituous, salty, sulfurous, and earthy. When blood passes through the heart, it is somewhat loosened; the spirits and sulfurous particles leap forth and by their deflagration impart heat to the entire body (1: 66, SP 59).

Blood, like wine fermenting in a tun, continually boils up. This kind of motion depends both on the heterogeneity of its component particles and on the various ferments, *which are breathed into the mass of the blood from the viscera* (1: 71, SP 64).[29]

Motion and heat in the blood depend chiefly on two things: first, being brought together with active components such as spirit, salt, and sulfur, the blood swells up; second, receiving ferment as it traverses the heart, it becomes rarefied and "leaps forth with a frothy heat" (*cum spumosa effervescentia exsilire cogit*) (1: 73, SP 65).

Effervescence, in wine or blood, is likely to be caused when anything extraneous and immiscible is added, or when some principle or element, such as salt or sulfur, "is carried forth beyond its natural temper, and becomes enraged." Thereupon "the Particles of this or that . . .

bring forth a heat . . . till the blood burns with the long fire of a Feaver."
Similar effects may be produced by coagulation (1: 75–76, SP 67).

In 1670, eleven years after the essays on fermentation and fevers,
Willis issued a treatise on hysterical and hypochondriacal diseases.
One of the two supplementary essays that accompanied this publication is titled "On heating or kindling of the blood."[30] In this work
Willis asserts that the heart is merely a muscle and does not heat
the blood. On the contrary, the heart borrows heat from the blood
(1: 663).[31]

We must now consider Willis's statements on the special subject of
the intermittent fevers (1: 76–102, SP 68–89). In these, he says, effervescence in the blood during the paroxysm is as intense as that which
occurs in a continued fever. Hence it must be concluded that, in both
of these conditions, the particles of the blood struggle against one another or against some "heterogeneous"[32] constituent, and intense fermentation arises. For this to occur, it is requisite that some principle
such as spirit or sulfur should be "exalted" (activated) to an excessive
degree, so that it comes to prevail over the others. *Continued* fever
arises from this cause. It is not readily quieted; and once quieted, it
does not soon return. In contrast, for an *intermittent* fever to occur, the
particles of the heterogeneous material that is mixed into the blood do
not become assimilated to it. Hence they produce ebullition until they
are vanquished and dissolved or extruded. Thereupon the paroxysm
halts until new "pullulation"[33] of the material produces a new seizure.

The origin, nature, and location of this foreign substance, says Willis, have been debated variously and vigorously. The long-accepted belief that it lodges in blood stagnating in the mesenteric veins has been
made obsolete by Harvey's discovery, since the blood never stagnates in
the vessels (1: 77, SP 69).[34] Willis offers a different explanation. He
says that if the nutritive juice that constantly restores the blood has not
been perfectly ripened by digestive processes, it enters the blood as a
heterogeneous substance, and its particles, although mixed with blood,
persist therein. On saturating the blood, they produce turgescence and
febrile effervescence in it (1: 78, SP 69).

In tertian fevers, Willis continues, the blood has a torrid constitution—*vulgo*, a parched makeup—caused by excessive impregnation
with particles of sulfur and salt. Hence the predisposing causes are a
hot and bilious temperament, a youthful age, and a hot diet (1: 87–88,
SP 77). These statements, derived directly from Galen,[35] are pro-
pounded without question. Also significant is the fact that they are presented without bibliographical reference, as if they were common
knowledge among physicians—which was presumably the case. Nor is

there any mention of possible incompatibilities between the particulate and the humoralistic components in the explanation.

Willis says, further, that when a tertian is protracted, it not rarely changes into a quotidian or even a quartan, and sometimes reverts subsequently to its original form (1: 88, SP 78). This statement has its antecedents in Hippocrates and Galen and may well have been supported by misinterpreted observation of complex cases.[36]

Of intermittent quotidian fever Willis says that when it is prolonged or is simultaneous with another chronic disease it may be accompanied by distention of the liver or spleen or obstructions in the mesentery; these changes are not causes of the fever but effects of it (1: 94, SP 82).[37]

In his discussion of quartan fever Willis emphatically rejects the ancient attribution "to a melancholick humour, heaped up somewhere in the first passages [the intestines], and there periodically putrefying" (*humori melancholico alicubi in primis viis coacervato, et periodice illic putrescenti*). Instead he asserts that in this disease the fluid part of the blood becomes acid and tart. It is deficient in spirits and its terrestrial or tartareous component is overactive (1: 96, SP 84).

The sickness is difficult to cure because the underlying atrobilious constitution of the blood is not readily removed and yields to almost no remedies (1: 96, SP 86). After the winter solstice the disease rages less [the symptoms are milder], but those who were of melancholic temper or whose viscera, especially the spleen, were severely affected, had no benefit from the change of season (1: 98, SP 86).

Willis's writings on fermentation and on fevers show that he was strongly interested in medical theory, etiology, pathogenesis, and pathologic physiology; his known interest in anatomy is not represented. Except for passages influenced by the discoveries of Harvey and Lower, most of his theory is merely the displacement of old imaginative suppositions by newer. His explanations involve particles and fermentation but do not exclude a noteworthy residue of Galenic humoralism. Galenic influence is probably represented also in Willis's references to putrefaction.[38] Other probable sources are Aristotelian: the *De generatione et corruptione*, the *Meteorologica*, and the *De generatione animalium*.[39] Bates (1981, esp. 53–55) has pointed to differences between Willis's concept of putrefaction and that of Helmont.

In addition, Willis's method of reasoning is strongly dependent on analogy, especially on analogy with familiar culinary or domestic processes.[40] There is almost no discussion of individual cases and almost no clinical description. Jaundice and labial "pustules" (now called labial herpes and well recognized as frequent in malaria) are mentioned.

Astonishingly, the spleen is not mentioned, except for the passage cited toward the end of the second preceding paragraph.

Descartes

It is to be regretted that the extensive anatomical and physiological researches of René Descartes (1596–1650) produced little by way of published writing on fever, although his work in physics and philosophy exerted strong influence on the development of pyretologic thought. Like Galileo, whose contributions he studied at the Jesuit college of La Flèche, he is regarded as a principal source of iatromechanical doctrine.

An early composition by Descartes, his *Le monde de Mr Descartes, ou le traité de la lumière,* is thought to have been written about 1629–33 but was suppressed by its author and was published posthumously in 1664 under the editorship of Claude Clerselier.[41] This essay is of interest in the present context because it describes a flame as dislodging and separating *particles* of wood, which *move* vigorously (11). The same text expresses the opinion that fire also is composed of particles. In other words, both wood and flame exhibit the traits that came to be recognized as basic in Cartesian philosophy.

The volume containing this treatise has a long title, which requires full quotation: *Le monde de Mr Descartes, ou le traité de la lumière, et des autres principaux objets des sens. Avec un discours du mouvement local, et un autre des fiévres* [sic], *composez selon les principes du méme* [sic] *auteur.* The last seven words show that the discourse on fever, which we are about to consider, was not written by Descartes but was intended to present Cartesian ideas. An introductory note by the book dealer, who was possibly the publisher, headed *Avis du libraire au lecteur,* states that the essay is the work of a philosopher and mathematician and was presented before the private group that met in Paris at the home of Henri Louis Habert de Montmor (1600–1679). This assemblage was ancestral to the Académie des Sciences.[42]

The term *fever* as used in the anonymous text does not refer to all elevation of body temperature but is limited to febrile diseases such as intermittent or continuous fevers. The author states that blood is rarefied in the heart and turns to vital spirit. It then departs impetuously from the heart and enters the arteries, which distribute it throughout the body (6). This part of the doctrine is Galenic, modernized by Harveian discoveries.

Several experiments supported by strong reasoning, the author continues vaguely, have shown that the body contains various fluids, other than blood, that travel along a regular route (7). The blood, he says, is made up of many little particles, which move in different ways. A considerable number constantly escape through invisible pores in the arteries and serve for nutrition and growth. The particles that escape are the most active and finest of all. The part of the blood that returns in the veins must be the coarsest, but it becomes finer on reentering the heart. The blood that flows to all parts of the body conveys heat acquired in the heart, while that which ascends through the aorta provides the means whereby the most active particles go through the carotid arteries to the brain, are separated from the coarser, and form the animal spirits, which advance into the nerves and muscles, producing motion, sensation, and wakefulness (9–10).

If for any reason, the author continues, a small portion of any humor stagnates in some part of the body, becomes corrupt, and then flows into the venous blood, which conveys it to the heart—if we suppose that this aliquot of blood is less suitable than the blood which physicians call laudable and which is comparable to green wood, less flammable than dry wood—the heart will expand very little. Hence the arteries will receive only a small amount of blood and will pulsate weakly. Further, the vital spirits will run in the body scantily and less actively than usual. The movement of the particles which they contain, and of which their natural heat consists, must cease. Then we must feel the sensation of cold, which is called the cold of fever (13–15).

In high fever the blood emerges from the heart boiling hot and runs very rapidly to the limbs. There is increased entry of spirits into the brain and thence into the nerves and muscles. These conditions must result in impaired sleep, headache, and hyperesthesia, and in the excessive strength that is observed in many diseases (18–19).

There is no doubt that fever arises in this way if we consider that it occurs while an abscess is developing and ceases when the pus is discharged. When the attack is over, the fever would not recur were it not that something resembling a yeast remains, or there is some arrangement that favors renewed assembly of corrupt matter. From this it must be concluded that the fever is quartan when the matter needs three days to ripen and to become capable of flowing with the blood. The fever is tertian when only two days are needed, and the sickness is a continued fever when the matter flows continuously (21–23).

These explanations, the author adds, gain in credibility when we consider the methods physicians use in treating fevers. For example, a reduced diet, commonly prescribed in such cases, thins the body. As a result the fibers become attenuated; they squeeze less strongly and the little channels in which the humors flow become dilated. The blood, reduced in amount, has less opportunity to be retained where it can support the illness (25–27).

The explanations are extensive, detailed, and almost totally mechanical but not really quantitative. Combining Galenic and Harveian doctrine with Cartesian mechanistic concepts, they rest also on a tiny amount of clinical observation, on a minimum of anatomical observation (probably derivative rather than firsthand), and on no new experiments. The reasoning is used to provide justification for traditional therapeutic methods.

A special problem, that of *cold* occurring in fever, is discussed prominently in the same *Discours*, but the presentation does not state clearly whether the author intended to consider the cold stage of common intermittents or the coldness that sometimes occurs in other fevers and that nowadays is usually attributed to shock.

Such are the main ideas presented in the *Discours des fièvres*. They can certainly be designated as Cartesian, although the essay was written by some other author than Descartes.

In 1637, Descartes issued the famous *Discours de la méthode*.[43] Here he commended Harvey for discovering the circulation, but he offered a rival concept. Instead of holding that the heart by its contraction expels the blood into the arteries, Descartes asserted that the heat of the heart causes the blood to expand; this forces the blood to move.

It is interesting and necessary to recall that Galen repeatedly mentions cardiac heat. For example, in the treatise on temperaments (K1. 569–70), Galen says that the heart is the bloodiest and hottest part of an animal, and in a treatise on embryology he remarks that the heart is like a fireplace (K4. 671). These notions were not alien to the thinking of Descartes.

In April 1645 or thereabouts, Descartes wrote to William Cavendish (1617–84), marquis of Newcastle and a pupil of Thomas Hobbes, in reply to questions sent him by the nobleman.[44] Descartes stated that all animal heat consists of a kind of fire in the heart, unaccompanied by light. It resembles what happens in *aqua fortis* when a large amount of powdered steel is added; it also resembles what happens in all fermentations. The fire is maintained by the blood, which flows at all times in the heart, "as Harvey has discovered."

Fever is caused by a collection of corrupted humor, which is collected in the mesentery or elsewhere, flows into the veins and reaches the heart, which thereby is prevented from dilating as much as usual and from sending the usual amount of heat to the rest of the body. One result is the trembling that the patient experiences. Much of the discussion is almost identical with statements made in the anonymous *Discours des fièvres*, discussed above. As the reader will note, the occurrence of cold sensations during fever proved especially enigmatic, and hence attractive, to thinkers.

In the letter to Newcastle Descartes remarks, in addition, that a fever would always cease at the end of a paroxysm if supplementary humor could be prevented from arriving at the place where the first aliquot had become corrupted. Since there are many different ways of preventing this, *but they are not always successful,* the fever can be treated with an infinite number of different remedies, but all are uncertain. The letter does not consider individual drugs and does not mention the Jesuits' bark. The allusion to failure, and the failure to mention success, suggest the mishaps of precinchonal therapeutics.

In the spring of 1645, in a letter to Princess Elizabeth of Bohemia, who had had fever and cough for about three or four weeks, the great philosopher did not hesitate to pronounce that the commonest cause of slow fever is sadness.[45] In 1646, in another letter to the princess, Descartes described the hemodynamic changes that he believed to accompany emotion, a disturbance that allegedly involved not only the heart but also reserve supplies of blood in the liver and spleen.[46]

That Descartes accepted and modified the Harveian concept of the circulation is made evident in the foregoing brief discussion. To his combination of Galenic and Harveian ideas he added the mechanistic explanations that are also abundantly evident. That the writings of Thomas Willis exhibit Cartesian traits—especially the emphasis on matter and motion—will likewise be clear to the careful reader.

Necessarily the Cartesian and Willisian viewpoints differed. As is well known, Willis was a medical practitioner and a medical scientist, whereas Descartes was a philosopher and a basic medical scientist, but not a physician. Their common ground was anatomy and the science that we now designate as physiology. Both men used particles in the explanation of phenomena. Both referred to fermentative processes, which appear more often in the writings of Willis than in those of Descartes.

In view of the rather close relation between the opinions of Descartes and those of Willis, and also in view of the contrasts, it is surprising that the ample writings of the latter rarely mention the former. An exception is the first chapter of the *De anima brutorum,* in which Willis discusses the mechanistic Cartesian concepts of the soul.[47]

Zacutus Lusitanus

Zacutus Lusitanus (1575–1642),[48] one of the last outstanding Galenists, was succeeded by a host of greater or lesser believers and caliphs, who tagged along for a full hundred years at the tail of a dwindling procession and repeatedly testified to the practical use and usefulness of their increasingly obsolete beliefs. The sixteen hundred

folio pages (6.1 kg) of Zacutus's *Opera* allow us to see Galenic concepts, including Galenic explanations of observable facts, applied in
daily medical practice. Yet it would be a gross error to view Zacutus as
totally or narrowly or fanatically a Galenist, and it gradually dawns on
the reader of the *Opera* that Zacutan Galenism applied mainly to fundamental principles, to categories, and to methods. It did not automatically exclude the admission of new facts. This is most clearly evident
in his discussion of drugs imported from the Indies.

Zacutus had read very widely—indeed, he comes close to giving the
impression that he had read everything—and he had seen much, but
his great knowledge had not stupefied him. He was therefore able to
add large experience to long tradition, his pages being rich in new
comments interspersed occasionally with original observations. Hence
his writings, including both his explanations and his case reports, are
well worthy of our esteem.

Notable clarity of exposition combined with systematic arrangement
confer the special advantage that the Zacutan treatises can be used as
an introduction to Galenic doctrine.[49] For this purpose they at times
are better than the writings of the ancient prototype. Since Zacutus's
habitual retrospect included the principal post-Galenic physicians (and
did not exclude philosophers and poets), his intelligent, intelligible,
and well-indexed writings are especially suitable for explaining ancient, medieval, and Renaissance concepts to twentieth-century seek-
ers. To the considered results of reading and experience he added the
bonus of common sense.

These traits can be observed in his discussion of the behavior of the
spleen in severe quartan fever. After giving a brief excerpt from Galen
on dropsy complicating quartans, Zacutus presents a *paraphrasis*,
which reads as follows:

Although, as I have said above, the quartan is very safe and kills no one, because nature regains its strength during the two intervening days, it is often
fatal if it is complicated by great sicknesses. For when the spleen is swollen by
an abundance of melancholic humor, nature tries to expel the larger part outside the veins; and since this is coarse, earthy, and atrobilious, it produces a
quartan. Then, if the spleen becomes weak and cannot attract the coarse and
feculent humor, and it cannot separate pure blood from this black humor, and
it does not perform its function correctly, or because the dregs of the blood
cannot pass from the liver into the spleen because the passageways are stuffed
with sticky fluid, this humor is regurgitated into the liver and by its abundance
and coldness chokes the natural heat. The consequence is dropsy, a fatal disease indeed, certainly terrible,[50] since in this protracted sickness the forces
weaken, and the liver, inadequately purged of this black humor, decays, weak-
ens, and cools. Thus the natural heat, overcome by an abundance of sticky

fluid, is reduced and finally extinguished. Hence Avicenna stated correctly
[book 3, fen 1, tract 2, chap. 61] . . . that a quartan which comes from an impostume of the spleen, or in which there is an impostume of the spleen, very
often leads to dropsy and destruction. But you may rightly ask, "How should
such great sicknesses be treated?"

Say: in complicated sicknesses the physician's attention should be directed
to the most urgent. Therefore if the signs of dropsy are conspicuous, the helpful
hand should be applied to it. If however the quartan produces only weakness of
the spleen, then the spleen should be strengthened, the body should be purged,
the visceral obstructions should be relieved, and aperient ointments and plasters should be applied to the affected structures (1: 731–32)

Another example is his comment on a case of splenic "scirrhus" that
had been reported by Alexander of Tralles (1: 379–81).[51] Previous physicians had treated the patient by "barbarous cauterization" (*barbaricis
ferramentis*) over the spleen; Trallianus obtained a favorable result by
milder treatment. The fascinating comments of Zacutus recognize the
dangers of refractory splenomegaly, explain the physiology of the
spleen (as stated by Galen, Amatus, and Fernel), expose a contradiction in Galen, and tend finally toward the use of mild medicaments.

Zacutus, the great-grandson of an astronomer who guided Vasco da
Gama and was useful to Christopher Columbus,[52] was born in Lisbon
in 1575 and received the doctoral degree at Sigüenza in Spain in 1595.
He then practised medicine in Lisbon for thirty years, but almost nothing is known about this period of his life,[53] nor has it been ascertained
whether his early education and early inclinations were Jewish, or Roman Catholic, or neither. It is at least possible that oppression had Ju-
daized him. Information on these matters might influence the interpretation of his literary style.

In 1625 a decree of King João III, the Pious, repersecuted the Jews
of Portugal. Thereupon Zacutus went to Amsterdam, where he practiced Judaism overtly and medicine successfully.

A major component of Zacutus's oeuvre is his *De medicorum principum historia* (1:1–984),[54] a work ultimately arranged as six books.
The first installment appeared in 1629. Then, after a seven-year hiatus
that included the year of his departure from Portugal, Zacutus issued
the remaining volumes and parts of volumes successively in almost
every one of the years between 1636 and 1642, when he died. These
facts imply a continued demand from publishers, based doubtless on
great popularity among readers.

In the final decade of Zacutus's life the febrifugal Peruvian bark
made its first transatlantic voyage. In 1649, seven years after his death,
his writings were gathered under the title of *Opera*. They were reissued
repeatedly thereafter.

His *De medicorum principum historia* contains 389 case reports. The first three books, arranged in the traditional head-to-foot order (*a capite ad calcem*),[55] are followed by chapter 4 on fevers, chapter 5 on envenomation, and a final chapter of miscellaneous cases. Each of the most elaborate reports starts with a case record taken from a Greek, Roman, or Arab author. This is regularly followed by a paraphrase, which explains the ancient or medieval record and then sets forth Zacutus's opinion. In addition, many of the discussions contain supplementary "Observations," which are reports of Zacutus's own cases; eighty-six of these are given. Often they are followed in turn by epiphytic questions and answers, and by additional *dubia*, which present unresolved or inadequately resolved problems.

Volume 2 of the two-volume *Opera* begins with the *Introitus medici ad praxin* (The physician's introduction to practice) (1–72). Next comes the *Pharmacopoea* (73–135), first published in 1641, and then the important *Praxis historiarum* (137–663), in which, says the title page, "the treatment of internal diseases is explained according to the opinion of the great physicians, doubts are aired and resolved, and, finally, very many case reports are interspersed in their places."

The *Praxis*, like the *De medicorum principum historia*, with its explanations, traditions, doubts, solutions, and case reports, is conspicuously systematic, but the origins of the distinctive system are beyond the scope of this history.[56] The popularity of the Zacutan writings is attributable to the fact that they were oriented toward clinical practice; that is, they were useful to the practitioner and consultant as well as the professor.[57] Although his successive chapters cover most of medicine, we shall concentrate on his observations of intermittent fever, taking the tertian as the principal example.

Zacutus's comments on exquisite or uncomplicated tertian fever (*Praxis*, book 4, chapter 22, 2:585–89) provide a good example of his opinions, his range, and his historical position. Restrictions of space limit us to a few excerpts.

As was his wont, he starts with Galen, who had stated the important distinction between the type of a fever and its period. Next, Avicenna's relatively elaborate classification of bilious fever is set forth, and Zacutus appends the caveat that it requires verification. He also disagrees with Aetius on this topic. Then, after this rapid survey of one and a half millennia, he puts a fundamental question (fundamental to Galenists): you may ask whether the exquisite tertian is produced by pure bile. He answers, judiciously, that pure bile is found in the gall bladder only; within the veins bile is always mixed with other humors (*sincera bilis solum in folliculo fellis reperiatur, in venis semper cum aliis humoribus sit mixta*) (2:585). This statement is professedly based on Galen.[58] It is

possibly a composite; the first seven words are perhaps based on anatomical observation, while the last eight come from Galen.

In addition, says Zacutus, in foci of putrefaction situated outside
vessels, bile is always mixed with a portion of blood or excrement and
hence it seems that no pure substances can be found there. Further, the
tertian is said to be exquisite both because it is combined with no other
disease and because only the biliary humor, pure and clear (*purus et
sincerus*), is at fault. Then, in thoroughly medieval fashion, he discusses
the qualities of purity and sincerity (clarity) and adds that "this is firm
Galenic doctrine" as is shown by a passage in which Galen drew an
analogy with wine (see above); even when diluted with a portion of
water, it does not lose its vinous qualities, such as color, odor, and taste.
Similarly, since bile, from which the tertian is generated, retains its
qualities, this fever is judged to be of the ardent kind. The exquisite
tertian and the causon [bilious remittent] are derived from the same
humor, but in causon the biliary humor is intravascular, whereas in
exquisite tertian it is conducted through the sentient structures.

Zacutus's discussion of cause supports the Galenic pronouncement
that in tertians the bile is inflamed or putrefied. If the bile remains
within vessels, it produces a continued fever; if it passes out of them, an
intermittent occurs.

The discussion of clinical signs brings up several questions. For example, is the chill in exquisite tertians always severe? Zacutus here
makes the interesting statement that in exquisite tertians the chills are
strongest in the earliest paroxysms and milder in the later ones, the
opposite being true in quartans (2:586). This notion is based in part on
an interpretation of a Hippocratic dictum and is attributed to peculiar-
ities of coction.[59]

The discussion of signs also raises the question whether the pulse is
unequal in exquisite tertians. Here Galen has contradicted himself and
Zacutus resolves the difficulty. Several other doubts, objections, and
opinions then complete the exposition of signs.

The discussion of treatment is only about a third as long as the discussion of signs. The relative brevity is probably due to the fact that the
basic principles of treatment are explained in earlier parts of the book.
As expected, the presentation is based on humoral doctrine: since the
cause of the disease is hot and dry, the recommendations are for things
that are cool and moist; moreover, the dyscrasia requires evacuation by
vomiting, defecation, and urination. After the peccant humor has at-
tained coction, a mild purge is given. Usually this is done as the fifth or
sixth paroxysm is approaching. Then cooling decoctions are given. Venesection from the right salvatella[60] is recommended.

The discussion of exquisite tertian fever ends with a brief *observatio,* which in this instance is not a case report but consists mainly of a recipe for an electuary designed to cool the liver and to produce gentle purgation. Its numerous ingredients include tamarind, barley, lettuce, seeds of gourds, and a conserve.

Of the very common false tertian (*tertiana notha*) we have only to add that it was considered to be a kind of tertian but was attributed to bile mixed with phlegm, or to thick "vitelline" (yellow) bile (2:589–93). The differences and distinctions, based not only on Galen but also on Averroes, need not be examined here, nor need we follow Zacutus onward into his chapter on semitertian fever (2:593–94), a disease that may appal the reader, since it is attributed to bile contaminated with phlegm and thus has perplexing resemblances to the false tertian.

The foregoing details are more than sufficient to describe the tenor of Zacutus's heavily Galenic outlook and presentation. We must now consider other facts that are hinted at in the initial paragraph of this Zacutan discussion and that point in another direction.

Zacutus's *Pharmacopoeia* was composed at least as early as 1641.[61] On first perusal, the text that is included in the posthumous edition of 1667 (2:73–135) does nothing to dispel the image of total Galenism, the drugs being arranged according to the humor that each medicament was believed to affect. However, into this framework Zacutus inserted the grossly Paracelsian powder of antimony (2:113–16).[62] He then made the following significant remarks:

Musk, amber, camphor, bezoar stone, ebenum [gray millet],[63] china [Smilax], sarsaparilla, and very many other oriental and occidental drugs were unknown to ancient physicians yet are highly useful to patients and quite often block the pathway to death. So day unto day uttereth speech, and night unto night sheweth knowledge.[64]

Gutta gamba [gamboge] is a noble drug, recently brought to us.[65] Many testify that by its use obstinate diseases are dispelled and I, an ocular witness, make and confirm the same testimony. . . . Some call it Peruvian or Goan gum . . . ; from which plant it originates is unknown.

And for fevers Zacutus repeatedly advocated a Brazilian botanical drug called maracaju-açu,[66] which he considered to be a prime febrifuge and which also strengthened the heart (2:101–2; 1:777).[67]

A difficult question arises at this point. If cinchona bark is suspected of having caused the fall of Galenism, or at least of having contributed to its decline, why did the very same suspicion not arise against maracaju-açu, the powerful febrifuge, or against ipecacuanha, which is effective against severe (amebic) forms of dysentery? It is quite clear that new drugs were accommodated in the structure of Zacutus's Galenist beliefs but did nothing to weaken them. We can see also that

Zacutus was not totally resistant to new facts. Moreover, he could not deny that some patients recovered after taking the new exotics.

It is observable that some great writers—and probably some lesser authors—acquire credit or discredit for discoveries that they never made. These are the barnacles of time. Friedenwald (1944, 312) made the surprising statement, which he credited to Fielding Garrison, that Zacutus Lusitanus was "one of the first to describe blackwater fever." The association, well known but not invariable, between blackwater fever and quinine, a drug unmentioned by Zacutus and unknown to him, at once threw suspicion on this claim. It was then noted that Garrison, the alleged source, wrote: "According to Garrod, black urine (alcaptonuria) was observed by . . . Zacutus Lusitanus (1649)."[68] Evidently Friedenwald, an ophthalmologist, confounded blackwater fever with black urine.

Zacutus's report on the subject is titled *De urina. Urina nigerrima, citra noxam excreta* (On urine. Extremely black urine emitted harmlessly) (2:138). It tells of a boy aged seven years who passed black urine. After many kinds of treatment had failed, he bade farewell to therapeutics and lived happily ever after. Zacutus cites an earlier report, brief and questionable, by the obscure Henricus Petraeus of Marburg (1589–1620).[69]

Isaac Cardoso

Isaac Cardoso (1615–80), sometimes designated, because of historical vicissitudes, as Ferdinandus Cardoso, was well but not widely known in his country and era. He has long been overlooked by medical historians. For this circumstance the reader is invited to consider several explanations—first, that Iberian medicine, like Iberian culture in general, tended toward partial isolation from the rest of European culture; second, that Jewish authors have not rarely been ignored by others;[70] third, that Cardoso's contributions lacked outstanding merit; and fourth, that his writings had a small press run. Despite the obscurity that resulted from one or more of these causes, his work deserves renewed examination because it exemplifies several aspects of medical thinking in his era.

Cardoso, a graduate of Valladolid, held a professorship there and was a protegé of the count-duke of Olivares, prime minister of Philip IV.[71] Like Zacutus Lusitanus, he recorded very little about his personal life, but it was almost certainly persecution that, about 1648, caused him to leave Spain. Later he worked in Verona. His writings include a book on the usefulness of snow and ice, and a large but apparently undistinguished treatise on philosophy.[72]

The contribution that brings Cardoso to our notice is his book *On Syncopal Fever*, published in 1639.[73] It is based on a severe outbreak that occurred in Madrid in 1637–38, causing many deaths.[74] This disease, or approximations thereto, had been mentioned, clearly or obscurely, since antiquity. Galen, for example, had written of syncope occurring during fever but had not established a special category for the combination. Avicenna and others had recognized two subclasses. Amatus Lusitanus and some authors of lesser note had discussed the disease also. A more recent writer, the famous Ludovicus Mercatus, had classed the disease as a continuous quotidian that belonged among the pituitous fevers and, like Avicenna, had divided it into two subordinate categories.[75]

Cardoso, reflecting the scholastic tradition that was so prominent in his double heritage, devoted much attention to the definition and classification of the disease. Significantly, he emphasized the dissension that existed: "In these years these fevers have infested the Court, to the regret of many and the confusion of all. The physicians differed as to its recognition and treatment; some characterized it as syncopal, others as malignant" (dedication to Olivares). Cardoso's deliberations, which occupy most of his text, necessarily relied on the humoralistic concepts that were then dominant. He emphasized such problems as the difference between syncopal fever and fever that is merely accompanied by syncope (3r ff.). He quoted, with apparent approval, authors such as Mercatus and Pedro García, who had held that the actual presence of syncope was not essential to the diagnosis; a mere tendency to syncope was sufficient. At the same time he accused Mercatus of having confused syncopal fevers with malignants (19v).

Special embarrassment was caused by the famous Hippocratic statement that "intermittence of any kind indicates that there is no danger."[76] If this pronouncement is correct, why did so many people die of syncopal fever?

These examples illustrate the perplexities which existed in the absence of reliable etiology and physiology and which are paralleled by the debates that characterize the history of semitertian fever.[77] It is to be noted additionally that, eleven years after the *De motu cordis*, Cardoso failed to mention William Harvey or to evince knowledge of the Harveian circulation.

Cardoso explains that syncopal fevers start like ordinary tertians but during the third or fourth paroxysm are complicated by fainting, absence of the pulse, and weakness of the faculties, especially the vital faculty (1v–2v). The last-named deficiency is the principal cause of death. In some instances there is mild chilliness or severe rigor or suffocation. There is no delirium since the humors mainly attack the abdomen and heart but not the head. At the time of death a cold or warm sweat appears over the forehead and neck. Men are more often affected than women, and the disease occurs mainly in summer and autumn. The concomitant fevers are for the most part intermittents.

Cardoso's four clinical reports, which occupy ten printed pages (35r–40v) allow the reader to formulate an independent opinion as to diagnosis. Even if we admit that this kind of retrospective identification verges on futility or impossibility, a few facts stand out and a few inferences are warranted.

In all four cases the pattern of tertian intermittent fever emerges. Most of the patients had sweats, which usually were profuse and often were protracted; thirst was usually intense. Vomiting and abdominal distress occurred. Anxiety, restlessness, jactitation, and headache are mentioned, but there is only one record of coma (37r).[78] A conspicuous sign was weakness or irregularity of the pulse; in one patient the pulse was absent for periods as long as ten to eleven hours (37v).[79] All four patients died.

The clinician's first inclination would be to regard these as cases of malignant tertian fever caused by *Plasmodium falciparum*. At least three of the four are not well-marked examples of cerebral malaria. It would be rash to designate the series as exemplifying a special syncopal kind of malaria in view of the fact that phlebotomy was used freely in all four cases and in no case is the quantity of blood reported.

In the first case, for example, death occurred on the fourth day; phlebotomy had been done twice. In the other cases the procedure had been used three, seven, and five times respectively, not always with Cardoso's approval. In addition, all four patients had had laxatives or purges, and some had vomited. These losses of fluid are more than sufficient to explain syncope, profuse sweats, and arrhythmia.

Abandoning inconclusive speculation of this kind, we may prefer to view Cardoso's study as an effort to isolate, define, and explain a clinical syndrome that he had investigated and that had been noticed by earlier physicians. It should be recognized that he did about as well as was possible in the existing state of knowledge.

Giacinto Gigli

Just as any procession of dignitaries may be accompanied or paralleled by random characters who scamper along beside it, the important personages whose writings and deeds contribute the bulk of the present analysis were not the only individuals who took note of the fevers. In July 1645 one Giacinto Gigli, a middle-class Roman layman, noted in his diary that "at this time a large part of the populace began to sicken, and many died of malignant fever. Of those who were opened after death, it was observed that they had inside them a live worm, which did not die even if it was touched with theriac but died only if it was treated with wine. It was attributed to the water that people drank. For this reason the physicians gave the patients no [un-diluted] wine but had them drink water well mixed with wine" (270).

At this point the reflective reader will wonder: What did the early autopsies contribute to understanding of the problem? Did they contribute anything beyond confirmation of preexisting misconceptions? In the remarks of Gigli we can at least observe postmortem findings being used as a guide to treatment.

Patin

Far from Giacinto Gigli on the educational scale we find Guy Patin (1601–72), a Parisian medical professor and dean, whose erudite opinions and prejudices are discussed in Chapter 5. Here I merely note his comment on quartan fever: sufferers from the quartan are usually melancholic and obstinate and do not readily believe in physicians. This is what often makes the disease last for several months or even years. Patin remarked also that taxation is an ill not curable by Peruvian bark.[80]

Sydenham

The great Thomas Sydenham (1624–89) is traditionally and correctly called the English Hippocrates. As his writings show, he leaned strongly toward clinical observation. Disliking and mistrusting theories, he strove in vain to avoid them. It is not surprising that the passages in his writings which undertook to cope with etiology, patho-genesis, and physiology are difficult and obscure, in sharp contrast to the simple clarity of his observational reports and his practical descriptions of therapeutic methods.

In his biographical essay on Sydenham Dr. Donald G. Bates discusses Sydenham's relations with Locke and Boyle. He considers it "highly improbable . . . that the works of Charles Barbeyrac [1629–99] had any influence on him, as has been claimed."[81]

Bayle and Thillaye state that Barbeyrac left no writings, not even case reports (il n'a laissé aucun écrit, ni même des observations).[82] A posthumously and anonymously edited collection of his prescriptions contains a chapter on the use of cinchona, commending it for both treatment and prophylaxis.[83] An anonymous collection of notes, be-lieved to have been assembled about 1770 and bound with a lecture by

Barbeyrac on syphilis, contains sixteen leaves of prescriptions. Among these are four prescriptions for tertian, double tertian, and malignant fever, and one for obstruction of the spleen. None mention the Peruvian bark.[84] All these bits of negative evidence tend to confirm Dr. Bates's comment in that they show nothing that points to a relation between Sydenham and Barbeyrac.

Sydenham's earliest published work, issued in London in 1666, bears the title *Methodus curandi febres propriis observationibus superstructa;*[85] this wording leaves no doubt that the text is based on what he had seen at the bedside. The dedicatory epistle, addressed to Robert Boyle, informs the reader that the book is not stuffed with materials taken from other authors (*neq[ue] spoliis Authorum . . . sufferta*). The brief treatise, which its author designated as *tratiuncula*, discusses, in separate sections, continued fevers, the symptoms of such fevers, the intermittent fevers, and smallpox. Sydenham states that the paroxysms of intermittents are divided into a period of shivering, a period of ebullition, and a period of despumation (86). The two last named in this series suggest analogy with fermentation; obviously they do not directly represent the famous Sydenhamian observation but are imaginative constructs based on that observation. Overt mention of fermentation appears on a later page (107). In 1668 the *Methodus* was reissued in an enlarged edition that contains a chapter on plague. The third edition appeared in 1676 under the title *Observationes medicae circa morborum acutorum historiam et curationem.*[86] It contains Sydenham's most important writing on the fevers.

Since it has been impossible to extract from Sydenham's writings a complete, coherent, and systematic concept of either the fevers in general, or of the intermittent fevers, it has seemed best to select sequentially from his *Observationes medicae* the most important of the random comments in which he set forth his ideas.

At the outset he espouses atomism: "Nature is unable, from the continuous flux of particles, to remain unchanged." There is great need, he says, for a history of disease, that is, an accurate description. A praxis or methodus—a system of therapeutics—is needed also. The history should avoid "every philosophical hypothesis whatsoever"; it should note the natural phenomena of the disease only. Its purpose should be the detection of morbific cause and the indications of treatment for each disease (1:11, 12, 14, 15). Remote and ultimate causes are incomprehensible; only proximate, immediate, and conjunct causes can be known.

Humors may be retained unduly (1:18). They may also contract a morbific disposition from the existing atmospheric constitution[87] or from some venomous contagion (1:19).[88] They become exalted—intensified—into a substantial form or species, and every specific disease is a disorder that originates "from this or that specific exaltation." An example is quartan ague, which keeps to a regular course and preserves a definite type (1:19).

Although the causes of most diseases are inscrutable and inexplicable, "the question as to how they may be cured is, nevertheless, capable of solution" (20). Conjunct and immediate causes "are revealed by either the testimony of our senses, or by the anatomical observations" (20). In addition to the need for a true description of diseases and for a definite therapeutic method, there is need for the discovery of specific remedies (21). These considerations do not apply to chronic diseases because in such diseases the method of Nature for ejection of morbific matter is less efficacious (21).

Sydenham says that the only specific is the Peruvian bark (22). This unclear statement can be taken to mean that Peruvian bark is the only drug that destroys an acute illness directly without recourse to general (nonspecific) processes of evacuation, such as diaphoresis, diuresis, or expectoration.

A disease is "nothing more than an effort of Nature . . . to restore the health of the patient by the elimination of morbific matter" (29). This concept Benjamin Rush was later to list among Sydenham's nine principal errors.[89] Diseases, says Sydenham, arise "partly from the particles of the atmosphere, partly from the different fermentations and putrefactions of the humours" (1:29).[90] Epidemic acute diseases arise through atmospheric changes (31).[91] Sporadic or intercurrent acute diseases "originate from the particular anomalies of particular bodies" (1:32); probably this refers to individual susceptibility.

Constitutions—combinations of climatic phenomena—depend on changes in the bowels of the earth; they contaminate the atmosphere and they predispose people to acquire this or that kind of fever (1:33, 33), which may be prevalent for several successive years and hence is called stationary—that is, temporarily endemic.

All epidemics are either vernal or autumnal (1:35). The disease that is worst at the autumn equinox gives its name to the constitution for the whole year (1:37).[92] "Where any particular constitution engenders any species of epidemic . . . this species is generically different from the species of any other constitution, however much one name may be current for all."

Most of Sydenham's *Medical Observations* is devoted to the epidemic constitutions and the diseases encountered in the years 1661–75. He remarks in section 1, chapter 2 that he is unable to attribute them to "any perceptible quality of the atmosphere" (1:40). In chapter 4 he says, in a discussion of continued fevers: "I prefer the broad and general term *commotion*, to either *fermentation* or *ebullition*. . . . I have no desire to mix myself up with such controversies as these. Be the matter as it may, I shall, now and then, use the words *fermentation* and *ebullition*, inasmuch as they have been currently adopted by medical men of late years" (1:44–45).

Sydenham's pathogenesis of vernal intermittents (1:74) involves animal spirits evoked by the vernal sun and opposed by viscid humors accumulated during the winter. The struggle excites vernal ebullitions, which are paroxysmal and are comparable to phenomena that occur in beer barrels. Spring intermittents are far less dangerous than autumn intermittents, especially quartans, which may be complicated by dropsy. A quartan may change its type at any time.

In describing the pathogenesis of autumn intermittents (1:78) Sydenham says that from the high acme of its exaltation [intensification], prevalent in the early part of the year,[93] the blood declines, especially when accidental circumstances have existed, such as loss of blood or ingestion of cold and crude substances; the constitution of the blood is subjected to morbid impressions from the constitution of the atmosphere that then prevails. Ebullition lays hold of the humors of the blood, which are often "very degenerate" (1:79). The blood is in great measure deprived of its spirits since it has been parched by the heat of the preceding summer. Consequently its ebullition and despumation are retarded. Irregularities may occur because of slight errors in regard to the (Galenic) nonnaturals (1:80).

In attempting to describe the difference between intermittent and continued fevers Sydenham says that "by means of an effervescence limited to a definite period . . . Nature expels the matter of continued fevers" (1:81). To this he adds: "Consider this process, and you will find that those of intermittents accurately coincide with it." Apparently this means that each cycle of an intermittent fever represents a succession of events that is comparable to the entire course of a case of continued fever. The merit of this perception should not be belittled.

As has been shown above, Sydenham was averse to theories, but he used them, and used them inconsistently. His aversion must be attributed in part to his personal tastes, which leaned toward the practical and which in these respects were congruent with the famous British aversion to theory. It should be noted also that Sydenham, contrary to the usual perception, was not ignorant of the literature. Indeed, he was a man who had read widely. For example, his chapter, "The Pestilential Fever, and the Plague of the Years 1665 and 1666," says: "In truth, many authors (and those good ones) have all along perceived that bleeding is proper in the plague. The chief of these are, Ludovicus Mercatus, Johannes Costaeus, Nicolaus Massa, Ludovicus Septalius,

Trincavellius, Forestus, Mercurialis, Altomarus, Paschalius, Anderna-
chus, Pereda, Zacutus Lusitanus, Fonseca, and others" (1:110). He
then adds to the list Leonardus Botallus, and subjoins two quotations
from Botallus that run to twenty-six lines, accurately reproduced.[94]
Either he read diligently or he had a diligent assistant.

Sydenham repeatedly compared fever to fermentation, as Willis had
done, but he disavowed firm belief in the analogy. Probably his opinion
was really eclectic since he also referred occasionally to particles and
he was a close friend of Boyle. His comments also suggest Aristotelian
causes. Moreover, he retained the famous Galenic nonnaturals. But
throughout his writings observation took precedence over hypothesis.

His observations and his notions of constitution were influential in
western Europe and in North America. As can be seen in the writings
of Ramazzini, Baglivi, Ippolito Albertini, and Morgagni, his work was
also influential in Italy;[95] this aspect has received inadequate attention
from scholars of other countries.

Borelli

Giovanni Alfonso Borelli (1608–79), author of a concept
of pyretogenesis which was viewed with respect for a century but is now
deep in oblivion, was an astronomer, mathematician, and iatromechanical physiologist. His years of early maturity coincided with the
final years of Galileo's major pupils and with energetic activities of the
Counter-Reformation. He taught in Messina and Pisa and was in contact with major scientists including Benedetto Castello and Marcello
Malpighi. He participated actively in the doings of the Accademia del
Cimento.

In 1649, while he was professor of mathematical sciences at the University of Messina, Borelli published a valuable and charmingly digres-
sive epidemiological treatise, his *Delle cagioni delle febbri maligne di
Sicilia negli anni 1647, 1648* (On the causes of the malignant fevers of
Sicily in the years 1647 and 1648). At the time of writing the outbreak
was still in existence. Mention of petechiae suggests that the disease
was typhus.[96] Apparently Borelli's investigation was conducted independently of the government and the Church, but the book is dedicated, courteously, to the Senate of Messina.

Borelli observed that the sickness affected the rich and the powerful
as well as the poor and the beggars. Hence the cause could not be bad
food or bad water; the disease must come from corruption of the air.
This inference, based on social and economic distribution, he proceeded to test in the autopsy room. He found that although some patients died in delirium, there were no lesions in the brain. There were,

however, lesions in the lungs, and this was compatible with the presence of dyspnea. There were no lesions in the esophagus, stomach, or liver. Hence the noxious cause must have entered the body through the respiratory tract. Then, in consonance with the Harveian doctrine of the circulation[97]—a relatively recent discovery—the poisonous quality passed to the heart and was spread to the entire body by way of the bloodstream.

In a special appendix (157–79) Borelli discusses the nature of fever. He says that fever is not a disease but is a medicine *against* disease. Natural operations are conducted by the movement of spirits, humors, and solid components, reduced to tiny particles. The particles are capable of moving in a normal or a disturbed manner. If by some case the heart and arteries are greatly agitated, there is a great increase in the movements by which particles in the blood escape from the arteries. Hence oily, salty, and watery particles come to be retained among the muscle fibers and become rotten. This process produces abscesses, gout, and "other bad effects" (161). Furious agitation of the circulatory system can indeed produce heat, but one need not believe that this is what causes the heat in ordinary fevers, especially in those that are periodic (164).

Despite vagueness, which the reader will have observed, it is clear that in his treatise on the Sicilian fevers Borelli used the Harveian circulation to operate a combined iatromechanical and iatrochemical system that is reminiscent of Willis.

The work that requires principal emphasis in the present context is his posthumous book on the movement of animals; it first appeared, in two parts, in 1680 and 1681.[98] This treatise ends in a section of forty-five octavo pages devoted to the morbid movements that occur in paralysis, fevers, and old age (propositions 218–33, pp. 320–65). Most of the attention, appropriately, is given to fever.

At the outset Borelli declares that the most violent convulsive[99] tremors of all are those which occur during the paroxysms of quartan fever and which produce a very troublesome disease in the spinal cord[100] when salty fluids, secreted during previous fermentation, produce painful "mordications." He does *not* say that the spinal disease causes the fever, nor does he mention the cord again in his exposition.

He says that the traditional doctrine, which attributed fever to a focus in and near the mesenteric veins, is false since the Harveian circulation shows that intravascular stagnation is impossible; thus "this whole fable disappears" (prop. 110, p. 324). He shows, or purports to show, that fever is not caused by alteration of blood by heat, by putrefaction, or by admixture of salts or sulfur; this conclusion is based in part on miscellaneous observation and reasoning and in part on intravenous injections administered to dogs (prop. 224, pp. 333–36). He recognizes moreover that inferences can be vitiated by coincidences. He then proceeds to show that nerve fluids and nerve juices (*succi nervei*) which have fermented or have become acrid irritate the heart and are the primary immediate cause that produces the heat of fever (prop. 225, p. 336). "In order not to seem to be laboring under an imaginative and fantastic hypothesis" (prop. 226, p. 340), he finds it necessary to establish that from a distance effects can be produced which pass through the nerves to the brain and thence to the heart. Experiments performed with oil of tobacco and observations made in cases of snakebite showed that the brain was disturbed before any damage occurred in the heart. Borelli concluded that very rapid transmission of poisonous juices occurred by way of orifices in nerve twigs (*per ostia nervulorum*), which may be patent in ulcers and wounds. The noxious material goes to the brain and then to the heart. It shakes the latter and thereby arouses febrile "movement"; presumably this is the tachycardia of fever. Confirmatory evidence is derived from observations made in cases of purulent pleurisy and in several other kinds of fever, including that which accompanies arthritis.

Where does the alteration of nerve fluid occur (prop. 227, p. 343)? Autopsy experience—Borelli gives a rapid summary that includes a surprisingly perceptive explanation of agonal pulmonary congestion—shows that there is no observable alteration in the blood.[101] The nerve juices are intended to be expelled from nerves and deposited in glands. Gently sliding further into realms of hypothesis, he says it could be (*fieri potest*) that these juices are retained in the nerves, if the little passages and orifices in the neural twigs are obstructed by some kind of glutinous matter. The juices thereupon undergo a noxious fermentation and become degenerate. The resultant irritation could affect the brain; the vigorous disturbance, transmitted through nerves, would reach the heart (prop. 227, pp. 344–45) in the manner already suggested. At the end of a febrile paroxysm, says Borelli, the blood within arteries succeeds in removing corrosive materials that block orifices in nerves, and it opens up excretory channels (prop. 230, pp. 351–52). The contaminated portion of the nerve fluid is drawn off, while the healthy, clear part remains.

The periodicity, admittedly very difficult to explain, requires further resort to conjecture. Borelli envisioned the quotidian, tertian, and quartan fevers as comparable to a series of vessels in which different amounts of flour added to a standard amount of water cause different degrees of obstruction in channels from which wine is being drained (prop. 231, pp. 354–55). There is no reason to think that he was satisfied by this suggestion.

In proposition 233, the final part of his *De motu animalium*, Borelli says that remission in intermittent fevers is a temporary cure. The renewal is a new fermentation, which arises from residues of ferment hiding in glands. It is deduced that complete cure does not occur until the pyrogenic ferment is removed completely. He uses common catarrhal fever as an example. In the same manner other fevers are cured when the excretory vessels of glands in viscera and in the skin are opened (*deobstruuntur*) and the ferment in these glands is partly expelled in sweat or insensible transpiration, partly neutralized, partly expelled through veins and thence into urine, or neutralized by well-tempered chylous juice.

From this, he continues, it can be deduced that fevers can rarely or never be cured by profuse purgation or ejection of humors, since the pyrogenic ferment is apt to be of small bulk. This is shown by the cure of those fevers that start with chills. Such cure is produced by means of the febrifugal root that has been imported recently from the Indies; it removes the fever but causes no discharge by way of stool, sweat, or urine. The reader will be amused to observe that in quoting this passage in the third chapter of his treatise on fevers Francesco Torti was later to change "febrifugal root" into "febrifugal bark."

Borelli's treatise has much in its favor. It envisions problems clearly and approaches them systematically. The use of data obtained in experiments is especially notable, although the modern reader must often balk at the conclusions drawn. The experimental results are accompanied by observations made expertly in the dissecting room and by a variety of incidental comments and analogies. Conjecture is admitted, somewhat grudgingly. Humoral doctrine is attacked and massacred. The style is fluent, pleasant, and unencumbered by excessive quotation.

Borelli's concept of cerebral irritation in fevers was influential enough to last at least until the time of Cullen.[102] A curious sequel or reflection occurs in the work by William Cole, discussed later in this appendix.

Bellini

In 1662, Lorenzo Bellini (1643–1704), a pupil of Borelli—hence an heir of Galileo—and a leading protagonist of iatromechanical doctrine, made his most enduring contribution to medicine, the discovery of the renal tubules. This is recorded in his *Exercitatio anatomica de usu renum*. In the present context we are concerned not with this work but with a collection of writings published much later, in 1683, under the title *De urinis et pulsibus, de missione sanguinis, de febribus, de morbis capitis, et pectoris.*[103] As the title indicates, the volume includes a dissertation on fever (215–383).[104]

In the first section of this strange essay Bellini states that the nature of any disease must consist of that which is peculiar in whatever precedes the disease and of what accompanies and follows it, all these components being determined by physical observation. This system he proposed to apply in turn to each of the fevers. The reader soon learns that the promised observations are not forthcoming.

For the purposes of his investigation Bellini constructed a taxonomic system that would avoid the assumption of causes such as putridity, bubbling heat, poison, and fermentation. Instead, the causes and their manner of acting could be expected to appear by deduction. He felt that the older system must be rejected since it implies causes; that is, the ancients attributed ephemeral fever to the burning of spirits or blood, humoral fevers to putrefaction of humors or blood, and hectic fever to putrefaction of solid structures. Bellini replaced the venerable taxonomy by a simpler division into continued fevers and intermittents. From this attractively simple dichotomy he proceeded to consider subvarieties, the continued being divided into simple, periodic(!), and erratic, while the intermittents were merely bifurcated into periodic and erratic. Thus the total of categories and subcategories came to five; ancient kinds of fever, such as causus and synochus, were adapted to them.[105]

These considerations by no means represent the entire spectrum of febrile disease since Bellini in addition admitted that both continued and intermittent fevers might be legitimate, exact, and true, or spurious and illegitimate. Further, simple and periodic continued fevers and intermittents are sometimes mixed together. Moreover, wandering or erratic fevers may be continued as well as intermittent; this is true also of malignant and pestilential fevers.

On reaching the end of Bellini's exordium the reader is likely to have despaired of finding simplicity. He will also have noted that the entire introduction is devoted to taxonomy and devoid of observed fact; moreover, the reader is placed on notice that fermentation is excluded from consideration.

In the next four sections of Bellini's treatise four major categories of fever pass in review: (*a*) simple continued fevers, (*b*) continued periodic fevers, (*c*) intermittent periodic fevers, and (*d*) erratic fevers. In each category the antecedents, concomitants, and sequelae are considered.

The application of this system to the simple continued fevers (221ff.) provides a fair sample. In this category Bellini considers the daily fever or ephemera, correctly so called (*febris diaria, vel ephemera legitime et proprie dicta*), the ephemera of many days [*sic*], the nonputrid synochus, the putrid synochus or continent fever, the causos or nonperiodic burning fever, and the hectic. The reader at once observes that, contrary to the expectations aroused by the introductory discussion, the ancient terminology has not been discarded but is used repeatedly for reference.

The antecedents of the daily fever or ephemera are said to be: sadness, fear, anxiety, anger, wakefulness, disturbance of the mind, evacuations, exercise, excessive exposure to the fire or the sun . . . cold, inflammation of glands or buboes, especially if suppurated . . erysipelas, and plethora—to a total of thirty-one items. No evidence is presented and no description is given, despite Bellini's introductory salute to observation. It must be inferred that Bellini here intended nothing more than a concise summary.

The discussion of concomitants of ephemeral fever is longer but equally vague: it begins "from an evident and manifest procatarctic cause which immediately arouses fever, e.g., by reducing perspiration." The consequences are said to include a simple synochus or a continent fever, or a hectic, especially in hot youths in the spring.

The discussion of continued periodic quartan fever (228) is followed by a puzzling section headed, "A malignant fever, the cacoëthes (of bad character), and its several kinds, namely the Hungarian disease, the English sweat, a malignant fever with spasms. . . . See the medical writers." [106] This section is a composite presentation of typhus, epidemic influenza, and common exanthemata: "pain in the head, . . . the eyes very often look red, smallpox and measles break out over the whole body but most abundantly on the face, feet, and hands, and likewise purple spots or petechiae. . . . There is no bad thing that does not sometimes happen in malignant fevers. The pimples or petechiae that break out . . . are similar to fleabites of purple color." The antecedents of legitimate intermittent tertian fever are said to be all the things that can form excrementitious bile (235). This is obviously Galenic doctrine (K9. 652). Supplementary causes include youth, heat, hot foods, and overwork. The clinical description mentions no stage but the rigor. Nothing is said about the spleen or about labial herpes. Intermittent quartan fever is attributed, Galenically, to black bile (237). The semitertian is regarded as an especially dangerous combination of the tertian and the quotidian (238).

What has been described thus far is an introductory survey that occupies approximately one-seventh of the *De febribus*. The remainder is presented in the form of thirty-five propositions, [107] which are considered briefly in a later paragraph.

We must now digress in order to consider an important part of Bellini's pyretologic doctrine, that of *lentor*, a wholly original invention that did not long survive its author. Lentor is nowhere clearly defined in the *De febribus*; indeed, a clause in the text warrants the opinion that Bellini himself regarded it as hypothetical since he refers to "this lentor that is supposed in the blood." [108] The lentor was imagined as a coagulum that, in the course of fevers, affects part of the blood and causes it to resist the force of the circulation. Thereby it produces many of the signs and symptoms of fever, such as a sensation of heaviness, listlessness, chilliness followed by sensations of heat, and alterations of the pulse (prop. 18, pp. 281ff.). When influenced by heat, the lentor becomes stiff. If the coagulum has not been desiccated, it retains at least part of its viscidity.

Especially curious is the statement that a lentor which produces a feeling of cold by virtue of its adherence to capillary arteries may be carried away into the veins, the heart, the arteries, and the capillaries and may make many circuits of this kind (*atque ita deinceps ex ordine plures, ac plures circuitus ejusdem generis efficit*) (prop. 19, pp. 292ff.).

The lentor is subject to changes—including fermentation (prop. 19, p. 302), which Bellini, as stated above, has promised to disavow. Some of the changes may mutate the fever from quotidian into tertian or quartan, or conversely; lentor, moreover, can be produced by reduction in motion of the blood or by increase or decrease in its quantity.

The discussions of lentor occur, not in the introduction to the *De febribus* but chiefly in propositions 18 and 19. The total number of propositions, as already stated, is thirty-five. The first declares that there is no fever without some fault (*vitium*) in the blood, that every fever is attended by some fault in the pulse, and that every fault in the pulse is accompanied by some fault in the blood. The second proposition adds that fault of the blood can occur only by change in its motion, quantity, or quality; the third subjoins that there is no fever without some fault in the motion or quantity or quality of the blood. These three propositions, offered as declarations and unsupported by facts, are the heart of Bellini's pyretology and are a basic statement of iatromechanical doctrine. The remaining thirty-two propositions discuss in turn each of Bellini's nosographic groups in the light of propositions 1–3. The final or thirty-fifth proposition merely states that a fever is nothing else than a fault of the blood either in its motion, quantity, or quality. This statement repeats the doctrine pronounced in propositions 1–3.

Bellini's *De febribus* has the arrangement of a mathematical treatise in that the main body of the text is set forth as a series of propositions. Since this material consists of assertions rather than deductions and

because it is not truly quantitative, it can hardly be regarded as mathematical; because of its preoccupation with velocity and viscosity, it is
best described as iatromechanical. Very little of what is presented can
be regarded as evidence. This is especially conspicuous in the propositions that set forth Bellini's concept of lentor. No coagulum is described
from direct observation. Moreover, the alleged existence and travels of
coagula could have been tested experimentally, especially since Bellini
was in frequent correspondence with Malpighi, who repeatedly examined the circulation in living animals with the help of his microscopes.
Finally, the *De febribus* added nothing to extant knowledge and did not
recognizably lead to further investigation.

Pitcairne, Boerhaave, Castro Sarmento

It is appropriate to consider, however briefly, any consequences or influences that are justly ascribable to Bellini's writing on
fever. Bellini's principal admirer was Archibald Pitcairne (1652–1713).
Like Bellini, he had strong mathematical interests, and iatromathe-
matical concepts were prominent in his writings. Bellini dedicated his
Opuscula of 1695 to Pitcairne; the latter returned the favor in his *Dissertationes medicae* of 1701.

This contentious work, somewhat reminiscent of the acridity of
Dean Swift, contains an essay on the circulation of the blood through
the smallest vessels. It manages to avoid mentioning Malpighi's capillaries and Bellinian lentor and, at the same time, attacks Willis and
denies the presence of ferments in any part of the human body (14–
34). It contains another essay that deals with the treatment of fevers
(118–31). Here Pitcairne shows simultaneously his devotion to iatro-
mathematics and to Bellini and discusses the Bellinian measurement
of perspiration. Another essay, the last in the assemblage, commends
itself to our attention because it points out that the action of Jesuits'
bark is not explained by iatrochemical doctrine (136–37).[109]

Boerhaave wrote an introduction to the fourth edition of Bellini's
large treatise (1717).[110] In this good-natured statement he commended
Bellini highly but made no direct reference to the *De febribus*, which
constitutes more than a quarter of the volume. He stated, a little
vaguely, that in this book the reader very rarely finds anything mixed in
that can justly be called alien to nature, or dangerously asserted, or
doubtful because of obscurity. In his *Aphorismi* Boerhaave states that in
cases of fever bloody humors stagnate at the ends of vessels.[111] He refers only to accelerated cardiac contraction and increased capillary resistance in fevers. These statements are comparable to assertions made
by Bellini in proposition 18. Boerhaave says also that the proximate

cause of intermittents is viscosity of the arterial and nerve fluid, cerebral and cerebellar, that is intended to go to the heart.

I have mentioned among the sequels of Bellini's writing on fever the works of Pitcairne and the brief remarks of Boerhaave. It is relevant to intercalate here a surprising delayed statement that appears in the book on pharmacy by Jacobo de Castro Sarmento, which was published in 1735 (525) and reissued in 1758 (406–7). This author attributes intermittent fever to thickness and lentor of blood stagnating in capillary arteries. The malfunction, he proceeds to say, is relieved by *quina quina*, which acts as an alterant of both the solids and the liquids of the blood.

Much later than Castro Sarmento, William Cullen in 1778 wrote the obituary of lentor: "It has been supposed that a lentor or viscidity . . . is the cause of the cold stage of fevers and its consequences. But there is no evidence of any such viscidity previously subsisting in the fluids" (1:40).

Jones, Cole, Huxham

The year 1683, which witnessed the publication of Bellini's famous *De urinis*, also witnessed the publication of an obscure but instructive tractate, the *Novarum dissertationum* by the equally obscure John Jones (1645–1709).[112] This author derides those who believe in four humors; he replaces them by three, which he derides likewise. He states that all the alleged causes indicate a single fundamental origin, namely, crude matter arising from bad composition of the blood and chyle. Yet to humoralists (designated pejoratively as *humorum patronulis*) he concedes that the crudities are weightiest in quotidian fevers, that the blood is more sulfurous in tertians and less sulfurous and spirituous in quartans.

He points out that all protracted intermittents that do not come to a proper crisis (*malé judicatis*, 10) turn into sicknesses made horrible by "crudities."[113] Examples are anasarca, ascites, leukophlegmasia, and pituitous and serous swellings of the spleen, legs, abdomen, "and other parts." Sometimes they even produce a pituitous mania, described by the illustrious Sydenham. These conditions yield to febrifuges and moderately warm cardiac remedies. The most effective and faithful drugs for expelling these fevers are salts, especially the lixivials, as well as the rougher bitter drugs such as Peruvian bark, gentian root, lesser centaury, and likewise the warmer "discussants" (dispellents); all of them are diametrical opponents of crudities.

These remarks, as well as several encomia bestowed on Peruvian bark toward the end of Jones's book, show that the conspicuous effectiveness of this drug did not cause immediate abandonment of the other remedies. Peruvian bark was merely placed at the head of the old list. Jones's comments suggest also that iatrochemical and fermentationist opinions may have been more important than cinchona or any other drug in causing the decline of humoralism. It is to be noted also that Jones's extremely detailed discussion of symptoms suggests that his clinical experience with fever was very great, yet there is no justification for inferring that his opinions about pathogenesis were influenced thereby.

Less obscure than that of John Jones, and even more interesting, is the work of another independent thinker, William Cole (1635–1716), whose aberrant "new hypothesis excogitated to explain the type and symptoms of the intermittent fevers . . . and especially, on treatment by means of the Peruvian bark" (1693) commanded wide but brief attention.[114] The text leans strongly toward mechanical but not mathematical concepts. After summarizing the opinions and hypotheses of Sylvius, Jones, and Willis, Cole states that nutrition is conducted through the agency of nerves and that nerve fluid is the actual nutritive substance (35ff.). In intermittent fever the nerve roots in the cerebral cortex, relaxed because their pores become blocked or because other errors have occurred in the (Galenic) nonnaturals, admit unsuitable material to the brain (96ff.). In overcoming intermittent fevers, the Peruvian bark, "that famous remedy, confirmed by extensive trial in these diseases" (215),[115] acts exactly there, namely, in the "fourth region," which is the brain and nervous system (236). Further ratiocination, accompanied by clinical observation, explains why the fever is dispelled by the drug although no evacuation occurs (248); this had been a *crux* for half a century. And other reasoning, which I will not summarize here, reveals why the drug sometimes fails (247). The treatise ends with case reports.

Cole, a correspondent of Thomas Sydenham, is immortalized in the latter's *Dissertatio epistolaris*, dated London, January 20, 1681–82.[116] The *New Hypothesis*, like so many other works discussed in this history, exemplifies the struggle of strong minds against one of mankind's greatest afflictions. Cole used all the weapons that were within his reach: the medical literature (some of his ideas suggest the influence of Borelli), Willisian discoveries in neuroanatomy, a relatively new and obviously powerful drug, and current clinical observation.

John Huxham's *An Essay on Fevers* was one of the pyretologic treatises most often used in the second half of the eighteenth century. Originally published in English in 1750, it was repeatedly reissued in English and other languages during a period of eight decades. It makes repeated reference to Baglivi but mentions Bellini only once (119), and this unique reference does not deal with fever; mention of lentor, however, recurs in not a few passages. Despite this fact it is obvious that the enduring part of Bellini's contribution consists of his discovery of the renal tubules and his clinical observations on pulmonary disease. His pyretology disappeared with the subsidence and transformation of iatromechanical doctrine.

Morton

Richard Morton (1637–98), a clergyman ejected from his living in 1662 because of theological nonconformity, turned to the vocation of medicine. In 1692 and 1694 he issued treatises on fever.[117] At the start of the first volume (1692) he announced that therapeutic intentions, toward which his writing was clearly directed, can be derived only from a true etiology, which in turn could be based only on the certainties of anatomical demonstration (3). After this impressive statement of aims and hopes he declared that the entire structure of the body, its viscera, and its vessels, comes from a spirit that originates in the brain. In abnormal conditions the animal spirit, like the entire blood mass, is stained by exogenous ferment; thereby it acquires a morbid character, which is the cause of all diseases, acute and chronic. By this concept, clearly marked as a hypothesis—*juxta hanc hypothesin* (5)[118]—the pathology of such diseases, he said, is put together more reliably, and in a manner much more congruent to reason, than is possible by the use of humoralist doctrine. In addition Morton offered as postulates the propositions that (a) animal spirits exist in all fibrils of the mechanism; (b) these spirits, coming from the brain and spinal cord, are channeled through nerves; (c) they unite intimately with the blood; and (d) the crasis of the blood is always altered by disease of the spirits, a process that causes universal diseases.

In contagious diseases, Morton added (16, 31), the spirits become contaminated and infect the entire mass of humors. Indeed, it would be impossible to imagine that the relatively coarse and sluggish congeries of humors could become contaminated by exogenous effluvia unless the spirits had become contaminated by them previously.

Changes that occur in blood are analogous to changes observed in wine and beer in consequence of thunder (23).[119] The effect of spirits on the blood is shown in acute fevers. In acute diseases the nervous structures are affected before the rest of the body, as is shown by the fact that headache occurs at the onset of the attack[120] and is often accompanied by mild dizziness, while the pulse indicates that the entire drama is being enacted in the nervous system before the blood is affected (28–29).

General diseases, including acute fevers, are often caused by cold entering the pores of the skin (34).[121] The effect goes to the brain, the workshop of the spirits, and affects the body much more easily than if the cold were impressed on the humors first.

In discussing the causes of the paroxysms that occur in intermittent fevers, Morton ridiculed the older notions of a *fomes* or focus of bile or black bile or phlegm situated at some place in the viscera, such as the mesenteric veins; the discovery of the circulation had shown that no such stagnation occurs in the vessels. As was shown earlier in this appendix, the same objection had been voiced by Willis. Morton argued also against the *primae viae* (alimentary canal) and other visceral structures being regarded as primary sites (37–39).

Morton set up two taxonomic groups, designated as universal and partial, for all the diseases that are of internal origin—*qui intus nati, corpus humanum affligunt* (43). His phrasing involves an inconsistency since, as we have seen, he had already referred to exogenous effluvia and miasmas as causes of disease (16, 31) and he had attributed pathogenic properties to cold that entered the body through pores in the skin (34). It is at least possible that he would have refuted these objections by defining miasms and cold as remote causes and by limiting his bipartite classification to proximate causes.

Of Morton's two main classes[122] I here consider only the first, that of universal diseases. These arise immediately from a preternatural (abnormal) diathesis of the animal spirits, which ruin the blend in the blood and which, in their first attack, affect the body's entire system. This process is not caused by any sickness in any single bodily structure.

Among universal diseases Morton recognized a subgroup of *primary diseases*, which arise directly and can be either acute or chronic. The acute are those that are terminated by crisis, whether favorable or unfavorable, within a few days. The chronic do not threaten destruction as promptly as the acute and include hectic fever, chlorosis, scurvy, scrofula, and rickets. The second subgroup of universal diseases consists of *secondary diseases*, in which a single part of the body is affected and immediately thereafter affects the blood and the spirits; the process therefore must be included under universal diseases. The reader will observe that this subcategory conflicts with Morton's specification for universal diseases as stated in the second sentence of the preceding paragraph.

Using an expression reminiscent of Galen, Morton says that acute fever in general is preternatural heat (50).[123] To this he adds that it comes from blood kindled by animal spirit that has been contaminated by a deleterious miasm and has been irritated and hence has expanded unduly. This miasm cannot be described since it is beyond the scope of all our senses. Acute fever does not come merely from abuse of the Galenic nonnaturals (approximately, bad hygienic practices); not rarely it arises from inhaled contagious effluvia, from snakebites, or from mental disturbances. One may conjecture that the causative poison, whatever its nature, is so fine as to resemble spirit rather than appreciable matter.

In intermittent fever the heat is kindled in the blood by undue expansion of the spirits at regular intervals in accordance with the character of the causative poison (*pro genio veneni eam efficientis*) (71). The identity of this poison—whether generated internally or admitted from the exterior—is as difficult to explain as are the spirits that are imbued with it. Hence its reality, says Morton, must be judged by its effects, that is, by the symptoms that are produced. In intermittent fevers the poisonous ferment apparently is milder than that in any other kind of fever since it is rapidly overcome by Peruvian bark; nor would anyone now assert, as older authors did, that the ferment is situated in receptacles, viscera, or recesses (72).

The most obvious predisposing causes of the intermittents are cold (73) and exposure to the open air. Inspired air, especially autumnal air and the air of swamps, is often full of foreign and poisonous particles. For this reason in swampy and coastal areas intermittent fevers arise endemically; in autumn they become epidemic almost everywhere. The causative poison is intensified by badly cooked food and by emotional disturbances. Moreover, bad hygienic practices, followed for a long time, may cause the poison to be formed within the body.

Morton felt that intermittent fevers are usually to be classed as chronic, although the individual paroxysms are acute. He believed that, whatever his predecessors may have thought, all intermittents are produced by the same ferment—*omnium intermittentium fermentum est ejusdem generis* (78)—since, without apparent cause, they may change their type. This remark is difficult to reconcile with his earlier statement that the timing of the paroxysm depends on the character of the causative poison (*pro genio veneni*) (71). Moreover, Morton judged that identity rather than diversity is shown by the fact that all kinds of intermittent respond equally well to an ounce of Peruvian bark, without the fanfare of deobstruent decoctions and evacuations advocated by previous authors.

The foregoing pages describe Morton's concepts of the acute fevers, especially the intermittents, as presented in the first six chapters of the *Pyretologia* of 1692. The straightforward text is devoid of rhetorical flourishes. The opinions show the independence expected in a religious nonconformist and are based as far as possible on Morton's own observations and his own hypotheses, with relatively little mention of the writings that he can be assumed to have read.

Morton did not refrain from stating hypotheses but he freely and distinctly marked them as such. They impress the modern reader as fanciful and they have not proved durable.[124] Nondogmatic and occasionally self-contradictory, they are best regarded as provisional attempts to explain observed phenomena.

Morton attributed great importance to animal spirits, an entity or concept found repeatedly in Galenic writings. In stating that these spirits are capable of expansion when they are contaminated by miasm, Morton may have reflected iatromechanical influences and, specifically, the work of Boyle.

The humors, as Morton mentioned them, are not really the famous Galenic humors and differ little from ordinary fluids. Moreover, Morton made no claim that yellow bile causes the tertian fever or black bile the quartan.

Morton accepted the Harveian circulation as axiomatic. Using it as a basis, he rejected the old opinion that attributed intermittents to a visceral focus, situated usually in the mesenteric veins. Rightly or wrongly, he judged that according to Harvey's discovery visceral vascular obstruction does not exist. He therefore rejected also the use of drugs that were alleged to be deobstruent.

He referred to the body, incidentally, as a mechanism, but he did not elaborate this opinion.

He stated that fever comes from the heating of blood that has been kindled by animal spirits contaminated by miasm. He referred repeatedly to ferments as important causes of fever; his statements in this respect are not significantly different from those of Willis. He also regarded noxious particles as important causes of diseases such as intermittent fevers; especially in autumn the air might be rich in these pathogens. He did not discuss the relation between particles and ferments.

Morton held that the skin might be a portal of entry for some diseases since cold might come in through the pores. He did not consider the alimentary tract a portal of entry, yet he wrote that badly cooked food might intensify the poison that causes intermittents.

It is not surprising that Morton's speculations should contain components derived from antiquity, from early modern anatomy, and from diverse seventeenth-century sources. The school least represented in his thinking is the iatrochemical. The physician whom he resembles most closely is Sydenham. The resemblance emerges more distinctly in Chapter 4 of this history.

Muralt and Tozzi

In 1689, less than a decade before Morton reached the end of his valuable life, Johannes von Muralt (1645–1733), an eminent Swiss anatomist, surgeon, and professor, issued a note on the successful treatment of fevers by means of Peruvian bark (Muraltus, 1689). This article is significant beyond expectation. Muralt had observed that the symptoms of intermittent fever tended to be alleviated by phlebotomy and catharsis; when these procedures were omitted, treatment by means of drugs was apt to be difficult. For these reasons, and also because of the prominence of such symptoms as nausea, vomiting, anorexia, and eructation, many notable observers had inferred, not without the appearance of correctness—*non sine veritatis specimine* (4)—that the cause of the intermittent fevers must be harbored near the precordia. Muralt did not agree with this opinion.

His essay is valuable to us because it shows, more clearly than a great many writings, that to innumerable competent physicians the old doctrines—humoral, Galenic, and Fernelian—provided a satisfying explanation of observed phenomena. It shows no less clearly the unemphatic dissent of an independent thinker.

Luca Tozzi (1638–1717), professor of medicine in Naples and Malpighi's successor as papal physician, is one of the best of the many good medical writers who have fallen into oblivion. His commentary (1693) on the aphorisms of Hippocrates is both a careful evaluation and a valuable "update" or modernization. Especially close to our theme is his comment on *Aphorisms* 2.25 (1:243–46), in which the ancient sage had observed that summer quartans are apt to be brief, whereas the autumnal ones are long and those of winter are longest.

Tozzi's comment shows that he was a fermentationist, but his use of the expression *fermentorum, sive peccantium humorum* (ferments or peccant humors) (1:243) could be interpreted to indicate either that he considered ferments equivalent to peccant humors or that he was in doubt as to the equivalence.

Like older authors, including Galen, he believed that abdominal viscera are involved in the intermittent fevers. He felt that fevers of this kind might be caused by one kind of humor. He believed also that autumnal fevers tend to be long because pores tend to become clogged; consequently excretion is retarded.

To this collection of opinions that were for the most part antiquated he added that quartan fevers formerly lasted so long that they were classed as chronic diseases but nowadays they are quickly dispelled; this shows how greatly modern medical practice surpasses that of earlier times (1:246). And in the next sentence he says that the Peruvian bark can be given with theriac!

Additional Comment

It is appropriate now to review rapidly a few of the developments that have been mentioned in this appendix and to offer some additional observations concerning them.

The seventeenth century witnessed a high prevalence of war, famine, and fever. Tuberculosis and malaria were widely and heavily endemic. Even Whitehall in London was malarious; the disease was notoriously common among royalty and high ecclesiastics. Superimposed upon the endemicity were epidemic outbreaks of malaria, and also of typhus, typhoid, and influenza. The total incidence of febrile disease was therefore very great.

During the seventeenth century, Galenism was arousing disbelief and opposition, but it had not come to an end. Evidence of contra-Galenic observation and opinion is found in Harvey, Helmont, Willis, Sydenham, and many other authors. Yet Galenic observations could not be discarded wholly; indeed, some have been verified by succeeding ages. Moreover, Galenic humoralism continued to be useful since it offered convenient explanations or convenient frameworks for many phenomena observed in daily clinical practice. For example, as late as 1751 Richard Mead was to state in his *Monita et praecepta medica* that, as Galen had declared, semitertian fever was due to combined obstruction produced by bilious humors and tenacious lymph (40–42). Peruvian bark, he stated, might increase the obstruction and thereby cause a hectic fever. Translated into modern terms this probably means that a fever thought to be a simple tertian and treated with inadequate doses of the bark might come to reveal itself as a malignant tertian or as sepsis or typhoid. Mead's comment, couched in Galenic concepts and terminology, offered a convincing explanation of the clinical sequence.

A special aspect or corollary or concomitant of humoral doctrine, usually overlooked, is its relation to the employment of abdominal palpation in cases of fever. This unexpected concatenation, evident in the writings of Spigelius, outlasted the vicissitudes of iatrochemical and iatromechanical contention and has left its mark on the diagnostic procedures of our own time. In addition it appears almost certain that *general* palpation (as distinct from special abdominal palpation) was also favored by Galenic doctrine. For example, Zacutus Lusitanus, in his paraphrasis (which here is also a scholium) on a case of tertian fever recorded by Galen, mentions equality of heat all over the body as a sign of exquisite tertian fever.[125] Indeed, Galen elsewhere discusses at length the palpatory findings in various kinds of fever.[126] Interesting brief observations on the behavior of the spleen are in the writings of Sydenham[127] and are scattered through the writings of other clinical authors.

The emphasis that historians have justly placed on Galenic influences has tended to reduce the attention paid to the influence of Aristotle, which is exemplified in the writings of Harvey. Much better known to general readers of medical history is the Hippocratic tendency, well represented by Sydenham and Morton.

During the period that is being summarized in these paragraphs a few discoveries proved outstandingly important in the study of fever. The first is William Harvey's discovery of the circulation. An early example of its use or misuse is the Willisian *non sequitur*, repeated by Morton and mentioned earlier in this appendix, that Harvey's discovery had proved intravascular stagnation to be impossible. Important, too, were the discoveries made by Lower, which also influenced Willis.

Another major discovery was the recognition that the Peruvian bark is effective in intermittent fever. The important achievement forms a principal subject in several chapters of this history. Neither discovery produced the immediate overthrow of Galenism,[128] but both assisted in its demise. Also to be mentioned is the discovery of the lymphatics, which I have not undertaken to study in detail. These and other discoveries in physiology, anatomy, and therapeutics stand in contrast to the meager advances that were made in clinical observation of the intermittent fevers during the period under consideration. Many of the clinical descriptions are unimpressive.[129] Labial herpes, a common concomitant of malaria, is rarely mentioned. Malarial splenomegaly, also known to the ancients, often fails to appear in seventeenth-century case reports of fever, although it is found occasionally under the disguise of "splenic obstruction." The distinction between exact and spurious tertians, set forth by Galen and discussed by Mercatus, was mentioned by Piquer as late as 1751 but was soon to disappear from the literature. The syndrome of pernicious tertian fever, described by Mercatus, was discussed by Piquer and is a permanent part of clinical medicine.[130] Necessarily new was the observation of cinchonal tinnitus. The epidemic and exanthematic fevers described by Sydenham are outside the scope of this history.

Since neither the malarial fevers nor the great continued fevers (typhoid and typhus) yield large harvests of conspicuous gross lesions, increase in the number of autopsies produced little advance in the understanding of these diseases. An interesting example, already discussed, was furnished by Spigelius, whose postmortem examinations merely confirmed his Galenic and Fernelian preconceptions. In his cases and in many others, progress was impeded by confusion about postmortem coagula ("polypi"). Probably the most important gross anatomical advances in the study of fever are in Morton's observations of tuberculosis.

It is not surprising that clinical observation should be accompanied by clinical theory, since many physicians abhorred the vacuum of the unexplained. Occasional medical authors, such as Sydenham and Bellini, disliked theories but used them. The seventeenth century, moreover, witnessed the contention between iatrochemical and iatromechanical concepts, just as the eighteenth witnessed repeated efforts to construct medical systems. The literature of both centuries is replete with bold assertions unsupported by evidence, and it is observable that in both centuries many physicians actually used an eclectic approach, reminiscent of ancient eclecticism.[131] Confronted by a bewildering succession of phenomena, the practitioner needed explanations, order, and rationale. He had at his disposal few means of establishing truth. Autopsies were becoming increasingly numerous, but the findings they yielded could not always be interpreted correctly or applied usefully. Statistics was a novelty, not yet in extensive use. Clinical experimentation had hardly begun. In the presence of these deficiencies, reliance was necessarily placed on impressions. Some were crude, others astute.

Appendix B The *Schedula Romana*

THE EARLIEST KNOWN DESCRIPTION of the manner of administering the Peruvian bark is the *Schedula Romana*. The original text was written in Italian, probably in Rome, and almost certainly no earlier than 1647, the year in which Pietro Paolo Puccerini began his service as director of the pharmacy at the Collegium Romanum. Occasional commentators such as Hernándo y Ortega state that two versions appeared, in 1649 and 1651, but no documentation has been given. As the reader will observe, textual analysis shows that more than one prototype existed. Heinrich von Bergen (1826, 92, no. 23) stated that the first edition of the *Schedula* appeared in 1649; he wrote a German translation (see below). Ernst Gotfried Baldinger (1778, 997) stated, without documentation, that a *Schedula medicorum Romanor[um]* was published by Roman druggists on February 17, 1651, and is an instruction for physicians on how to use china bark (Peruvian bark) in intermittent fevers. He added: "It seems to me that two such *Schedulae* appeared."

Among the possible authors are: Gabriele Fonseca (d. 1668), archiater to Pope Innocent X; Cardinal de Lugo; Honoratus Fabri, S.J.; and Pietro Paolo Puccerini. No specimen of the original imprint is known to be extant.

Following is a list of editions of the *Schedula*, including translations and excerpts; probably it is incomplete. The entire Italian text is given below, under Sturmius. The full Latin translation is presented in the earliest available edition, that of Chifletius, 1653; this version was reproduced pseudonymously by Antimus Conygius (Honoratus Fabri) in 1655. An English translation was published by Jaramillo Arango in

1949, and a Spanish translation was published by Hernándo y Ortega in 1982 (see below).

List of Editions, Translations, and Excerpts

Chifletius (1653, 4–5), examined in photocopy kindly furnished by the Wellcome Institute for the History of Medicine. The complete text is as follows:

Adfertur cortex iste ex Peruuiano Regno, vocaturque China febris; exhibetur contra febrem tertianam & quartanam, quae cum frigore aegros prehendunt, & quae per multos dies sunt confirmatae. Praeparatur autem in hunc modum: Corticis drachmae duae tunduntur subtiliter, ac per setaceum traiiciuntur. Tribus horis ante paroxismum puluis maceratur in vini albi potentis cyatho dumque frigus febrile incipit, vel sentitur aliquod leue accessionis principium sumitur tota dosis praeparata, aegerque se componit in lecto. Constat experientiâ omnes ferè, qui eo puluere sunt vsi, à febre liberatos fuisse, purgato benè priùs corpore, et quaternis à sumptione diebus abstinendo ab omni alio medicamento. Sed non est assumendus nisi praeuio Medici consilio, qui iudicet de modo & tempore quod sumptioni sit opportunum.

Comparison of Chiflet's text with the Italian and Latin texts given by Sturmius shows not a single omission, although the clause *et quae per multos dies sunt confirmatae* appears in Chifletius immediately after *exhibetur contra febrem tertianam & quartanam quae cum frigore aegros prehendunt*, whereas in Sturmius the equivalent appears later, namely after *aegerque remandatur ad lectum*. This difference in arrangement defines two different textual traditions. Moreover, Haggis erred when he wrote (1941, 443) that Chiflet in 1653 "gives excerpts from the *Schedula*, translated into Latin." The Chifletian text is complete.

A copy of Chiflet's version, lacking only the first sentence and showing a few tiny changes, is in Larrieu, 1889, 104.

Conygius [Fabri], 1655.

This work includes (45–88) a complete reprint of Chifletius, 1653. Chiflet's complete Latin translation of the *Schedula* is preceded by an introductory statement (51): *prodiitque typis Romae Schedion, quod ex Italico sic Latinum feci.* The translation proper appears on pages 51–52 of the book and is an accurate reproduction of that given by Chiflet.

Sturmius, 1659, part 1, 146–50. (Italian text of *Schedula*, 146–48; Latin translation, 148–50.)

Sturmius (145) introduces the Italian text with the words, *Primò igi-*

tur hìc offero Schedam Authenticam, quae talis est. This is followed (146–48) by the text proper:

Modo di adoprare la Corteccia chiamata della Febre.

Questa Corteccia si porta dal Regno di Peru, e si chiama China, o vero China della febre, laquale si adopra per la febre quartana, e terzana, che venga con freddo: s'adopra in questo modo, cioè:

Se ne piglia dramme due, e si pista fina, con passarla per setaccio; e tre hore prima incirca, che debba venir la febre si mette in infusione in un bicchiero di vino bianco [147] gagliardissimo, e quando il freddo commincia à venire, ò si sente qualche minimo principio, si prende tutta la presa preparata, e si mette il patiente in letto.

Avertasi, si potrà dare detta Corteccia nel modo sudetto nella febre terzana, quando quella sia fermata in stato di molti giorni.

L'esperienza continua, hà liberato quasi tutti quelli, che l'hanno presa, purgato prima bene il corpo, e per quattro giorni doppo non pigliar' niuna sorte di medicamento; ma avvertasi di non darla [148] se non con licenza delli Sig: Medici, acciò giudicano se sia in tempo à proposito di pigliarla.

In the Latin translation by Sturmius (148–50), the wording differs from that of Chiflet. For example, in Sturmius the first sentence after the caption reads, "Cortex hic advehitur ex Regno Peruvii vocaturque China, sive China febris qui adhibetur ad febrem quartanam & tertianam, quae cum frigore invadunt, paraturque hoc modo," whereas Chiflet reads, *"Adfertur cortex iste ex Peruuiano Regno, vocaturque China febris; exhibetur contra febrem tertianam & quartanam, quae cum frigore aegros prehendunt, & quae per multos dies sunt confirmatae. Praeparatur autem in hunc [52] modum."*

Sturmius's Latin translation ends: "Cave tamen, eundem exhibere absque consilio Medicorum, qui judicent an tempus assumtioni sit opportunum," whereas Chiflet ends, "Sed non est assumendus nisi praeuio Medici consilio, qui iudicet de modo & tempore quod sumptioni sit opportunum." These differences are sufficient to indicate that the Latin translation of Chiflet and that of Sturmis were made independently.

Joncquet, D. 1659.

On page 29 a discussion of cinchona bark begins, "Romam, vnde dumtaxat prodijt Italico idiomate schedium illus Latinum factum." This is followed by a slightly condensed translation, which begins, "Adsportatur ex Peruuiano Regno cortex dictus China febris, laudatur aduersus febres." The wording differs from that given by other authors listed in the present census. The authorship of the translation is not stated, hence it can be assumed that the version was written by Joncquet.

Bartholinus, 1661, 108–9. The schedule is introduced by the words, "Schedion Romae Italica lingua prodiit . . . cujus hic sensus: Cortex hic ex Peru Regno affertur . . . qui febribus . . . cum frigore invadetibus adhibetur." It lacks the words "& quae per multos dies sunt confirmatae," which occurs at this point in the translation given by Chiflet, 1653, but not in that of Badus, 1663, or in the Latin and Italian presentations of Sturmius, 1659. It also contains, at the end of the sixth sentence of the text, the expression, "nec assumatur nisi elapsis 25 vel 30 diebus, ex consilio dominorum medicorum," which is not in the authors just cited. In addition it contains a final cautionary sentence not found in these authors, "Observandum, opus non esse forti alia purgatione ad hujus pulveris usum, si per morbi necessitatem corpus satis sit expurgatum: sufficiet pridie alvum fuisse laxam quocunq[ue] leniore medicamento vel clystere."

These differences show that the Bartholinus translation is a distinct and original product. At the same time it should be noted that Bartholinus followed Sturmius's order of sentences.

Brunacius, 1661, 17. The first chapter of this book is titled "De Cinae Cinae Historia" and contains, on page 17, an explanatory sentence: "Vt autem tutius eius vsus adoleret, & ad febres omnes frigidas dictas, seu quae cum frigore, & rigore inuadunt securiori pacto vsurparetur Schedion fuit." This is followed by a two-sentence Latin excerpt from the *Schedula:* "Corticis dracmae duae tunduntur subtiliter, ac per setaceum traijciuntur. Tribus inde horis ante paroxismum maceratur puluis in vini albi meracioris ciatho, dumque frigus febrile, seu rigor irrepere incipit, in eo leui, ac primo accessionis principio vinum, & puluis praebetur, & aeger se in lecto pannis coopertus componit."

The excerpt is limited to the dosage, preparation, and administration of the drug. It lacks the first one and a half sentences and the last two sentences that appear in the Latin of Chiflet. In the passage presented by Brunacius the expression "in vini albi meracioris ciatho" replaces the less pretentious "in vini albi potentis cyatho" of Chiflet, and "dumque frigus febrile, seu rigor irrepere incipit" is given where Chiflet reads simply "dumque frigus febrile incipit." Further, Brunacius says "aeger se in lecto pannis coopertus componit," whereas Chiflet simply says "aegerque componit in lecto."

These and a few smaller differences, found neither in Chiflet nor in any of the other versions, show that Brunacius's excerpt was based on the text given in Chiflet but introduced a few small variations and elaborations, at least two of which were in the direction of elegance.

Badus, 1663, 119–20.

Badus reproduced Chiflet's translation, which he prefaced with these words: "Formulam exhibendi corticem latine dedit Chifletius, exceptam ab ea, quae Romana lingua, scilicet Italica series latinae est ista."

In Badus's presentation the first sentence of the text proper ends with the words, "quae cum frigore aegros praehendunt" (Chiflet reads *prehendunt*). Badus omitted the immediately subsequent clause, "et quae per multos dies sunt confirmatae." In both the Italian and the Latin versions given by Sturmius, and likewise in the version given by Bartholinus, this passage is transferred to a subsequent part of the *Schedula*. This difference allows us to infer that Sturmius and Bartholinus did not copy Chiflet but used the original handbill, while Bartholinus translated either the handbill itself or the Italian text reproduced by Sturmius. Curiously, the clause omitted from Badus's presentation of the *Schedula* appears elsewhere in his book (108).

In addition to quoting the text given by Chiflet, Badus (123) states that he had obtained a copy from the Collegium Romanum.

Two minor deviations by Badus, his use of *ex Peruviae Regno* where Chiflet reads *ex Peruuiano Regno* and his *aliquod accessionis principium* where Chiflet reads *aliquod leue accessionis principium*, probably signify carelessness or haste; we know from the *Anastasis* (2) that Badus was a very busy man.

In sum, Badus's version is close to being what he announced in his introductory sentence, namely a copy of Chifletius.

Rothmann, 1663, fols. [374]–[383].

Rothmann presents a complete version of the *Schedula*, which differs notably from that given by Chiflet. For example, the opening sentence reads: "Cortex hic advehitur ex Regno Peruviano vocaturque China s[eu] China febris, qui adhibetur ad febres, tertianam et quartanam." This text differs from that of Chiflet and from the condensed version of Ioncquet (Joncquet), 1659. These deviations are somewhat surprising because Rothmann precedes his version by the words, "Patefacit has nobis schedium Romanum Italicô idiomate prius ad nos allatum, quod Chifletius et ex eo Joncquetus ita verterunt (These [precautions] are set forth for us in the Roman leaflet which first came to us in Italian and which Chiflet, and Joncquet, following him, rendered as follows)."

Bergen, 1826, 92, presents an accurate and slightly condensed German translation of the Latin version given by Chiflet. Where Chiflet reads, "contra febrem tertianam & quartanam quae cum frigore aegros prehendunt, & quae per multos dies sunt confirmatae," Bergen says simply, "wird gegen das Tertian- und Quartan-Fieber gebraucht, doch muss dieses sich schon gesetzt haben." And where Chiflet reads, "Corticis drachmae duae tunduntur subtiliter, ac per setaceum traiiciuntur. Tribus horis ante paroxysmum," Bergen omits mention of filtration and merely says "Zwei Drachmen der Rinde werden fein gestossen, dieses Pulver wir dann drey Stunden vor dem Paroxismus." These are the only deviations.

The omissions in Bergen's version are different from those in Brunacius.

Flückiger, and Hanbury, 1874, 304, n. 4, 1879, 343–44, n. 5. These authors refer to the *Schedula Romana* as "the handbill of 1651" and reproduce accurately the Italian text given by Sturmius.

Suppan, 1931, 29–138. On p. 35 Suppan reproduces, from the second edition of Flückiger and Hanbury, the Italian text given by Sturmius (see above). Suppan's version contains at least eighteen errors, for example, *cive* for *cioè*, *Si* for *Se*, *ore* for *hore*.

Jaramillo Arango, 1949 (plus plates 10–21). On pages 306–7 there is a slightly inaccurate transcription of Sturmius's Italian text and on page 297 an English translation.

Hernándo y Ortega, 1982, 194–95. A complete Spanish translation is probably based on Sturmius since the preceding sentence reads, "Reproducido por Rolando Sturmio." Hernándo y Ortega says also (194) that two texts are known, one of 1649 and one of 1651, but fails to document this statement.

Summary

The comparison of texts described in the foregoing pages shows that at least *two* slightly different texts were in use, the difference consisting mainly in the translocation of the words, *quando quella sia fermata in stato di molti giorni* (Latin: *quae per multos dies jam confirmata est*).

One version of the *Schedula* appeared in Latin in 1653 in Chiflet's book and was reproduced, with or without variation, in the Latin editions of Fabri (who used the pseudonym Antimus Conygius, 1655), Badus (1663), Brunacius (1661), and Bergen (1826). It is impossible to determine whether the dislocation that characterizes the texts in this group was introduced by Chiflet or was present in the Italian original that he used.

The second tradition is represented by the Italian of Sturmius (1659), his Latin translation (1659), the independently fashioned Latin version of Bartholinus (1661), the Italian of Flückiger (1874, 1879) and Suppan (1931), and Jaramillo Arango's English translation. The abbreviated Latin translation by Joncquet (1659) is not assignable to either tradition.

Both traditions include examples of independent translation into Latin, namely those by Chiflet, Sturmius, Bartholinus, and Joncquet. This is hardly surprising in an age when Latin was the language of the learned in the Western world.

The present review mentions eight editions, transcriptions, and excerpts published between 1653 and 1663. In addition the literature contains occasional references to the *Schedula*. The most important are those in Richard Morton's *Pyretologia* (1692, 174–76), which reveal that Morton had exact knowledge of the dosage prescribed in the leaflet and that, because available supplies of the bark were adulterated, he had been obliged to increase the dose from two drachms to one, two, or even three *ounces*.

At one point in his extensive discussion Morton added that, according to another rule in the *Schedula*, immediately after ingesting the entire dose of cinchona the patient should go to bed and should be covered by the bedclothes. This statement, like the rest of the *Pyretologia*, is written in Latin but is set in italics, which suggest that it is a quotation. Mention of bedclothes is not found in Badus's version of the *Schedula* but occurs in the brief and differently worded version by Brunacius (1661). From these fragments of evidence it appears probable that Morton's statement is an independent translation or paraphrase that could have been based on any of the texts discussed in this analysis.

Morton's remarks demonstrate that the *Schedula* was in active use for at least four decades. Probably its withdrawal from practical usefulness should be ascribed to his influence. Confronted by the need to use samples of cinchona that were adulterated or otherwise impaired or falsified, and confronted also by the resultant clinical relapses and failures, he was obliged to go beyond the modest dosage recommended in the *Schedula*.

Subsequent mentions of the leaflet show a transition from the pharmaceutical and posologic to the historical. This trend is evident in remarks made by Sir George Baker (1785, 202), followed by those of Sprengel (1821–38, 4:519) and Bergen (1826, 92), to which we may justly add the texts and translations given by Flückiger (1874, 1879), Suppan (1931), Jaramillo Arango (1949), and Hernándo y Ortega (1982).

The *Schedula Romana* was far from being the only pharmaceutical handbill circulated in the seventeenth century. An interesting parallel is furnished by the Electuarium Orvietanum, a modified theriac alleged to be effective against plague. Its formula is given in Schröder, 1649–50, 184. According to a handbill that is said to have been extant recently, the drug was popular in the time of Urban VIII. Later it was hawked by one Antonio Theodorich in a booth in Venice and continued to be sold at least until the end of the seventeenth century. Additional information is in Schelenz [1904] 1965, 522, 524.

Appendix C Torti's *Synopsis*—The Latin Text

Synopsis
Libri, Cui Titulus, Therapeutice Specialis
Ad Febres Quasdam Perniciosas, inopinatò, ac repente lethales, una verò
CHINA CHINA *peculiari methodo ministrata sanabiles*

Aucta Curationum Historiis, Quaestionibus, ac Animadversionibus practicis, aliisque plurimis variam hujusmodi Febrium habitudinem, Intermittentium omnium, quin & Continuarum naturam, & Chinae Chinae praestantiam, actionemque respicientibus, nec non usum, & abusum illius in singulis Febrium speciebus. In gratiam Juniorum praesertim & Candidatorum Artis Auctore FRANCISCO TORTO MUTI-NENSI Sereniss. Raynaldi I. Mut. Reg. &c. Ducis Medico, & in Patrio Lyceo Pr. Med. Professore.

Licet propositum, seu primaria intentio hujusce Tractatus sit tradere minus tritam, & vulgari praxi, atque notione semotam FEBRIUM quarundam EXITIALIVM, in extremo etiam earum periculo, curationem, ope CHINAE CHINAE peculiariter administratae: complectitur is nihilominus considerationem quoque, ac examen integrum CVIVSCVMQVE oblationis ejusdem Chinae Chinae in QVIBVSVIS Febrium speciebus, juxta id, quod suadent Ratio maturior, & Experientia comparata usu non interrupto hujusce Febrifugi per triginta annos, & ultra; ut ideo Tyronibus praecipue inter oppo-[2]sitas saepe opiniones fluctuantibus nil desit ad completam cognitionem practicam, tum Febrium omnium (praesertim PERNICIOSARVM quarundam) in quibus convenit China China, tum Remedii ipsius hic, & nunc congruenter, atque utiliter administrandi.

Dividitur propterea totus Tractatus in quattuor Sectiones, quarum series compendiose hic exhibetur.

Prima Sectio, caeteris, quibus praeludit, universalior, & in decem rursus Capita subsecta, usumque COMMVNIOREM Chinae Chinae in DIVTVRNIS tantùm Intermittentibus respiciens, patefacit quomodo innotuerit primum FRASSONO Practico eximio, & Auctoris Praeceptori, statim ac appulit in Italiam, imò in Europam Peruvianus Cortex, & successive postmodum ipsi Auctori. V VLGATIOR illius oblatio in Intermittentibus BENIGNIORIBVS, selectioresque illum praescribendi formulae obiter recensetur. Consideratur praestantia, & innocentia Remedii in concursu complurium satis celebrium supereminentis, etsi omnem metum recidivae non semper excludat. Examinatur per extensum Antipathia Eorum, qui Corticem criminose reprobant, refelluntur objectiones, & recividatum inhibendarum certiores modi indicantur. Ostenditur Virtutem illius, etsi absque sensibili evacuatione saepius (non tamen semper) exercitam, non ideo infidam esse, ac respuendam. Inquiritur per varia experimenta, in quo consistat ineffabilis illius vis, probaturque usum ejusdem, sensibiles licet evacuationes non inducentis, cohaerere vel ipsi Galenicorum, ac Humoristarum Doctrinae. Expenduntur cursim celebriores quoque Neotericorum opiniones circa Intermittentium Causas, iisque pariter omnibus operatio Corticis nil sensibile evacuantis adaptatur. Eliciuntur deinde ex opinionibus istis magis receptis verosimilia quaedam Theoremata generalia circa naturam, & causas Intermittentium Febrium, juxta quae statuitur, & dirigitur VVLGARIS oblatio Corticis. Circa abstrusas verò, & penitiores istarum Causas solùm nutante gressu conquisitas, informis quaedam se prodit Auctoris Idea, cui propterea vel Ipse nequaquam acquiescit. His praemissis proponitur Quaestio, An in principio earundem Intermittentium VVLGARIVM, hoc est periculo de morte carentium, [p]ossit, aut debeat exhiberi Cortex, ut in ipsarum progressu: & solvitur cum distinctione. Quaeritur pariter, An ante illius oblationem debeat praemitti Purgatio aut Venae Sectio, & pariter cum distinctione respondetur, ostenditurque, quam parum proficua generaliter sit in ipsis Intermittentibus (ncdum in Continuis) aluina dejectio, tum maxime artificialis, tum non rarò etiam spontanea, ni morbus jam simul declinet; Quod quidem dimissa etiam ratione, & auctoritate, peculiaribus tantùm Casibus in hanc rem adjectis, atque descriptis, sola experientia, fit palam. Denique ad normam distinctionum supradictarum, pro tempestivo, moderato, & congruo Corticis usu in iisdem ORDINARIIS Intermittentibus, Historiae aliquot afferuntur, opportunis animadversionibus identidem respersae, quae Distinctiones easdem supra enunciatas in omnibus earum partibus illustrant, atque confirmant.

Secunda Sectio, octo Capitibus comprehensa, nil aliud exhibet, nisi descriptionem earum Febrium PERNICIOSARVM in communi, ex natura sua, & primo saltem ortu Intermittentium, quae vel tertia, quarta, quintave Accessione Aegrum, caeteroqui diebus vacuis bene se habentem, inopinatò, & quasi repente tollunt de medio, vel ad acquirendam continuitatem, acutiem, ac malignitatem proxime vergunt, cum Vitae periculo minùs quidem praecipiti, sed non minùs gravi. Quia verò de his omnibus Febri-[3]bus, & de singulis, vel saltem praecipuis, earum speciebus, unus inter Antiquos luculenter egit (easdem ut periculo, & terrore plenas graphiche delineans) LVDOVICVS MERCATVS: inter Recentiores verò, pressiùs licet, ac subobscuriùs (feliciùs tamen eas curans, China China inventa) RICHARDVS MORTON, Primi ideo Auctoris Tractatulus integer, Secundi vero peculiare quoddam Caput recusa exhibentur, quae breviorem hanc Sectionem magna ex parte constituunt. Vtrique autem Auctori fusiora, ut congruum visum est, adjuncta sunt Scholia, Illi quidem ad aliqualem castigationem veteris Doctrinae, atque ad indicanda quaedam notatu digniora. Isti verò ad clariorem explicationem rei, & ad moderamen aliquod tum usus liberalioris Chinae Chinae, tum hypotheseos Febrium ab eodem adstructae.

Tertia Sectio, quae potissima est, duodecim diffusis Capitibus PECVLIAREM Chinae Chinae administrationem in praedictis PERNICIOSIS complexa, exponit Naturam, Morem, Diagnosim, atque Prognosim ipsarum Perniciosarum, juxta observationem Auctoris, Dividuntur illae, juxta Eundem, in octo Species singillatim descriptas. Earundem Perniciosarum, qua talium, Causae generaliores superficie tenus considerantur, ut & varia illarum actio in triplicem nostri corporis regionem. Adducitur denique ipsarum Curatio per usum Chinae Chinae minùs tritum, aperiturque METHODUS PECVLIARIS, certis regulis, modis, atque cautionibus, ex praxi rationali deductis, constituta, qua mediante plurimi ab Orci faucibus evidenter erepti sunt, atque identidem eripiuntur, sanati videlicet, non modò priusquam res ruant in praeceps (tunc enim quaelibet Methodus, etiam vulgaris, apta est, dummodo Cortex tempestive offeratur) verum etiam (atque in hoc consistit summa rei) postquam actum videtur de Aegri Vita inopinatò iam corruente dummodo ad vigintiquatuor horas circiter ea sit protrahenda; Quam Curationem in talibus circumstantiis caeteroqui sperare non licet, nisi aliquando fortu[i]tò, ab ullo a[lio] Remedio, neque ab eadem China China qualibet alia Methodo administrata. Comparatur ideo in universum haec Methodus cum Methodis celebrioribus Aliorum, puta TALBOTII, HELVETII, nec non ipsius MORTONI, cujus Methodo licet ista propior sit,. . . . eadem tamen non parum discriminatur, quippe certior, ac industrior, inventaque ab Auctore, & exercita, priusquam Genevae cusa forent Opera MORTONI. Revocatur postmodum ad examen particulare Eadem Methodus, perpenditur illius

praestantia, utilitas, & quiquid habet singulare, ac novum in caetera-
rum, quae prostant, concursu: siquidem quicquam novi allatura est Ex-
teris, ut attulit in Patria Auctoris, ubi antea nemini nota, sive spectemus
peculiarem dispositionem, & administrationem Remedii, sive Febres
ipsas vim illius eludere, quin & respuere creditas, sive circumstantias
caeteroqui lethales, in quibus nihilominus felicissime usurpatur. Defenditur itaque ab objectionibus facilè excogitabilibus, & a vulgi dicter-
iis, tandemque determinantur circumstantiae ipsae, in quibus ea lo-
cum habet, & in quibus non. Recensentur idcirco fideliter, &
describuntur ingenue Casus omnes infausti (pauci quidem) quibus in-
sons China China prodesse non potuit. Contra subnectuntur plurimi
inter quam plurimos vere mirabiles Casus, singulis octo Perniciosarum
Febrium Speciebus abunde correspondentes, Personarum cujusc-
unque ordinis, & conditionis, sanatarum hac methodo in hanc usque
diem, exordio ducto ab anno 1695, quo primum ab Auctore excogitata
fuit, & in usum, feliciter deducta eadem Methodus, quin & pluribus
statim Vr[4]bis Medicis in publicam utilitatem candide communicata.
Denique clauditur Sectio arduo, & maximi ponderis in praxi Quaesito,
Num scilicet quando Perniciosae octavae Speciei, quae nempe de Intermittentibus, vel QVASI, degenerant in Continuas essentiales, atque
malignas, id moliuntur citissimè, ac in ipso statim PRINCIPIO (cujus
phaenomeni haud infrequens est occursus in praxi) expediat, aut liceat
ILLICO Peruviano Cortice oblato intercipere cursum illarum, & inhibere
effervescentiam febrilem, forsan depurativam, ut licet quanto peden-
tentim id fit, ac in earum PROGRESSV: etsi febres hujusmodi non tam
certum, & praeceps exitium, ut Perniciosae reliquarum Specierum, sed
anceps tantummodo, ac serius periculum minitentur, quod idem est ac
quaerere, An certò servanda periclitantis Hominis Vita cum suspicione
incerta novi morbi, an reliquenda in discrimine. Examinatur serio
Quaesitum, nec plane enodatur; Distinguitur tamen utiliter, dum ana-
lytice pertractatur, ac subinde adducuntur nonnulla exempla felicia sic
sanatorum in ipso talium Febrium principio, ubi, etiam ex tunc, ratione
vehementiae Symptomatum, metus longe praevalebat spei: quae quidem Exempla fidentiam aliquam circa hoc (non sine magna tamen,
prudentique cautela) perito, ac circumspecto Medico possunt exhibere.

Quarta denique Sectio stans quasi Corollarii loco, & sex tantùm
Capitibus absoluta, consideratis obiter, quantum sat est ad intentum,
Febrium omnium CONTINVARVM speciebus, aut differentiis, resolvit
Quaestiones nonnullas circa usum Peruviani Corticis, An scilicet illum
liceat offerre cum fructu, & utilitate sensibili in Febribus, ut quiunt,
Putridis CONTINVIS CONTINENTIBVS, seu NON REMITTENTIBVS, tum PRIMA-
RIIS, ac ESSENTIALIBVS, tum SYMPTOMATICIS, aut COMITATIS, INFLAMMA-
TORIIS videlicet &c, iisque tam MALIGNIS, quam ACVTIS simpliciter; &

negatur; multòque magis negatur in HECTICIS veris. In Hecticis autem, ut aiunt, Puerilibus, seu potius LENTIS Hecticas aemulantibus Chinam Chinam posse prodesse, videntur suadere nonnulli Casus felices Auctori comperti, atque descripti. Quaeritur pariter an Ea conveniat in Febribus per SVBINTRANTES accessus CONTINVIS redditis, item in COMPLICATIS, ut ajunt, puta HAEMITHRITAEIS &c. & asseritur. In Continuis autem simpliciter dictis, seu CONTINVIS PROPORTIONATIS, hoc est NON CONTINENTIBVS quidem, sed periodice RECRVDESCENTIBVS, ET REMITTENTIBUS, distinguitur. Et hic explicatur, atque ex parte defenditur MORTONVS, qui caeteroqui, ut nimius in pluribus aliis casibus circa usum Corticis, non plane potest admitti. Denique ad dispiciendos generaliter Casus omnes, in quibus China China conveniat, aut non, universalis categoria Febrium, earumque varia Metamorphosis illam modò admittens, & modò non, ob oculos ponitur. Disquiritur tandem, An idem Remedium congruat aliis Morbis, praesertim periodicis, praeter Febres: nec satis creditur; & an per clysteres injectum, vel carpis appositum quicquam curationi Febrium confere valeat; neque praxis hujusmodi, utut imbecilla, plane contemnitur.

MVTINAE, Typis Bartholomaei Soliani Impress, Duc[is] 1709. SVPERIORVM PERMISSV.

Appendix D Editions of the *Therapeutice Specialis*, 1712–1928

SOURCES: the holdings of the National Library of Medicine and a computer printout dated March 9, 1989; the *National Union Catalog, pre-1956 Imprints*, vol. 225 (Washington, 1978, 226). Each of these entries has been checked by S.J. Supplementary information was obtained from Di Pietro, 1958, 469–71, and by visits and correspondence with libraries in Italy, England, Scotland, Spain, Belgium, and Holland.

The significance of the data is discussed in Chapter 9.

Editions

Modena: Soliani, 1712, 736 pp. First edition. Dedicated to Raynaldus I, Duke of Modena, Reggio, Mirandola, &c. Preface by author; five books of text, divided into 36 chapters.

Modena: Soliani, 1730, 576 pp. Second edition ("editio auctior"). Characterized correctly by Di Pietro as the fundamental edition of the work, reproduced in subsequent editions.

New dedication, to Hans Sloane, "Baronetto," replaces earlier dedication to Raynaldus I. Extensive new preface to the reader (v–vii).

Book 1, chap. 5, has amplified chapter title (52); two new paragraphs on obstruction of chyliferous ducts and on Bellini's lentor, both of which had been falsely alleged to cause intermittent fever (56–57).

Book 1, chap. 10, pp. 126–30, contains five new paragraphs, in which there are three case reports; the first is dated 1709, the others date from 1728.

Book 5, chap. 6, has new statement containing refutation of Morton's opinions on usefulness of Peruvian bark in cases of hemoptysis

(516–28). Extensive insert, titled *Quaeritur Tertio,* on indiscriminate use of the bark (530, line 1 to 542, line 10).

Venice: Basilus, 1732, 526 pp. Third edition. Reproduces the *Responsiones
jatro-apologeticae* of 1715.

Venice: Basilius, 1743, 520 pp. Fourth edition. Reproduces the amplified
text of 1730, the *Responsiones jatro-apologeticae* (1715), the epistolary
dissertations on the barometer (1695, 1698). Also contains three letters
from Torti to Muratori (xxii–xxxvii) and Muratori's biography of Torti
(ix–xxi). The three letters to Muratori are part of a series of four; the
second letter is missing.

Venice: Basilius, 1755. 496 pp. Fifth edition. For Italian translation of this
edition (Lega, 1928), see below.

Frankfurt and Leipzig: Fleischer, 1756, 496 pp. Fifth edition [*sic*]. 2 vols.
in 1. Includes the *Responsiones jatro-apologeticae* (1715) and the two
epistolary dissertations on the barometer (1695, 1698).

Venice: Basilius, 1769, 484 pp. Sixth edition. In National Library of Medicine; not listed by Di Pietro.

Louvain, 1781, 2 vols. (cited by Di Pietro, 471).

Louvain, 1821 (cited by Di Pietro, 471).

Liège (Leodii): Bassompierre, 1821. New edition, edited by C. C. J. Tombeur and O. Brixhe. Latin introduction by editors, two pages not numbered; two introductions to the reader, reproduced from the editions of
1730 and 1732, written by Torti (xxiv–xxxviiij); and the biography by
Muratori from the edition of 1743 (i–xxiii). Includes Torti's explanation
of his diagram, the Tree of Fevers, but does not include the diagram
itself. Vol. 2 (1–254) reproduces the *Responsiones jatro-apologeticae*
(1715).

Rome: Camera dei deputati, 1925. Reproduction of "sixth" edition (Venice,
1769) under editorship of Professor Vittorio Ascoli. In National Library
of Medicine and Biblioteca Nazionale Centrale Vittorio Emmanuele II,
Rome.

Rome: Pozzi, 1928, 308 pp. *La terapia speciale delle febbri perniciose.* Italian
translation, by G. Lega, of the fifth edition, Venice, 1755.

Holdings in Major Libraries

The National Library of Medicine in a computer printout dated March 8, 1989, reported the following: Modena, 1712; Modena, 1730; Venice, 1732; Venice, 1743; Venice, 1755; Frankfurt, 1756;
Venice, 1769; Liège, 1821.

The *British library general catalogue of printed books to 1975,* London, 1986, 328:65, lists three editions: Modena, 1712; Modena, 1730;
Frankfurt and Leipzig, 1756.

The general catalog of the Bibliothèque Nationale (Authors), vol.

191, column 1069, lists: Modena, 1712; Modena, 1730; Frankfurt and Leipzig, 1756.

The library of the New York Academy of Medicine lists: Modena, 1712; Modena, 1730; Venice, 1732; Venice, 1743 (microfilm); Liège, 1821.

The card catalog of the Biblioteca Apostolica Vaticana lists no printed work by Torti.

The Biblioteca Estense of Modena possesses: Modena, 1712; Modena, 1730; Venice, 1743; Rome, 1928.

The Biblioteca Nazionale Centrale V.E. II lists: Modena, 1712; Venice, 1732; Venice, 1755; Rome, 1925.

Notes

Unless otherwise indicated, references to Galen are to the 1964–65 edition of C. G. Kühn. Citations use the letter K, followed by volume and page numbers.

Preface and Acknowledgments

1. Linnaeus, 1742, 527.
2. La Wall, 1932, 24.

Chapter 1. Two Rival Historical Traditions

1. This part of the discussion is based chiefly on Badus, 1663. Additional information is available in Baldus, 1656. See also [Badus], 1656. The last-named volume is a collection of essays by several authors, some of them anonymous. It contains an anonymous introductory letter, pp. 3–36, which is shown by internal evidence to have been written by Badus, who also collected the other component essays; Badus makes brief mention of the *China china* (Peruvian bark) on p. 16 of his introduction. An apparently unique copy of the volume is in the Biblioteca Civile of Genoa. Additional details are given in Chapter 2. Public-health reports and other papers signed by Badus are in the Archivio di Stato in Genoa.

See also Rompel, 1932. The change from Baldus to Badus is recorded in Badus, 1663, 4–5.

2. "Verum, ne quid dissimulem, suspicor de aliqua antilogia inter Bollum, et Pharmacopaeum Rom[ani] Collegii." Badus, 1663, 19.

3. Badus, 1663, 1. In 1985 the archdiocese of Genoa, at my request, graciously instituted a search for information about Rev. Federicus Conti. Don Luigi Alfonso reported that no records of this person were found. It is possible that Conti was of Genoese birth but worked elsewhere. The Pammatone Hospital, founded in 1423, was partly destroyed by bombardments in 1942 and 1945. See Carpaneto da Langasco, 1953, 400–401; Manno, 1898, 309–10; and Pescetto, 1846, 1:273–84.

4. Badus, 1663, 16–17. I have been unable to find the text of Bollus's letter or

any biographical information about him. Dr. Aldo Agosto, director of the Archivio di Stato, Genoa, has sent word (letter, 18 July 1986) of the following facts, recorded in *Notizie di famiglie liguri*, MS. Bibl. 169, p. 90: the Bolli, an old and noble Genoese family, came to live in Genoa in 1188 A.D.; one member was among the citizens who were involved in relations between Pisa and Genoa in that year.

5. Loxa, now called Loja, is situated at 3°59′S and 79°16′W. During the period of this history it belonged to the *audiencia* or presidency of Quito, which was part of the viceroyalty of Peru. Nowadays it forms part of the Republic of Ecuador. S.v. "Ecuador," *Encyclopaedia Britannica*, 1953, 7:936–45 (esp. 942). *Encyclopedia of World History*, 1968, 532.

6. Trousseau and Pidoux, 1858, 2:334.

7. Ruiz López, 1792, 2.

8. The reader may enjoy the elaborate essay by Leo Suppan, 1931, 29–138 (see esp. 33). A more recent repetition of the tale is in Bastien, 1987, 144. Of Markham, the *Dictionary of National Biography*, 1975, 2781, states significantly: "It was inevitable that much of his published work should show signs of over-hasty production. . . . He was in all things an enthusiast rather than a scholar." See also Markham, 1874 and 1880. Humboldt, 1807, 1:57–68, 104–20 (see 60).

9. Rompel, 1905, 1–64; 1929; 1931, 416–51. (Rompel [1931, 418] lists the contents of a second part of this work, but it was never published; see also a review in *Archivum Historicum Societatis Iesu* 2 [1933]: 169.) Vargas Ugarte, 1928, 291–301; 1963–1965, 2:29–33. Haggis, 1941: see esp. 448 for critique of Badus: "Singularly destined was the work of Sebastiano Bado to mislead posterity. His compatriots of the seventeenth century almost without exception were equally unreliable, yet the works of these early Italians assumed an authoritative ascendancy which, on the score of accuracy, they did not merit." This strong pronouncement does not do justice to Badus's frank recognition of discrepancy in the statements that were available to him (see Badus, 1663, 19, and note 2 above). Jaramillo Arango, 1949, with twelve plates and one text figure, is more easily accessible than its Spanish counterpart, *Estudio crítico acerca de los hechos básicos de la historia de la quina, Anales de la sociedad peruana de historia de la medicina* 10: 31–88, 1949. Valuable but less extensive are the documented contributions of Blanco Juste, 1935, and Zegarra, 1879.

10. Cobo's *Historia del nuevo mundo* (1956) was completed by 1653 and first published in 1890. The copy of Calancha (1638, vol. 1) in the New York Public Library contains a series of permissions dated from Lima and Barcelona, 1633–37. Two of them are dated 1633; if we allow Calancha at least three years for the writing of his book, we may guess that he knew of the bark by 1630. The suggestion made by Vargas Ugarte, 1963–65, 1:29, n. 2, that Calancha probably copied from Cobo is not supported by comparison of texts.

11. Haggis, 1941, 570–82. The dates are based on the *Municipal Archives of Chinchon* and on the Archivo General de las Indias in Seville.

12. Suardo, 1935. In the final official report of his tenure as viceroy the count of Chinchon mentions the laborious record compiled daily by Suardo: "encargado lo mas prolixo de ese cuidado al Doctor Don Ioan Antonio Suardo." Chinchon, 1640 (see fol. 14r.).

13. Badus, 1663, 202. This is discussed in Rompel, 1931, 428, and Haggis, 1941, 581–82. Guerra (1977b, 117) points out that the name is Villarroel, not Villerobel. (N.B. The Madrid telephone directory for 1984–85, 2:1283, shows fifty-three entries under Villarroel and not one under Villerobel.)

14. Misdesignated as Juan *de Vigo* by Garrison, 1929, 290, and as Juan *del Vigo*, ibid., 824.

15. Condamine, 1740, 226–43 (see esp. 234–45).

16. Haggis, 1941, 582. I have been unable to find any published work by de Vega.

17. Heredia, 1689–88 [*sic*], 1:554. As Guerra (1977b, 117) has pointed out, this statement does not appear in the first edition (1665 [copy in Koninklijke Bibliotheek Albert I, Brussels]). Guerra has found it in editions of 1673, 1679, and 1680.

18. Caldera de Heredia, 1663, 155–56. The *Medicus politico catholicus* of Hieronymus Bardus (1634) announces on its title page that its author is a philosopher, physician, theologian, and professor of Aristotelian and Platonic philosophy at the University of Pisa. The statement that he was pharmacist at the Jesuits' college in Rome (Guerra, 1977b, 116) is apparently a mistranslation of Badus (1663, 18): *in iconibus, quas . . . habui a Cl. Hieronymo Bardi, & a peritissimo pharmacopola Rom. Collegii.*

19. Valdizan, 1915; see esp. 78 and n. 10. Pardal (1937, 357) adds that the corregidor had been treated successfully with *quina* and in 1638 sent a package of the powder to his physician, Juan de Vega in Lima, for treatment of Countess Ana, first wife of the viceroy.

20. Arcos, 1933, 77. Paredes Borja, 1947, 19 (fully warranted criticism is found in Jaramillo Arango, 1949, 283–84). See also Paredes Borja, 1963, 1:310.

21. Badus, 1663, 12–14. Guerra, 1977b; 1977a, 7–26 (same as 1977b plus illustrations); see also Guerra, 1982, 1:383–84. Great as is the literary and historiographic separation of Italy from other Western countries, that of the Iberian culture is even greater and has been affected only to a small extent by the recent acceleration of travel and communication. The learned Rompel remarked significantly (1905, 55, n. 1) that he was not taking the Spanish literature into consideration.

22. Caldera de Heredia, 1663, 155–61. See also Badus, 1663, 13.

23. Part of this narrative was to reappear a decade later in the book by Raymond Restaurand (1681), discussed in Chapter 5.

24. Caldera de Heredia, 1663, 157.

25. See the excellent concise exposition in Granjel, 1978, 220–22.

26. Bravo de Sobremonte, 1671, 312; also 1654, 402. Badus, 1663, 111–12.

27. Heredia, 1689–88 [*sic*], 554. More readily accessible is the extensive excerpt in Hernández Morejon, 1842–52, 6:28. The name *quarango* appears especially in early Spanish writings. Other terms are *china, china-china, quinquina, cascarilla,* and *gannanaperide*. The terminological confusion is discussed amply in Haggis, 1941, esp. 421ff.

28. Kühn edition (1821–33) 1964–65, 11:619–703.

29. The brevity of the notice about this author in August Hirsch's *Biographisches Lexikon,* 1962, 5:759, does not suggest importance.

30. Whoever seeks to judge this man's opinions and historical position should not overlook his remark (*Opera medica,* 1670, 2:16) that if the heart is the "principle" for the distribution of vital heat throughout the body, it is likewise the principle for the distribution of febrile and abnormal heat.

31. Salado Garces, 1678, 1.

32. Salado Garces, 1678, 2–3.

33. Salado Garzes [*sic*], 1679, 4–5, 10. It is not certain that the patients in the three cases discussed were treated by Salado.

34. Borghesi, 1705, 15–18.

35. See note 27 above. I have not undertaken to investigate whatever developments may have occurred in the Basque region. Such investigation should start with Granjel, 1983, esp. 117–22.

36. It is to be noted as a useful incidental that Portuguese authors are included in Hernández Morejon, 1842–52.

37. Da Orta, 1913 (colloquy 46), 373. Boxer, 1952, 11; Boxer quotes Diogo do Couto's *Decadas* (Lisbon, 1616).

38. Bagrow, 1964, 105–19.

39. Morão Simão Pinheiro, [1677] 1965.

40. *Ratio atque institutio studiorum Societatis Iesu. Auctoritate septimae congregationis generalis aucta*, 1635, 76. This manual was set forth in 1584, revised in 1599, and survived until 1832. S.v. "Roman Catholic Church," *Encyclopaedia Britannica*, 1953, 19:420.

41. The curriculum of the famous Jesuit school, the Collegium Romanum, is discussed in Heilbron, 1979, 160–92.

42. For analogy, consult the following sources: (*a*) *Ancient.* Lloyd, 1973–74, 1:60–63. Nutton, 1983 (esp. 2–4). Galen (Kühn ed.), 1: 126–32 (nature and uses). Galen: (Kühn ed.), 7:276–77 (the famous analogy of the cauldron and the bellows). Scarborough, 1985 (Galen misled by use of analogy). (*b*) *Early modern.* Lacuna, 1553, 28–30 (much used in the sixteenth century). Willis, 1681a, 1: second page of preface (an example of Willis's extensive use of analogy). Dewhurst, 1966, 179–80 (John Locke). (*c*) *Recent, general.* Leatherdale, 1974. (*d*) *Recent, special.* Higby, 1986. (*e*) *Attacks on the use of analogy.* Suárez de Ribera, 1726, 41. Baglivi, 1704, 26–32 (*falsum genus analogiarum, sive falsae similitudines*).

43. Hernándo y Ortega, 1982, p. 173.

44. Guerra, 1977b, 135. It is not easy to sweep aside the bit of word-of-mouth testimony preserved by Condamine (1740, 233n.) to the effect that "avant que le Quinquina fût connu à Lima, ce remede étoit d'un usage commun à Loxa." See also the comments of Condamine's fellow traveler Jussieu (note 15 above).

45. Goodman et al., 1985, 1043.

46. Satinoff, 1977, 539–43.

47. Wunderlich, 1857, 11; 1868, 371–73 and fig. 7; Wunderlich and Seguin, 1871.

Chapter 2. Peru, Italy, and the Low Countries

1. Jussieu, 1849, 15, n. 1. Weddell introduced the Latin text of Jussieu's unpublished note with the following statement: "Voici textuellement la note qu'il jeta sur le papier à ce sujet lors de son voyage à Loxa; elle fait partie de son mémoire sur le quinquina, resté inedit."

2. Vargas Ugarte, 1928, 293–94.

3. In his 1935 edition of Suardo's diary he is designated as "Catedrático de Historia Crítica del Peru en la Universidad Católica, Miembro del Instituto Histórico, Correspondiente de la Academia de la Historia de Madrid." See also Vargas Ugarte, 1928 and 1963–65.

4. Vargas Ugarte, 1928, 293–94.

5. Vargas Ugarte, 1935, viii. At this time Vargas Ugarte was evidently unaware of the writings of Caldera de Heredia and Pedro Miguel de Heredia, discussed in Chapter 1.

6. A critique of this explanation is given in Jaramillo Arango, 1949, 278.

7. Vargas Ugarte, 1963–65, 2:30–31; 1928, 294. Torres Saldamando, 1882, 178–94 (esp. 191). Jaramillo Arango, 1949, 181–83, has pointed out what appears to be a citation of part of the letter in Canezza, 1933, 89–90. This proves to be a

translation into Italian of the paragraph given by Torres Saldamando and is presented without documentation.

8. Canezza, 1925 and 1932. Per la storia della malaria nell'agro Romano, 1926, 532–34, has a summary of Canezza, 1925.

9. Canezza, 1925, 7. In addition to its errors the article quoted (Sheridan, 1922) provides no assurance that the tree in question was in fact cinchona. Haggis, 1941, was later to expose numerous instances of botanical confusion.

10. Canezza, 1932.

11. Ogg, 1960, 1.

12. In histories written in our own century they become statistics.

13. Rompel, 1905, 63–64: "besondere Verbindungen Tafurs mit dem Kardinal de Lugo—es handelte sich um theologische Schriften—in Rom nachweisen lassen." A biographical note on Tafur is found in Torres Saldamando, 1882, 294.

14. Conygius [Fabri], 1655, 16. Sturmius, 1659, 86–87. Bartholinus, 1661, historia 50, p. 109. See also Rompel, 1905, 1–64.

15. Hirsch, 1962, 2:560. Friedenwald, 1944, 724–25. Mandosio, 1696, 79–81. Marini, 1784, xlij.

16. *Inventario dei manoscritti delle biblioteche d'Italia*, 100: 122, item 502, no. 10(7).

17. Mandosio, 1696, 81. It is not certain that these consultations were ever published.

18. Fonseca, 1623, 117–19.

19. Conygius [Fabri], 1655, 7–8, 16.

20. Benedictus, 1649. Unhappily, the same is true of Benedictus, 1650. Nine consultations on fever are on pp. 355–401.

21. Badus, 1663, 239.

22. This center of learning, and much of Jesuit science, are discussed in Heilbron, 1979, esp. 101–13, 160–97.

23. This discussion is based in part on Rompel, 1931, and on Canezza, 1925, 1932. Additional sources consulted include: de Backer, 1890–1932, 5: col. 176–80; de Lugo, 1751; Migne, 1857, 31: cols. 1161–62; Nieremberg, 1890, 5: 221–44 (biography by P. Andrade); Brinkman, 1957; Cardella, 1792–97, 7:47–49; Astrain, 1916, 5: 81–88. Rompel, 1931, 428, 444, gives evidence that de Lugo had never seen the drug or known of its action until a later time, namely 1644.

24. Duran-Reynals, 1946, 40–41. The article "Lugo (Jean de)" in *Biographie Universelle*, 1843–65, 25:457–58 has a vague hint: "On prétend qu'il renouvela dans ses oeuvres philosophiques l'hypothèse des *points enflés* pour remedier aux difficultés que présentent les points mathématiques et la divisibilité de la matière à l'infini."

25. Canezza, 1925, 20. The result of his investigation was "nulla, proprio nulla." Abad, 1943.

26. This event is mentioned by Guy Patin (see Chapter 5), in a characteristically nasty way, in a letter to Charles Spon, Paris, 18 Jan. 1644. See Patin, 1907, 364, letter 101, n. 4. De Lugo's letter of thanks to Urban VIII, Seville, 9 May 1644, is preserved in the National Library of Madrid; see *Inventario de manuscritos de la Biblioteca Nacional*, 1953–70, 3:102. Rompel, 1931, 427. Canezza, 1925, 8–9, 19.

27. Schreiber and Mathus, 1987, 215.

28. For example, Brunacius, 1661, 16. See also the expressions of praise in Badus, 1663, 25.

29. Sturmius, 1659, 11–12. A physician's holograph request, dated 19 Sept. 1653 and addressed to Cardinal de Lugo, is reproduced in Canezza, 1932, 593.

30. Canezza, 1932, 596. The hospital, which was established by Innocent III, is still active. It contains murals (unmentioned in Baedeker's *Italie Centrale, Rome,* 1909) that show Cardinal de Lugo distributing the drug.

31. Rompel, 1931, 447.

32. Two spellings appear in the literature: Puccerini and Pucciarini. The former is to be favored, since it appears in the apothecary's letter to Badus, reproduced in Badus, 1663, 240.

33. Badus, 1663, 240–41 (in Italian); Latin translation by Badus, 241–43.

34. [Bado], 1656. The copy in the Biblioteca Civile of Genoa bears on its title page an inscription in ink "*cioe dal sigr Sebastiano Baldo*" (this is by Sig. Sebastiano Baldo). The quoted material is on p. 16 and 21.

35. Rompel, 1929. Part of his information is found in Badus, 1663.

36. Badus, 1663, 119–33.

37. Condamine, 1740, 226–43 (esp. 232); Haggis, 1941, 421. The criticisms of Haggis, which are valuable insofar as they relate to botanical and taxonomic matters, must be accepted by the modern reader, but their tone is harsh and their historical perspective is intermittently faulty.

38. Monardes, 1565, 8r.

39. Arnobius, 1949, 46, 133–37, 301, 317–18. See also the memorable tests instituted at the behest of Croesus (Herodotus 1.47).

40. Migne, 1844, 5: cols. 840–49.

41. Badus, 1663, 207–8.

42. Ibid., 208–12.

43. Ibid., 212–13.

44. Ibid., 245–46.

45. Ibid., unpaginated prefatory material.

46. It is interesting that De Renzi, [1845–49] 1966, 4:397, attributes the adulteration to Spaniards: "Italy had then become the prey of Spanish merchants."

47. Riddle, 1985, 74–77; Stieb, 1958.

48. He is Doughi in Morton, 1692, 125; Lange, 1704 (pt. 3) 364; Sprengel, 1821–38, 4: 524; and De Renzi, 1966, 4:398. This misspelling did little to help the present investigation. Biographical information about Donghi can be found in Gams, 1957, 695, 702, 764; and Katterbach, 1931, 289, no. 82.

49. Pastor, [1938] 1955, 29:163–64.

50. Rocco Casati, Christoforo Paravicino, and Giorgio Serponti. See Argelati, 1745, Appendix: col. 1346, no. 1558; col. 1898, no. 2214. See also Corte, [1718] 1972, 113–15, 176.

51. For example, the last of the twelve prefatory items (unpaginated) in the *Anastasis* is a sonnet dedicated to Badus, "to whom Cardinal Donghi owes his life and the entire populace owes its health." The case report is given on pp. 93–95; discussions are on pp. 95–103; other notices are on pp. 251 and 270–71. Filippo Argelati (see preceding note) refers to opinions expressed in writings on cinchona prepared by Parravicinus and by Serponti at the request of Cardinal Donghi. It is not certain that these were ever published.

52. Badus, 1663, 95.

53. Valentini, 1696, 41–60 (esp. 54).

54. Badus, 1663, 250.

55. Ibid., 109; Fernel, 1554, bk. 4, chaps. 9 and 10.

56. Rompel, 1931. See also Padberg, 1974.

57. Padberg, 1974, 23.

58. Brunacius, 1661.

59. The text is given in full in Menéndez-Pidal, 1944, 8–9. The probable author of the questionnaire was Juan López de Velasco, cosmographer; multiple authorship cannot be excluded.

60. For example, see Rompel, 1931, 416–52 (esp. 424).

61. Fletcher, 1969.

62. Zendrini, 1715, 7–8 (second pagination).

63. Chifletius, 1653, 5, examined in microfilm. Transmission of the bark from Rome to Flanders is mentioned also by Puccerini in his letter to Badus; see Badus, 1663, 240. Curiously, the mention of Flanders is omitted from the Latin translation of the letter on p. 242.

64. Padberg, 1974, 22–27.

65. Chifletius, 1653, 5. Pedro Toledo y Leyva was first marquis of Mancera, fifteenth viceroy of Peru. Valega, 1939, 68–69.

66. Rompel, 1905, 61, 63–64.

67. Archivo de Indias, Sevilla, 1980–86.

Chapter 3. Continental Developments, 1653–1675

1. Soers, 1641. In a letter (1 Feb. 1987) Dr. J. Germain, *conservateur* at Louvain, informed me that the thesis is no longer in the collections of the library there, but apparently was destroyed by a fire in 1974. The thesis has been made available through the kindness of the British Library. See also the comments of Rompel, 1905, 47–48.

2. Soers, 1642 (in National Library of Medicine, Bethesda).

3. Barba, 1642?. Detailed discussions are in Rompel, 1905, 43–47, and Guerra, 1977b, 137.

4. Garrison, 1929, 824. See also Suppan, 1931, 40.

5. Barba, 1642?, 11, 14, 15.

6. Plempius, 1642, 5–49 [only]. The copy I consulted is at the National Library of Medicine, Bethesda, and lacks the first four pages. There is no reason to think that the deficiency is significant.

7. The final sentences translate as follows: "You, Peter Barba, have my permission to wallow lifelong in the foul mud and filth of your barbarity and solecisms. Farewell." A more famous example of Plempius's contentiousness is his fight against the Harveian discovery of the circulation; he later recanted. See Beverovicius, 1641, 118–49, which records the correspondence between Plempius and Descartes on the circulation. See also Osler, 1969, item 722, pp. 76–77, and item 2030, p. 190.

8. Van der Heyden, 1643, 97. This designation for cinchona is not rare in the older literature. For example, in Nieremberg, 1890, 5:239, Cardinal de Lugo is said to have distributed "los polvos de la India para las cuartanas." See also Sturmius, 1659, 3 (*praeter pulverem Indicum, non aliud extare remedium*). The quaint biography of van der Heyden by Malcorps, 1853, 449–61, states (460) that "à cette époque on ne connaissait pas encore la précieuse écorce du Pérou."

9. This is the fibrosis of prolonged infection and is manifested clinically as induration. See Bruce-Chwatt, 1985, 76. For detailed discussion of the anatomical changes see Seyfarth, 1926, 1 (pt. 1): 178–248 (esp. 202–8).

10. Rompel, 1905, 64. Jaramillo Arango, 1949, 296, 301. *Antidotarium Gandavense*, 1663, 134, 220.

11. Chifletius, 1653, 9.

12. Ibid., 21, 23; *diuturni et exitiales morbi a viris magnis memorati*, p. 29.

13. Ibid., 24–30. The comment from Rome is dated 25 Nov. 1652. That from Madrid, 8 January 1653.

14. Rompel, 1907, 55.

15. Chifletius, 1653, 4–5. The statement in Haggis, 1941, 443, that Chifletius gave "some excerpts" of the *Schedula*, is erroneous; he includes the entire document. Additional information is given in Appendix B.

16. Conygius [Fabri], 1655. A description of Jesuit rules concerning anonymous and pseudonymous publication can be found in Harris, 1988. 103–4. What may be interpreted as exceptions to Jesuit practice are recorded in Sommervogel, 1884.

17. Conygius [Fabri], 1655, 10–12. 16.

18. Ibid., 20–24.

19. *Mirifici huius pulveris effectus*, ibid., 29–34.

20. This is Fabri's order of categories.

21. Conygius [Fabri], 1655, 30–33.

22. Fabri's curious role as (non) discoverer of the circulation is summarized in Eloy, 1778, 2:177–78. Eloy wrote, "Il s'est approprié, la découverte de la circulation du sang, et il a trouvé des gens assez crédules pour l'en croire sur sa parole." Conygius [Fabri], 1655, 45–88; the scarcity of Chiflet's original treatise adds to the usefulness of the reprint.

23. Rompel, 1905, 50.

24. Plempius's biographer says of his contributions, "D'ailleurs dans le nombre de ces écrits il en est plusieurs presqu'entièrement remplis de polémique médicale." Haas, 1845, 209–32 (esp. 215–16).

25. Protimus [Plempius], 1655, 27, 20.

26. Ibid., 2, 8, 9, 12.

27. Ibid., 17, 16, 9–11.

28. Ibid., 16.

29. We may guess that the author was Jean Bissel, S.J. (1601–82). See de Backer, 1890–1969, 1: cols. 1513–17. See also Sommervogel, 1884, col. 1272.

30. Biss[el?], [1653?], 4.

31. Ibid., 8.

32. Ibid., 13–14.

33. Ibid., 14–16.

34. Steele, 1964, 19.

35. Guitton, 1953, 183.

36. Protimus [Plempius], 1655, 10.

37. Bartholinus, 1663, 529–32 (centuria 2, epist. 42). The letter of Langelottus, 22 July 1654, is epist. 43, pp. 533–35.

38. Bartholinus, 1654, 246–47 (centuria 2, historia 56). While the description strongly suggests plague, who can say that malaria was absent?

39. Bartholinus, 1661, 107–16 (historia 50).

40. Von Moinichen was a Danish surgeon who came from Schleswig. Interesting observations by him are recorded in Haller, [1774–77] 1969, 1:458–59.

41. Obviously it is not impossible that examination of commercial records would reveal earlier shipments of the drug.

42. This opinion appears, for example, in the entry for Castelli in the *Dizionario biografico degli Italiani*, 1978, 4:747–50.

43. Rompel, 1905, 38–42. Haggis, 1941, 446–48.

44. Malaria in Italy, especially but not exclusively in Rome, is described in inter-

esting detail by Anna Celli-Fraentzel, 1928, which includes valuable archival material, such as a statistical record from the Hospital of the Holy Spirit in Rome.

45. The principal biographical sources are Rompel, 1905 and 1929. Supplementary sources, not totally reliable, are Soproni, 1667, 253; Mazzuchelli, 1753–63, 2 (pt. 1): 29–30; Pescetto, 1846, 273–84; and the *Dizionario biografico degli Italiani*, 1963, 8:87–88. Additional biographical fragments are found in Badus's writings.

46. Badus, 1663, 37, 99.

47. See Chapter 1, note 3.

48. Baldus, 1656, 1–5.

49. Ibid., 40, 41–43.

50. Ibid., 1656, 40; Conygius [Fabri], 1655, 16; Protimus [Plempius], 1655, 9.

51. Badus, 1663, 250–51. See also Chapter 4.

52. This college was one of several created by the energetic Federigo Borromeo (1564–1631), Archbishop of Milan and a leader in the Catholic Counter-Reformation. See *Storia di Milano*, 1953–66, 10:108, 456; 11:695.

53. The present (secular) owners, whom I visited on 17 June 1987, are little interested in the history of their shop. See, however, Notizie storiche sull' antica farmacia di Brera, in *Notiziario dell' antica farmacia di Brera*, vols. 1–3, 1924–26. Note especially 3:129–35, on Andrea Castoldi (d. 1826), the last of a family of owners. I learned from Signora Lelia di Domenico, a scholarly librarian at the Brera library, that his heirs have divided the eight volumes of early records. See also Bigatti, 1926.

54. Rompel, 1929, 136. I have been unable to obtain a photocopy of the thesis.

55. See *nox sexta*, 445–48.

56. Haller, 1776–78, 2:609–10.

57. Hoefer, 1657, 256–57. The statement of Glantz is accompanied by no bibliographic information, nor is Glantz's name included in major North American, British, or French medical bibliographies.

58. Rompel, 1935, 56 (*die erst Erwähnung der Rinde für Österreich*).

59. Confusion is compounded by the marginal annotation, which reads *Chin. Chinae*, the abbreviation of a term often used for Peruvian bark.

60. Biographical information on Sturmius is in Broeckx, 1855, 5–24. See also Hirsch, 1962, 5:446–47.

61. Sturmius, pt. 1: 146–51. François de Cleyn (1608–69), a Jesuit, was professor of sacred theology in Louvain (1643–52), rector of Malines (1652–56), and provincial (1661–64). De Backer, 1890–1960, 2: cols. 1240–42.

62. According to Broeckx, 1855, 14, these two physicians were from Louvain.

63. Sturmius, 1659, pt. 1: 15, 17–28.

64. "Ex quibus sane posse concludi videtur, singularem in eo latere virtutis causam, quae soli temperamento non possit." Ibid., 49.

65. The heading of the section (ibid., 51) contains a significant turn of phrase: "it is shown by repeated observation."

66. *Instructione schedae Romanae ad amussim observata* (ibid., 70). The influence of Rome extended to Delft and included posology.

67. Ibid., 146–51, 87.

68. Broeckx, 1855, remarked acutely: "Since modern writers are scarcely in agreement on this matter, is it astonishing that Sturmius found explanation to be very difficult?"

69. Brunacci's biography mentions many historical, literary, and other works; some remain unpublished, including a *Theatrum magnum medicinae*. S.v. "Brunacci, Gaudenzio," *Dizionario biografico degli Italiani*, 1972, 14: 517–18.

70. Brunacius, 1661, 17.

71. "Ab Eminentissimo de Lugo receptus, experimentis nec non plurimis existimatione adeo habitus, ut inde magnum et nomen, et pretium fuerit adeptus." Ibid., 16.

72. See the censures issued by Haggis, 1941, 443–45.

73. See Ackerknecht, 1967, on the role played by the hospitals of Paris in the advance of medicine.

74. Brunacius, 1661, 19, 17, 114.

75. Ibid., 108, 109.

76. Rompel, 1905, 57: "He [Brunacius] attempted to establish the new drug on the doctrine of the old school."

77. Sylvius, 1679.

78. Ibid., 904.

79. Dekkers, 1673, 198.

80. Barbette, 1675. A Dutch edition was issued in Leyden in 1669. A posthumous edition, with appendix by Mangetus (Geneva, 1704, 113) says that the bark cured many quartans but not as safely, quickly, or pleasantly as various salts.

81. *Pharmacopoea Amstelredamensis*, 1636. *Pharmacopoea Amstelredamensis*, 1639. *Pharmacopoea Ultrajectina*, 1656. *Pharmacopoea Belgica*, 1659. *Pharmacopoea Hagiensis*, 1659. *Pharmacopoea Amstelredamensis*, 1660.

82. Letter from W. K. Gnirrep, Amsterdam, 6 June 1985. Enclosed with this letter is a photocopy listing under *Cortices*, . . . Casia lignea, China China [handwritten], Cinamomum . . .

83. *Pharmacopoea Harlemensis*, 1693, 2.

84. Barckhausen, 1696. The preface is dated 1695. I have not seen the 1690 edition, *Synopsis pharmaceutica*, published in Frankfurt.

Chapter 4. England after 1650

1. Burton [1651] 1838, 436. See also 456.

2. Sydenham 1848–50, 2: 3–4. Latham, who edited this edition, dated the letter 30 Dec. 1670 (2:4) and 30 Dec. 1679 (1:lxxvi). Since Sydenham's reply is dated 7 Feb. 1679 (2:28), we may skeptically assign 1670 as the date of Brady's letter. In any case, it is evident that Brady's "twenty years" were an approximation only.

3. Baker, 1785, 188. In Sydenham (1848–50, 1:lxxv), Latham's biographical preface states, without documentation, that in 1655 the bark "appears to have been first introduced into England." I have been unable to find the source that Baker used at this point.

4. Baker, 1785, 190.

5. Issues reviewed are the *Publick Intelligencer* no. 117 (22–29 Mar. 1658) to no. 168 (14–21 Mar. 1659); *Mercurius Politicus* no. 1 (6–13 June 1650) to no. 149 (14–21 May 1653), no. 343 (1–8 Jan. 1656) to no. 396 (24–31 Dec. 1657), and no. 409 (25 Mar.–1 Apr. 1658) to no. 559 (17–24 Mar. 1659). The advertisements appeared in *Publick Intelligencer* no. 131 (21–28 June 1658); *Mercurius Politicus* no. 422 (24 June–11 July 1658), no. 426 (22–29 July 1658), no. 439 (21–28 Oct. 1658), no. 545 (9–16 Dec. 1658), and no. 553 (3–10 Feb. 1659).

6. Some of the advertisements use the spelling *Thompson*.

7. Letter dated Antwerp, 14 Jan. 1985. The other dates recorded in Baptismal Register no. 16 are 31 Aug. 1654 and 30 Jan. 1657.

8. S.v. "Somerset, Edward," *Dictionary of National Biography*, compact ed. 1975. Dircks, 1865, 211, 212, 232.

9. The activities of English Catholics in Europe, especially in Belgium, are described in Watkin, 1957, esp. 73–78.

10. Badus, 1663, 240.

11. Public Record Office, London, 1960.

12. Plomer, 1907, 57.

13. Belon [also Bellon], 1681.

14. De Meeüs, 1962, 197. See also Watkin, 1957, 73–78.

15. Bruce-Chwatt, 1982. See also Jarcho, 1982.

16. Some facts about Cromwell's final illness are given in Morton, 1692, 416.

17. Dewhurst, 1981.

18. Baker, 1785, 192.

19. Willis, 1660, 143–44. In Willis, 1681b, this appears on p. 82.

20. Willis, 1660, 152–57.

21. Dewhurst, 1981, 49–51, n. 36–38.

22. I have used the version in Willis, 1681, vol. 1.

23. Morton, 1692, 136.

24. Several Osleriologists have been unable to discover when or where or whether Sir William said this.

25. Baker, 1785, 206–9. And s.v. "Tabor or Talbor, Sir Robert," *Dictionary of National Biography*, compact ed., 1975.

26. His first contact with the king is described in Siegel and Poynter, 1962, 82–85.

27. Sydenham, 1848–50, 1:lxxx.

28. Probably confusion with the so-called ague cake. Talbor, 1672, 22.

29. *London Gazette*, no 1593, 21–24 Feb. 1680.

30. Wooton, [1910] 1971, 1:100. Wooton remarks misleadingly that this document was part of a "collection of quack advertisements." I have been unable to find the original.

31. Talbor, 1682, 49, 19–20, 29.

32. Ricani, 1694. Castro Sarmento, 1758, 403–4. Baker, 1785, 206–9, 215–16.

33. S.v. "Sydenham, Thomas," *Dictionary of Scientific Biography*, 1970–80, 13: 213–15 esp. 214.

34. See note 2 above.

35. See note 23 above.

36. Sydenham, 1666, 107–8.

37. *Philosophical Transactions* 1 (7 May 1666): 210–13. Reprinted in full *Sydenham*, 1848–50, 1:xxvii–xxx.

38. This discussion is based on the version given in Sydenham, 1848–50, 1:1–276.

39. Ibid., 1:76, 83, ci.

40. Ibid., 1:84–85.

41. Ibid., 1:92.

42. Ibid., 2:9, 119–84, 238–39; see also 161–62.

43. Dewhurst, 1966, 58.

44. *Index-Catalogue of the Library of the Surgeon-General's Office, United States Army*, 1893, 1st ser., 14: 22–24.

45. Browne, 1946, 24.

46. *Pharmacopoeia Londinensis*, 1678, 20, 22.

47. Morton, 1692, 96. Morton says, concisely and beautifully, *cum magno Reipub[licae] (praesertim literariae) detrimento.*

48. Morton, 1692, 162. The letter of Sir Thomas Browne quoted above implies possible adulteration of the powder.

49. Davis, 1971. See also note 30 above.

50. To the modern reader such effects may indicate adulteration of the drug.

51. Dewhurst, 1962, 491–92. Sydenham's dedicatory letter is in Sydenham, 1848–50, 2: 187–89.

52. Dewhurst, 1962, 493, see also 495.

53. Harris, 1683, 166, 169, 176, 179–80, 190.

54. Raius, 1686–1704, 2:1796–97.

55. Not intended as a pun. Ray wrote (p. 1797): *non intra scrupulos subsistebat, sed ad drachmas et uncias ascendebat.*

56. Harvey, 1678, 140–43. Also s.v. "Harvey, Gideon," *Dictionary of National Biography*, compact ed., 1975.

57. Harvey, 1683, 181, 151, 215. Haggis, 1941, 451–52, has presented evidence that Harvey, like many others, was unaware of the difference between the new *quina-quina* (cinchona) and the old (Peruvian balsam).

58. Ibid., 185–86.

59. Harvey, 1689, 5, 7, 95–96.

60. Haggis, 1941, 452.

61. Morton, 1692, 59, 72, 120, 162.

62. Ibid., 121, 123–35, 188, 174.

63. Haggis, 1941, 452–53.

64. Slightly more than half are dated. Of these the three earliest are from 1672–79, and thirteen are from 1682–90. A few fatal cases are included.

65. Morton, 1692, 81.

66. Ibid., 81–82. His own hemicranial attack is described in case 27, pp. 259–60.

67. For example, cases 16–18, ibid., 228–36.

68. Ibid., 342–50.

69. Morton, 1689, 131.

70. Dewhurst, 1963, e.g., 176, 177, 196, 206. These entries date from 1679 to 1681; the total span reproduced in the volume is from 1675 to 1698. See also the discussion of Monginot in Chapter 5.

71. Vogel, 1764, 287–91.

72. See Lister, 1697, 1–2. See also Lister, 1684 (second discussion l[1] verso).

73. Lister, 1697, 269, 272 (an interesting footnote mentions the destruction of the Indians of Maryland by smallpox), 188, 32–33.

74. Ibid., 3, 125–27, 219.

75. Warren, 1729. The final page is dated 6 Dec. 1728. Blake, 1979, 482, records a treatise in English (London, 1733) with similar title.

76. Houghton, 1727–28, 4:163, 2:335.

Chapter 5. France, Germany, and Switzerland

1. Mettam, 1988, 1–10, 309–22.

2. Hirsch, 1883–86, 1:215–17. Bruce-Chwatt and Zulueta, 1980, 67–71.

3. Héritier, 1987, 61–71.

4. Lévy-Valensi, 1933, 1.

5. The most recent extensive work on Renaudot is Bailly, 1987. This book is useful but bibliographically exasperating. Also valuable is Brown, 1934, 17–40. The range of Renaudot's interests and activities is suggested by [Renaudot], 1664. See

also Renaudot, 1665. Renaudot's journalistic activities, which have bearing on his iatrochemical leanings, are discussed in Hatin, 1853, 1–26.

6. Galen (K 13.501), with simple quaintness, defines *polychreston* as a drug of multiple use. Gothofredus Held, 1715, 383–86, later applied the term to the Peruvian bark.

7. Bailly, 1987, 35–36. These broad claims are regarded nowadays as characteristic of quackery. However, Renaudot's virtues are undeniable.

8. It is hardly necessary to state that this was not the faculty of a college; it consisted of all the regular medical practitioners of Paris.

9. Delaunay, 1906, 66–67.

10. This involves the interesting story of the "gray eminence," Père Joseph (François Leclerc du Tremblay), a Capuchin. See Dedouvres, 1932.

11. Hazon, 1778, 99. The system of (nonmedical) patronage in France and the extensive activities of Richelieu and Mazarin as patrons are described in Kettering, 1986.

12. Granel, 1964, 18. A confirmatory statement appears in Chomel, 1732, 2:212: "Barbeyrac, eminent physician of Montpellier, and one of the most famous physicians of the last century . . . contributed greatly to making it [*quinquina*] popular."

13. Dousset, 1985, 161.

14. Adam and Milhaud, 1934–63, 6:217. Descartes's replies to Cavendish are discussed in detail—as far as physiological fundamentals—in Appendix A.

15. [Chomel], 1762, 2.

16. Moreau, 1647a and 1647b, were examined in microfilms provided by the Bibliothèque Nationale.

17. It would be profitable for such an investigation to include the records of the Hôtel-Dieu de Québec, which was founded in 1639. Information about the practice of pharmacy by religious groups, including the interdiction in Toulouse in 1691, can be found in Bouvet, 1937, 301–5.

18. Patin, 1907, 347. Correspondence with well-informed Lyonnais scholars has yielded no additional information about this, but in a personal letter (23 June 1987) one eminent author has suggested that the Jesuits' bark apparently was introduced into Lyon by André Falconet (1612–91), a graduate of Montpellier and physician of the Hôpital de la Charité.

19. Guitton, 1953, 183. Honoratus Fabri, S.J., is mentioned repeatedly in this volume (esp. 48 and 55–56) because of his work in Lyon and his later role as long-term papal advisor. He appears also in Chapter 3 but is not known to have had a role in the transmission of the Jesuits' bark to Lyon.

20. Patin, 1718, 2:87.

21. Rompel, 1905, 63. Condamine (1740, 226–43) states without documentation that "ce même Procureur de la Société passant par la France pour se rendre à Rome, guérit de la fièvre avec le Quinquina, le feu Roi Louis XIV, alors Dauphin" (p. 234).

22. Riverius, 1690, 538–50, 536.

23. Riolan, 1651, 228–54.

24. After describing Patin's repulsive traits, summarized in the statement that Patin was a man who cannot be either esteemed or loved, Lévy-Valensi stated, with Gallic astuteness, that we must credit Patin with having fought against the pharmacopoeia of his time and with having preferred hygiene. See Lévy-Valensi, 1933, 505. The bust of Patin by Etienne Leroux shows a diabolical face. It is reproduced as the frontispiece of Coquerelle, 1901.

25. Patin, 1707, 1:68 (letter no. 23), 75 (no. 25), 170 (no. 58), 200 (no. 70).

26. "Ces bon pères passefins."

27. Larrieu, 1889, 102.

28. Patin, 1707, 1:217 (no. 78). Chiflet and his book are mentioned again, favorably, in letters dated 3 Feb. 1654 (Delaunay, 1906, 66) and 21 Sept. 1655 (Patin, 1707, 262, no. 100). According to a Spanish proverb, God creates such people and the Devil brings them together.

29. Packard, 1925, 154. Canezza, 1925, 16. Packard, 1925, 154–55.

30. Protimus [Plempius], 1655, 2. Moreau's statement conflicts with the testimony of Sebastianus Badus (1663, 200), who cites the case of a cardinal's nephew, which, unfortunately, is both isolated and undated.

31. Chapter 3 noted the thesis of Bovonier (1656), which is reported by Rompel (1929). It apparently discusses the use of *pulvis chinchinae* in intermittent fevers. I have not had access to this publication. Some sources give the author's name as Bovionier.

32. Patin, 1707, 1:283 (no. 110).

33. Raynaud, 1862, 218. Bergen, 1826, 17, gives a variant version of the title, taken from Baldinger, 1778, 1006. I have not seen the original thesis.

34. Delaunay, 1906, 49–64, esp. 55–56. Dieuxyvoie was councillor and physician-in-ordinary to the king and in 1682 was dean of the Faculty. Delaunay, 1906, 59, 61 states that the only known printed work by Dieuxyvoie is a scrawl (*grimoire*) on silphium.

35. *Croton eluteria*, family Euphorbiaceae; cascarilla. (Caution: the term *cascarilla* has also been used for cinchona.)

36. Sur le chacril, [1719] 1723, 68.

37. Patin, 1707, 2:301, Bartholinus, 1667, letter 98, 559–62, Patin, 1707, 3:21.

38. Patin, 1707, 2:238ff.; 265.

39. Dewhurst, 1963, 59, 1966, 41–42.

40. Nolhac, 1911, 1:108; 2:50–51, 249. Pluchon, 1985, 60–61.

41. Sévigné, 1972–78, 2:632.

42. Delaunay, 1906, 67–69.

43. Sévigné, 1972–78, 2:1415.

44. Blegny, 1680. Belon, 1681. Blegny, 1682. *The English Remedy,* 1682. Blegny, 1685. Blegny, 1687, 1–48.

45. A typical example appears in the biographical dictionary of Bayle and Thillaye, [1855] 1967, 2:413–14: "a strange man who played every sort of role to gain credit with the public."

46. Blegny, 1685, 3.

47. Sévigné, 1972–78, 2:696, 725, 743. Michel Emery (1888, 29, n. 1) made the undocumented but not incredible statement that d'Aquin had previously written against the use of the bark.

48. Sévigné, 3:28, 30, 56, 317, 320, 342. See also Le Roi, 1862, 171, 194, 431.

49. Lévy-Valensi, 1933, 514.

50 Le Roi, 1862, 431.

51. Jarcho, 1989b, 221.

52. Torti, 1730, 538. This statement, or an equivalent, does not appear in the first edition (1712) but is repeated in later editions.

53. Le Roi, 1862, 183.

54. Monginot is the pseudonym of François de La Salle.

55. Wolfart, 1695, 3 (*ob constantem Religionis Reformatae cultum carceri famoso, la bastille dicto inclusus erat*).

56. An English translation by Peter Belon was published in London in 1681 under the title *A New Mystery in Physick Discovered, by Curing of Fevers and Agues by Quinquina or Jesuites Powder.* A Latin version, prepared by T. Bonnet, appeared in *Zodiacus Medico-Gallicus* 2, 1682. Another Latin edition was included in [Nigrisoli], 1687, 49–86, and in the second edition, 1700. A curious review of the earlier edition appeared in *Acta Eruditorum,* Leipzig, 1688, 87–88.

57. These comments are based on the edition of 1680.

58. Monginot, 1680, 142, 20–21, 34, 35.

59. See note 38 above.

60. Monginot, 168c, 142–43. A discussion of these conditions can be found in Jarcho, 1984a, lxv–lxvi.

61. Monginot, 1680, 19–20.

62. Monginot erred. As we have seen, Morton used the drug for many different sicknesses.

63. Monginot, 1680, 143–45.

64. La Fontaine, 1682, 1–56.

65. This fact was recorded by the invaluable Mme de Sévigné, 1972–78, 2:1415.

66. La Fontaine, 1682, 9, 32, 36.

67. Fonssagrives, 1859.

68. See La Fontaine, 1883–92, 2:454–80 (Discours à Madame de la Sablière); 9:390–401 (Lettre XXII à Madame la Duchesse de Bouillon, Paris, Nov. 1687).

69. Spon, 1682, 2 (emphasis added). The original, *Observations sur les fièvres et les febrifuges,* was published in Lyon in 1681. A second Lyonnais edition was issued by Amaulry in 1684. A Latin translation, bearing Spon's initials but not his name, appears in [Nigrisoli], 1687, 139–84 (see 143–44).

70. Restaurand, 1681. Reference will be made to the Latin translation in [Nigrisoli] 1687, 87–138. An Italian translation was issued also (*Ippocrate dell'uso della kinakina per la guarigione delle febbri.* Parma: Pazzoni e Monti, 1695).

71. [Nigrisoli], 1687, 115–16 (and footnote).

72. Lémery, 1683 (5th ed.), 416–22; many editions and translations were issued. Lémery, 1716 (3d ed.), 287; an earlier edition appeared in Paris in 1698. Lémery, 1707.

73. Charas, 1730, dates from 31 May 1692. On p. 64, Charas states that he had been using the new preparation *for about fifteen years.*

74. *Acta eruditorum,* 1685, 333–34.

75. Delaunay, 1906, 69–70 mentions J. Desprez, 1680, and R. Maurin, 1683 (affirmative); M. Pichonnet, and Bailly, 1683 (negative). Waring, 1878–79, 1:339–40, mentions Lombard, 1695; Poisson, 1696; Lelong, 1696; and Vesou, 1696.

76. An anonymous review appeared in *Acta eruditorum,* Leipzig, 1688, 87–88. A second edition was published by Lilius in Ferrara in 1700.

77. Bernier, 1689, xcvi–xcvii.

78. Bayle and Thillaye, [1855] 1967, 2:132.

79. Unconvincing attribution to Fagon is found in Bayle and Thillaye, [1855] 1967, 1:534. These authors mention an edition dated 1703; the author catalog of the Bibliothèque Nationale, 49: col. 427, gives the date as 1705.

80. *Les admirables qualitez,* 1689, introduction and 1, 11, 39. A *sol* was reckoned at a twentieth of a *livre.*

81. In 1686 the Swiss physician and teacher, Johann Conrad Peyer, wrote clearly enough: *nuperrime rursus increbuit à multo tempore neglectus cortex Peruvianus, Anglis Gallisque de novo concelebrantibus* (very recently the Peruvian bark, neglected

for a long time, has become popular again, with the combined approval of the English and the French).

82. Bouley et al., 1982.

83. Minot, 1691. I have not had opportunity to consult the smaller first edition of 1684, which is registered in the author catalog of the Bibliothèque Nationale, 115: col. 711, nor have I succeeded in finding a biography of Minot.

84. Ibid., 108–12, 253, 260.

85. Ibid., 321.

86. Ibid., 327, 353.

87. Waring, 1878–79, 1: 339–42.

88. The *index rerum* in Schröder's *Pharmacopoeia medico-chymica* of 1649–50, for example, has twenty-four main entries under *antimonii* and thirteen under *mercurii*.

89. Guiart, 1947, 141–50. Dulieu, 1975, 236–41, 444–48. Bouvet, 1937, 266–72. Emery, 1888, 34–67, 113–26. Debus, 1977, 1:148–73. Fischer, 1988.

90. Counterblasts to his early writings (De Launay, 1564, 1566) were written by Jacques Grévin (1538–70).

91. The condemnatory document is reproduced in Emery, 1888, 113. See also Perreau, 1655. Condemnation by the Parlement of Paris in 1560 is mentioned in Granel, 1964, 18–19.

92. For full biographical details see Durling, 1967, 446–47 (items 3477, 3481).

93. Astruc, 1767, xxviij. The reader is reminded that the word *Faculté* designated all the physicians of the area and not merely a limited body of academic medical teachers.

94. Schelenz, [1904] 1965, 417, points out that in Lille, at some time earlier than 1573, the use of antimony had been forbidden.

95. See, for example, Patin, 1707, 1:223, 226, 328–29.

96. Bouvet, 1934, 268; 1937, 266–69. Dulieu, 1975, 237.

97. Salmon, 1671, 366; 1680, 892.

98. Some details can be found in Cheylud, 1897, 66–67.

99. Hoffmann, 1729–34, 4:23–24, 69. Flores, [1698], 71, 72, 77, 113–17. Huxham, [1757] 1988, 229–30; 1765, 190–92. Huxham, 1756, 73, mentions the use of antimony "particularly in slow fevers, low irregular intermittents and remittents, in catarrhal fevers."

100. Jüngken, 1732, 866. Boerhaave, 1757a, 327–28. Suárez de Ribera, 1724, 159.

101. Snapper, 1946.

102. The twentieth-century use of antimonials in tropical medicine is outlined in a Bordeaux thesis by Boisseau, 1933.

103. Waskin, Harpaz and Navin, 1987. Badaro, 1990.

104. Schneider, 1968–75, 5 (pt. 1): 262–64.

105. Latham, 1848–50, 1:83.

106. Goodall, Letter to Mr. H, in Davis, 1971 (see 297). Stisser, 1687, 99, Fonseca Henriquez, 1714, 138. Boerhaave, 1757, 300–304.

107. Jarcho, 1972.

108. Haller, 1758, 5: items 151–89.

109. Schröder, 1649–50, contains two title pages, dated in successive years. The dedications are dated 1641–44. An edition marked Ulm, 1641, is recorded, as are many later editions.

110. Rolfincius, 1658, 314–15.

111. See Chapter 3, note 55.

112. Rothmann, 1663, fols. [374]–[383], 376r.

113. Schelenz, [1904] 1965, 506 (n. 9), 507, 523. I have had access neither to the original documents nor to Schelenz's source, namely, articles by B. Seybold, *Apotheker-Zeitung* 10 and 12, 1895 and 1897.

114. Tschirch, 1907–25, 1(pt. 2): 810–35. I am indebted to Prof. Dr. Erika Hickel of the Technische Universität Braunschweig for directing me to this and other valuable information on the subject. The interpretations are my own; Prof. Hickel is not responsible for any errors that they may contain.

115. A sampling of *Taxen* beginning in 1601 is given in Schelenz, [1904] 1965, 506–8.

116. Tschirch, 1907–25, 1 (pt. 2): 916.

117. The full text of this letter appears in Boccabadati, 1833, 125–47 (see 145).

118. Bayle and Thillaye [1855] 1967, 51–52.

119. Sprengel, 1821–38, 4:535, 538. See the brief commendation of Sprengel in Garrison, 1929, 371.

120. Brunner and von Muralt, 1969, 177.

121. Peyer, 1686. The manuscript of this article was sent to its editor in 1685. See also note 81 above.

122. Haller, 1776–78, 3:422. That Haller himself was cured of a very violent fever by means of the bark is related by Morgagni, 1761, 68.2.

123. Muraltus [von Muralt], 1689. Von Muralt's opinions are discussed in greater detail and from a different point of view in Appendix A.

124. Hoffmann, 1687, 649–702.

125. Schondorff, 1694, sect. 12, fol. 6v.

126. Hoffmann, 1695, chap. 3, paragr. 54; chap. 1, paragr. 27. King translation, 1971, 52, 116.

127. Schelhammer, 1693, 132–33.

128. See Chapter 2, note 51.

129. I have been unable to identify Faustus. Possibly this is a misspelled allusion to Johann Caspar Fausius (1601–71); see Stübler, 1926, 84.

130. Langius, 1704, 361–75.

131. Fluctuations in the reputation of the drug are described in a brief and interesting passage in Berger and Stieler, 1711, 46.

132. Stahl, 1726, 144: "so sehr *mode waren.*"

133. Ibid., 157. Some countervailing favorable comments appear on pp. 314–17.

134. Cramer, 1713, for example, emphasizes the alleged constrictive action of the bark.

135. See also note 34 above.

136. Duhr, 1907–28, 3:298–302; 4 (pt. 1): 426; 4 (pt. 2): 495.

137. Badus, 1663, 240–41 (Italian), 242–43 (Latin translation). The letter is discussed in Chapter 2.

138. Duhr, 1907–28, 3:302, n. 2. According to this source the letters are in the Staatsbibliothek in Munich.

139. See note 112 above.

140. S.v. "Bohn, Johannes," in Hirsch, 1962, 1:606–7.

141. Bohn, 1710, 619–40; see esp. 624–29. (Haller, 1776–78, 3:88, mentions an edition dated 1709.)

142. I have not seen this rare edition; instead, I have consulted the second edi-

tion, 1745. Of less interest is Werlhof's diatribe, *De limitanda febris laude et censura corticis Peruviani*, 1759.

Chapter 6. Russia, the Orient, and the Americas

1. Rowell, 1978. Rowell here quotes *Akty istoricheskie*, 1841, 473.
2. Appleby, 1983, 295). Appleby cites Novombergskiy, 1905.
3. *Dictionary of National Biography*, compact ed., 1975, 414.
4. Richter, 1813–17, 2:289–91. Gramann, 1666.
5. Ibid., 346r.
6. Gordon, 1859, Buxhoeveden, 1932.
7. The use of guaiac bark, as well as the wood and the gum, is mentioned in Schneider, 1968–75, 5 (pt. 2): 146–48. Novombergskiy, 1905, 52–53. Appleby, 1983, 295.
8. Peter the Great, 1887–1912.
9. Sollmann, 1948, 505.
10. *Materialy dlya istorii meditsiny v Rossii*, 1881, in Stakelberg, 1940–41 (item 5697), 819.
11. Richter, 1813–17, 2:185–88, 189–91, 80–95, 238–57. Several of the recipes call for antimonials, evidence of iatrochemical opinion among the prescribers.
12. Bruce-Chwatt and Zulueta, 1980, 151.
13. For abundant information on malaria in Russia, see ibid., 150–66.
14. Chapter 4, notes 70 and 71.
15. Vernadsky, 1959, 4:278–84; 1969, 5:227, 232, 339, 436, 450, 683–92.
16. Lutteroth, 1858, 2.
17. In Tschirch, 1910, 1 (pt. 2): 827.
18. Maclagan, 1932.
19. Madras Government, 1908–11. In Dutch, except for no. 13, which contains an English translation of nos. 1 and 2. In no. 13 (pp. 39–40) there is a bibliography.
20. Moens, 1911, 220.
21. Madras Government, 1909, 6.
22. Klerk de Reus, 1894.
23. Schouten, 1725, 1:16–17, 503, 586.
24. Sebastiani, 1672, 185–86, 204.
25. *Lettres édifiantes*, 1819, 6:29.
26. Johnston-Saint, 1929. Crawford, 1914, 1:37–57.
27. Crawford, 1914, 1:113–28.
28. Bruce, 1810, 2:433–34, 463–66, 518–19, 522–23; 3:174–81, 200.
29. Cook, 1989.
30. Madras Record Office (presidency), 1919, 16.
31. Madras Record Office (presidency). 1925.
32. Browne, 1698.
33. Reddy, 1947, 111. The term *Rez* is obscure.
34. Hedges, 1887–89. Collet, 1933. Hedges lived from 1632 to 1701; Collet was born in 1673.
35. Master, 1911, 1:240.
36. Freyer, 1698, 115.
37. Royle, 1839, 1:240; also s.v. "Royle, John F.," *Dictionary of National Biography*, compact ed., 1975. Markham, 1880, 86–89.
38. Pallegoix, 1854, 2:102–294. Pallegoix was bishop of Mallos and vicar apostolic for Siam. On p. 102, he says that these letters were written from Singapore.

Sommervogel mentions a letter by Xavier written from Singapore under date of 21 July 1552. See de Backer, 1890–1932, 8: col. 1329. Pallegoix is quoting a Portuguese historian ("un historien Portugais") whose name and date he fails to mention.

39. S.v. "Siam," *Encyclopaedia Britannica,* 1953 (see 20:592).

40. Pallegoix, 2:102. Again, Pallegoix does not provide the name of the Portuguese historian from whose writings he obtained this information, nor does he give the date of these events.

41. De Backer, 1932, 11: cols. 1245–46, nos. 2–8 (1664–90); col. 1250, no. 30 (1670); col. 1250, no. 34 (1687–1715); col. 1262, no. 46 (ca. 1655–89); col. 1262, no. 47 (1700).

42. S.v. "Paris Foreign Missionary Society," *New Catholic Encyclopedia,* 1967. Pallegoix, 1854.

43. Another example is the diplomatic tour made by Monsignor de Bourges. On orders of Bishop de la Mothe-Lambert, he left Siam in October 1663. He was well received in England in July 1665, went on to Paris and then to Rome, where he obtained approval from Pope Clement IX. Pallegoix, 1954, 2:120–21.

44. Ibid., 2:140, 163, 162.

45. Costa, 1961, 135. Early seventeenth-century hospitals are mentioned on p. 348 of this work.

46. *El archipiélago filipino,* 1900, 1:377–79.

47. Bantug, 1953.

48. This part of the discussion draws on Gicklhorn and Gicklhorn, 1954. See also Cullum, 1956.

49. *Webster's New International Dictionary of the English Language,* 2d ed. ("camellia"), states that Kamel is said to have brought the plant from the East. This is an error: Kamel never left the Philippines.

50. Gicklhorn and Gicklhorn, 1954, 74.

51. S.v. "Jesuits," *New Catholic Encyclopedia,* 1967 (see esp. 2:905).

52. Sebes, 1961, 88–94.

53. For example, the Franciscans had been in China during 1294–1368; Franciscans and Dominicans were there in 1632–33. The Société des Missions Etrangères de Paris, already mentioned in our discussion of Siam, first entered China in 1684 and worked mainly in southern and southwestern areas.

54. S.v. "Wang Hsi-Shan," *Dictionary of Scientific Biography,* 1976 (see 14:160).

55. Bouvet, 1697, 160–61. English, Latin, and Dutch translations have been published. A biographical note on de Fontaney appears in *Nouvelle Biographie Générale,* 1857, 18: cols. 116–17.

56. Peregrino da Costa, 1948, 1–236 (see esp. 46–48).

57. Peters et al., 1986.

58. Klayman, 1985.

59. Boxer, 1965, 24–57.

60. Boxer, 1957, 112, 151.

61. Piso, 1648, 15–16. Piso, 1658, likewise makes no mention of the Peruvian bark or tree.

62. Boxer, 1952, 7–15. See also Stepan, 1981, 16–22.

63. Leite, 1965, 169.

64. Leite, 1953, 83–89.

65. Cullum, 1956, 321–22.

66. Dominian, 1958, 130, n. 10.

67. Leite, 1953, 96, 99, 273. See also Leite, 1939–50, 1:578–79; 5:340; 8:133–34; 9:167.

68. Purchas, [1625] 1905–7, 16:417–503.
69. See Leite, 1938–50, 2:580, 584.
70. Leite, 1953, p. 91.
71. Santos Filho, 1977.
72. Valdizan and Maldonado, 1922, 3:10.
73. Those who contemplate doing research on the history of Jesuits' bark in Paraguay would be well advised to start with Jones, 1979. See also Streit, 1916–71 (especially vols. 2, 3, 25). Some useful hints can be gathered from Gicklhorn and Gicklhorn, 1954, 13.
74. Esteyneffer, [1712]. I have used the version edited by Carmen Anzures y Balanos. Mexico: Academia Nacional de México, 1978 (see esp. 514 and 524).
75. Wafer, [1699] 1903, 106–7.
76. Thwaites, 1896–1901.
77. Whittemore, 1713.

Chapter 7. Italy and Spain, 1679–1718

1. Adelmann, 1966, 169, n. 1, 429, 637.
2. Letter to Sig. Giambattista Tela, Florence, 19 Dec. 1682, in Redi, 1712–30, 2:69–73.
3. [Nigrisoli], 1687.
4. See Chapter 5, note 78.
5. [Helvetius?], 1694a, i.
6. Morgagni, 1761, 49.30 (1 paragr). Subsequent paragraphs contain detailed report of a cardinal who almost died of a periodic fever (1729). The bark, given by Morgagni and Vallisneri, rescued the patient.
7. This condition had been discussed in a special treatise by another Spanish author, Isaac (Ferdinand) Cardoso, in 1638. See Appendix A.
8. Cabriada, 1687, 207.
9. According to the equally pseudonymous Filiatro, 1688, "Aduanista's" onslaught was titled *Respuesta que la medicina dogmatica, y racional da al libro, que ha publicado el Doctor Don Iuan de Cabriada.* I have not had access to a copy of this work.
10. Corte, [1718] 1972, 193, lists the 1679 edition, which I have not seen. I have used the 1685 edition.
11. Mercatus, 1611, 526; see also the discussion in Appendix A. Heredia, 1689–88 [*sic*], 1:546–55, 593–630. Salado Garces, 1678, 9–10; see also Chapter 1. Cardoso, 1639 (discussed in Appendix A).
12. Flores, [1698], 93.
13. Juanini, 1685, 74, 92–93.
14. Colmenero, 1697, 10, 11, 17, 18. Colmenero refers to Cicero's *De natura deorum* and Galen's *De methodo medendi.*
15. Fernández, 1698, 70, 82, 87. The wise quotation from St. Ambrose appears on p. 69.
16. Suárez de Ribera, 1724, 162, 163; 1726, 41.
17. See Chapter 2, notes 53–55.
18. Collegium Physicorum, Milan, 1668.
19. Collegium Physicorum, Milan, 1698. The discussion of the Peruvian bark is on pp. 20–25.
20. Vallisneri, 1733, 3:143–46.

21. Ibid., 3:161 (the drug occasionally produces torpor), 415–17, 445–46, 513–14.

22. See note 6 above.

23. Morgagni, 1769, 30.5 (Alexander's translation).

24. *Dictionnaire des sciences médicales*, 1821, 4:542–44.

25. Colonne, 1929. Guglielminus, 1701, 79; 1719, 2:470–75.

26. Guglielmini, 1719, 2:471, paragr. 3.

27. Cogrossi, 1711, 9, 37–39. The experiment may have been inspired by Boyle, whose writings are mentioned by Cogrossi.

28. Ibid., 78.

29. In supplementary essays Cogrossi (1716, 17; 1718, 17) mentions a letter addressed to him by Torti on 16 Nov. 1716. This communication suggests that the pyrogenic ferment acts as a specific absorbent of the drug, not as a specific solvent.

30. De Tipaldo, 1835, 2:152–62.

31. Zendrini, 1715, 66 (second pagination). This work is dated incorrectly by De Renzi ([1845–49] 1966, 4:403) as 1615 and by Sprengel (1821–38, 4:540, 5:530) as 1705. De Renzi's error is an obvious misprint; Sprengel's might result in misinterpretations.

32. Corradi, [1865–94] 1972–73, 5:558.

Chapter 8. Antonio Frassoni and Francesco Torti's *Synopsis*

1. Di Pietro, 1952, 688–92.

2. Badus, 1663, 245–46.

3. Pastor, [1938] 1955, 29:163–64. Fantuzzi, 1781–94, 3:285–86. Dolfi, 1670. Katterbach, 1931, 277 (item 13).

4. Litta, 1819, 4:65.

5. Torti, 1712, 3–4. Torti uses the word *pharmacopoeas*, which perhaps could be interpreted to mean pharmacies rather than pharmacopoeias.

6. Di Pietro, 1952, 690–92 (the consultations are listed by title).

7. Gaddi, 1868, 9.

8. See Chapter 7, note 1.

9. Torti, 1712, 184–87.

10. The best modern biography of Torti is Di Pietro (1958), cited above. Also valuable is that by Muratori in Torti, 1743 and several later editions. Most easily accessible to North American readers is the biographical note in Hirsch, 1962, 5:613–14.

11. Ramazzini, 1964, 309 (letter 289).

12. Di Pietro, 1957, 81–87.

13. See the *List of the Royal Society, 1717*; from *Lists of Fellows, 1700–1774* (Royal Society Archives). In the *Journal Books of the Royal Society* 11:141–42, 8 Nov. 1716, it is recorded that "the President [Sir Isaac Newton] brought two Books of Dr. Torta [*sic*] of Modena about the Jesuits Bark which he desired some Gentlemen of the Society to look over, the Author being desirous of being a Member of the Society."

14. A list is in Di Pietro, 1958, 469–77.

15. Boccabadati, 1833, 125–47, esp. 139.

16. Torti, 1712, 502–3. Giambattista Davini (1662?–1733) was one of the physicians of the Modenese ducal family and author of *De potu vini calidi* (Modena,

1720), a work that had the honor of being mentioned in Morgagni's consultations (Jarcho, 1984a, 95); a biographical note on Davini appears in Tiraboschi, 1781–86, 2:204. By courtesy of the library of the University of Pennsylvania I was able to examine the entire run of *La Galleria* (in a copy that bears the signature of Albrecht von Haller), but I could not find the report by Davini. According to Torti (1712, 502) it was anonymous. Tiraboschi says it appears in vol. 4.

17. Torti, 1712, xv. The vagueness of this reference has caused much loss of time. Comparable experiences were reported by Di Pietro, 1981, 95–114, in his research on Ramazzini.

18. Sommervogel, 1864–65. I have examined issues of the *Mémoires* for 1709–12.

19. Dumas, 1936, 76.

20. *Miscellanea curiosa*, 1702.

21. These lists appear in the unpaginated prefatory materials included in successive volumes and are headed *Catalogus . . . dominorum . . . qui observationes communicarunt* (Catalog of the gentlemen who submitted observations).

22. Additional information about the *Galleria* is given in Kronick, 1976, 251. It is possible that this text of the *Synopsis* was submitted by Torti's colleague Giambattista Davini; see note 16 above.

23. Intending to convey a correct impression of the intricacy that characterized Torti's thinking and his style, I have abstained from dividing the supertortuous sentences of the original. Torti's inconstancy in the use of the terms *China* and *China Chinae* has been left unaltered. His frequent use of capital letters for emphasis has been preserved.

24. Puccinotti, 1842, 33 (no. 3). Sprengel, 1821–38, 5:530 (no. 20). Castiglioni, 1941, 648.

25. A copy is preserved in the University of Bologna Library, MS 2089, vol. 1 [consult. 40], 51–52, and is reproduced in Jarcho, 1989, 40.

Chapter 9. Torti's *Therapeutice Specialis*

1. Examples: Torti 1712, xxiv, l. 23; 14, 30; 547, l. 17. Morgagni, 1761, 28.2 (see the third sentence, *Praeterea si certas quasdam excipias . . . si illas, inquam, excipias*). As might be expected, the same trait is found in Torti's Italian writings, e.g., the fourth letter to Muratori (Torti, 1743, xxi): *Vi dico . . . dissi . . .*

2. Torti, 1712, 189. See also p. 574, ll. 19–21: *quám lubricae sint, ac fallaces conjecturae nostrae* (how slippery and deceptive our guesses are!).

3. Morton, 1692, 188.

4. We are warranted in surmising that Torti's numerous case reports were helpful to beleaguered practitioners and constituted a reason for the repeated reediting and reprinting of the book. He did not omit to mention his own instructive illness, judged to be a "diaphoretic pernicious tertian." Torti, 1712, 424–32.

5. Jarcho, 1989, 17–18: consultation 16, observation on *La China* [cinchona].

6. Bacon, 1624, book 4, chap. 2, page xvi.

7. Similar difficulties were reported by Ramazzini, 1714, 205–13.

8. A convenient concise summary appears in *Hippocrates*, 1923, 1:xlvi–lii. See also Hippocrates [1839–61] 1973–82, 1.619 (acute febrile illness terminated by evacuation of yellow bile); 2.627 (irregularity or failure of crises); 2.635 (contrast between successful and absent coction); 3.71 (absence of crises, difficult crises); 4.473 (relapse caused by residues after crisis); 6.217.8 (an unsatisfactory definition of crisis, in a tract intended for laymen).

9. *Hippocrates,* 1931, 4:147, 209. Of the former aphorism Galen explained (K 17/2, 722) that those fevers that intermit in an afebrile period are declared by Hippocrates to be free from danger, since they are not generated by any kind of inflammation or by putrefaction of malign humors.

10. Bruce-Chwatt and Zulueta, 1980, 19. The reader will find it interesting to study the entire Greco-Roman record, summarized on pp. 17–27.

11. Grmek, 1989, 276–77.

12. Henke and Lubarsch, 1926–70, vol. 9 (skeletal diseases), vol. 1 (pt. 1, Malaria).

13. Badus, 1663, 209–10.

14. A doubtful precedent is found in Avicenna, [1507] 1964, bk. 4, fen 1, tract 2, chap. 7, p. 400r: *Scias quod non est tibi possibile curare febrem nisi cognoveris eam* (Know that it is impossible for you to cure a fever unless you understand it).

15. Torti's taxonomy is described mainly in bk. 5, chap. 1, 577–90. Additional discussion is in bk. 3, chap. 1, 271–95.

16. *Communicans, coalternans*—these forms escaped inclusion in Torti's Tree of Fevers (see below).

17. See also Jussieu, J. de. 1779. Réflexions sur deus espèces de quinquina récemment decouvertes aux environs de Santa-Fé. *Histoire de la Société de Médecine de Paris,* 252–63 (cited by Weddell).

18. Condamine, 1740.

19. The tree diagram is explained in four Latin hexameters, which are inscribed at the foot of the tree:

> Quas jugulat Cortex, in Ramis Cortice tectis
> Inspicias Febres, quas jugulare nequit,
> In delibratis. Mediâ quae sorte fruuntur,
> Dimidio obductus Cortice Ramus habet.

These stately lines can be rendered in English as follows:

> Fevers that the Bark can quell
> Are shown as Branches covered well,
> But those the Bark cannot restrain
> Have nothing to protect their grain.
> The branches that between are placed
> With middling fate are partly graced.

20. "I say confidently that after daily use for twenty-five years . . . I have never known any harm to come from the use of the bark, except for deafness." Morton, 1692, 132. Torti, 1712, 467.

21. This of course suggests typhoid fever or the ingestion of iron.

22. For a Hippocratic precedent see *Prognostic IX,* in Hippocrates [1839–61] 1973–82, 2.132.

23. S.v. "Santorio, Santorio," in *Dictionary of Scientific Biography,* 1970–81, 12:101–4.

24. Cantù and Righini Bonelli, [1981?].

25. Ramazzini, 1716, 187–217 (see 190).

26. Torti, [1695] 1743, 487–500. Torti [1698], 1743a, 500–18.

27. Ramazzini, 1716a, 697–782 (see 713).

28. University of Bologna MS. 2089–1, Consultation no. 118, pp. 221–23 (esp. 2d paragr., p. 221), in Jarcho, 1989b, 192–94 (esp. 192–93).

29. Lindeboom, 1968, 294, 363–64. Boerhaave, 1757a, esp. aphorisms 563 (p. 208) and 673 (p. 216).

30. Wunderlich, 1857 (p. 6 refers to more than half a million observations on more than five thousand patients; p. 11 mentions intermittent fever with apparently continuous course). Wunderlich, 1868, 371–73 (fig. 7 shows graphs of tertian and quartan fever). Allbutt, 1870 (esp. 437).

31. *Consensu . . . universali rejecta est Humoristarum doctrina.*

32. See Appendix A, including note 105.

33. University of Bologna, MS 2089–1, p. 127, in Jarcho, 1989b, 111.

34. Morton, 1692, 174. See also Chapter 4.

35. Badus, 1663 (unpaginated prefatory material). See also Chapter 2, note 46.

36. Auda, 1740, 15.

37. Jarcho, 1989b, 221 (consultation 136).

38. Cinchona contains some twenty-five closely related alkaloids, the average yield being 6 to 7 percent, of which in the yellow barks from one-half to two-thirds is quinine, whereas in the red barks, cinchonidine exists in greater proportion; specimen pieces have yielded as high as 18 percent of total alkaloids. Gathercoal and Wirth, 1947, 600. Much earlier, Trousseau and Pidoux, 1855, 2:327, in an elaborate discussion of the different varieties, stated that no sample of yellow cinchona containing less than 15 grams of quinine sulphate per 100 could be accepted.

39. Morton, 1692, 174.

40. *Sydenham,* 1848–50, 2:5–28 (see esp. 13–14). Additional comment in 1:85–86.

41. Search for this doctrine in Avicenna, [1507] 1964, has been repeatedly unsuccessful. Sydenham, in the second chapter of *Processus Integri,* used the term *depuratory.* In his translation of Sydenham (1809, 417), Benjamin Rush used the explanatory expression, "the depuratory or cleansing fever."

42. Falloppius, 1606, 18. See also Falloppius, 1600–1606. I owe the discovery of this passage to the remarkable work by Jacob Wolff, 1907, 1:35 (English translation, 1989, 29). The identity of *unguentum Isidis* is obscure. Apparently it resembled the *unguentum aegyptiacum,* which was considered mild and which contained vinegar and copper oxide in a base of honey. See Falloppius, 1600–1606, 1:539, ll 30–41. See also Schneider, 1968–75, 3:39, 2:59; Estes, 1989, 113–14.

43. The heading continues with the remark, "Accurate writers on this subject are few."

44. "Non una tamen praecisè est Methodus in omnibus hisce casibus adhibenda."

45. Torti's statements on this subject vary slightly. On p. 333 he puts the total at two ounces (*duabus unciis ad summum . . . in totum absumptis*).

46. "I immediately gave the bark, the sacrament of the Eucharist having been administered" (434). "After the sacrament of the Church had been given, I prescribed the Peruvian bark by the strong method" (438).

Chapter 10. Torti as Seen by His Contemporaries

1. Morgagni, 1761, 5.13, 6.5, 10.21, 26.6, 41.5, 48.14. Jarcho, 1980b, 322–38; 1989b.

2. Both essays were reprinted, with a preface, by the illustrious Moritz Romberg in 1828.

3. Page references are to the 1748 edition.

4. Torti, 1712, 48–49.

5. Lancisi, 1717. Exposition is on pp. 213–91; comments by obscure correspon-

dents, on pp. 368–94, are not considered in the present discussion. A charming letter from Lancisi to Torti, dated 17 Feb. 1713 and acknowledging arrival of Torti's *Therapeutice specialis*, is in Boccabadati, 1833, 143–44.

6. Baglivi, 1704, 61–95 of second pagination (esp. 79–95).

7. *Oleum scorpionum magnum* Matthiolii. See *Pharmacopoeia augustana*, 1613, 249.

8. Morgagni, 1769, 49.1.

9. Crescimbeni, 1720–21, 1:270–76. Tiraboschi, 1781–86, 4 (1783): 240–50. Hirsch, 1962, 4:716. Wright, 1940.

10. Ramazzini, 1679, *Exercitatio iatroapologetica . . . seu, responsum ad scripturam quandam . . . Annibalis Cervi*, Modena: Dignus. I have not seen this work. One wonders why it is not included in *Opera omnia*.

11. Extensive documentation can be found in Haller, 1776–78, 3:483–85. A generous helping of the pamphlets is in the library of the New York Academy of Medicine.

12. Ramazzini, 1716, 364–469. Unless otherwise noted page references in the text to works of Ramazzini are to this volume.

13. Torti, 1712, 175–77, 181–83, 426, 562–65.

14. Torti, 1712, 637–40. Salado Garces is discussed in Chapter 1.

15. Salado Garces, 1678, 12. A search for the original text written by "Carlos Vallesius" has been unsuccessful; I have found no such author. Possibly Salado Garces intended to çite Francisco Valles Covarrubias (1524–92), whose Commentaria in prognosticum Hippocratis is in Valles Covarrubias, 1589, col. 252–396 (it does not contain the quoted passage).

16. He gave credit to Gulielmus Ballonius (1538–1616), a precinchonal physician, for suggesting that this determination was needed. See Ballonius, 1640, 120.

17. Jiang et al., 1985.

18. Torti, 1712, 564, 221.

19. Ramazzini, 1964.

20. Hirsch, 1962, 4:716, states that Ramazzini's blindness began a few years after the transfer to Padua. As to the severity of the visual impairment, which has possible bearing on the textual problems that are to be discussed, I have found no detailed information.

21. Torti, 1712, 368, 638–40.

22. Crescimbeni, 1720–21, 274.

23. Jarcho, 1989b, 17 (consultation 16).

24. Trousseau and Pidoux, 1858, 2:336. The reference is to De febribus malignis, et messentericis [*sic*] (Praxeos Medicae Liber I), in Baglivi, 1727, 33 ("usum damnabilem chinae-chinae").

25. Torti, 1730, 532 (*quas Responsiones . . . hortor, ne graventur legere Tyrones*).

26. Jarcho, 1989b, 18 (consultation 16), note 47.

27. Hirsch, 1962, 4:56. Bayle and Thillaye, [1855] 1967, 2:51–52.

28. Mangetus's introduction reappears in later editions.

29. Wright, 1940, 530.

30. Torti wrote: *me literariae concordiae quam maxime amantem et . . . ab hujuscemodi superuacaneis contentionibus . . . plane alienum*. Biblioteca Estense, Codice miscellanei (examined in microfilm prepared by the Biblioteca Estense). See also comment in Di Pietro, 1958, 460–78 (475).

31. This part of Mangetus's letter to Torti is discussed in Chapter 5; see note 117.

32. Mangetus, 1703, 2:695–98.

33. Mangetus, 1731, 2 (bk. 19): 387–88. See also *Acta Lipsiensia*, 1716, 220–23.

Chapter 11. Torti's Place in History

1. Torti, 1712, 580, referred to these fevers as "hermaphroditic."
2. Jarcho, 1984b.
3. Ramazzini's *Orationes iatrici argumenti* (Orations on medical subjects) was published in Padua in 1708. I have not seen this edition. It is recorded in Blake, 1979, 370. The *Oratio quarta* appears in Ramazzini, 1716, 45–55 (see esp. 53).
4. See Chapter 4 and Morton, 1692, 174.
5. Ramazzini, 1714, 207–8, 240.
6. Ives, 1773, 451.
7. Di Pietro, 1958.
8. Corradi, [1865–94] 1972–73. Pringle, 1752.
9. Huxham, [1757] 1988. Boerhaave, 1757a.
10. Haller, 1776–78, 4:433.
11. See also Morgagni, 1761, 68.2.
12. Sprengel, 1821–38, 5 (1827): 350.
13. Puccinotti, 1842, 37–206. Torti, 1712, 282.
14. De Renzi, [1845–49] 1966, 4:406–10, 435–36.
15. Renouard, [1846] 1856, 437.
16. Trousseau, 1869–72, 5 (1872): 32. Trousseau and Pidoux, 1858, 2:333–49.
17. Hernández Morejon, 1842–52, 4:36.
18. Welch [1897] 1920, 1:17–75 (esp. 18). Reprinted in Welch, 1920, 1:463–531 (see 464).
19. Thieme, 1916, 12:323.
20. The role of analogic reasoning at an earlier stage in the history of the bark is discussed in Chapter 1.
21. Weddell, 1849, 1 and note.
22. From M. Georges Colin of the Bibliothèque Royale Albert 1er it was learned (letter to S.J., Brussels, 13 Apr. 1989) that Tombeur, a native of Liège, presented a thesis, *De febre putrida*, at the University of Leiden in 1816. In the same year Brixhe, also Liegeois, submitted a thesis on dysentery at Utrecht.
23. See, for example, Duran-Reynals, 1946, 94.
24. Jarcho, 1989, xxvii. Boyd, 1949, 1:3–4, reports the findings of Scott and van Wesep. Russell, 1952, 94. Guarini, 1950, p. 296.
25. Quoted by permission of the Università degli Studi di Firenze, Dipartimento della Linguistica.
26. Details are given in Jarcho, 1970. An additional complication is that Jacopo Tatti (1486–1570), an eminent sculptor and architect, was a pupil of Andrea Sansovino (1460–1529), whose surname he assumed. *Webster's Biographical Dictionary*, 1948, 1310.
27. Celli, 1933, 156, 212 (n. 181).
28. Celli-Fraentzel, 1928, 101–19 (see esp. 110 and n. 3).
29. The document is numbered Medici F., 3377. Additional documents, ca. 1646, are mentioned in Celli-Fraentzel, 1928, 110, n. 4.

Chapter 12. The Bark: Botanical, Geographical, and Commercial Factors

1. Weddell, 1849; the previously unpublished Latin statement by Jussieu appears on p. 15, n. 1.

2. The observations (226–43) were made during an astronomical expedition designed to measure a meridian. It is rare indeed for medicine to benefit, however indirectly, from astronomical research. More often medical patients become involved with astrology.

3. Gray, 1737.

4. This statement does not appear in the 1712 edition of *Therapeutice specialis.*

5. Vesalius's *Letter on the China root* is discussed in O'Malley, 1964, 215–17.

6. Letter to S.J. from Miss H. Brenda Sutton of the Wellcome Institute, 17 Jan. 1989, with inclusion of an obituary (1946) by E. Ashworth Underwood and notes from other sources.

7. Haggis, 1941, 452–53.

8. Gathercoal and Wirth, 1947, 596.

9. Oliver, 1704. The *Dictionary of National Biography*, compact ed., 1975, 2:1542, mentions Oliver's presence at Cadiz in 1694 as physician to the Red Squadron. Further information in Keevil, 1958, 2:255–56.

10. Sollmann, 1948, 505.

11. Saunders, 1782, v, 2, i.

12. Gathercoal and Wirth, 1947, 600.

13. Senac, 1749, 2:524, 526.

14. Ramazzini, 1716b, 799.

15. Jarcho, 1986, 251, 297.

16. Interesting details, derived from archival study, are in Turrion, 1989.

17. Gray, 1737, 83.

18. S.v. "Zamora," *Webster's New Geographical Dictionary,* 1984.

19. Letter to S.J. from Col. Bolivar O. Arevalo, Quito, 23 Feb. 1989.

20. Oviedo y Valdes, [1535–57] 1944–45, 13:103–19, 14:104–60. Others give the date as 1541. Orellana preceded Padre Cristobal de Acuña by ninety-six years.

21. S.v. "Amazon," *Encyclopaedia Britannica,* 1953, esp. 730.

22. The original is in the Phelps Stokes Collection, New York Public Library. Reproduced in Deák, 1989, 2: no. 39; also in *Imprint* 13 (autumn 1988): 9.

23. Burger, 1989, 66–73; see especially the map on p. 69 and its caption. Keatinge, 1988, 279–300 (esp. 279, 287–88).

24. Riding, 1988.

25. Weiss, 1844, 2:226–31.

26. Spate, 1983, 204–7.

27. S.v. "Caribbean Sea," *Encyclopaedia Britannica,* 1953. Boxer, 1952, 74–77.

28. Jefferys, 1762, 35–39.

29. Ibid., 30.

30. Readers are likely to enjoy the stately descriptions and discussions in Raynal, 1780, esp. 4:228–31, 137–46.

31. Haring, 1918, 182–84. Some of the original documents are reproduced in *Relaciones históricas y geográficas de América Central,* 1908.

32. Boxer, 1952, 24.

33. Newton, 1933, 58. An amusing report, worth reading, is in De Leon, [1627] (see Levanto, Memorial).

34. For further details see the *New Cambridge Modern History,* 1970, 4:724–25.

35. Malvezin, 1892, 2:196, 3:234.

36. Jarcho, 1956.

37. Boxer, 1965, 25–27. Le Moine d'Espine, 1710, 127, 143, 145–146.

38. Sturmius, 1659, 15, 1.

39. *Archivo general de Simancas,* 1937, nos. 64, 85, 71, 112, 123, 127, 206, 207, 216, 232, 233, 428.
40. Ibid., vii, 2, 3, 13.
41. Ruiz Lopez, 1792, 24–26.
42. *Archivo general de Simancas,* 1937, experimentos, no. 141 . . . el buen efecto de la quina llamada inutil.
43. Braudel, 1982, 141, has pointed out the extensiveness of Dutch warehousing.
44. As to eighteenth-century transatlantic commerce, a concise authoritative summary (which does not exclude the seventeenth century) is given in Spain, Ministerio de Cultura, 1990, 63–69; for information on smuggling see esp. 67–69.
45. Condamine, 1740, 226–43 (esp. 234–35).
46. Sturmius, 1659, 15.
47. Cabanès, 1910, 317–54.
48. Dewhurst, 1963, 60.
49. Patin, 1707, 1:217.
50. *Les admirables qualitez du kinkina,* 1689, 11. Torti, 1712, 20, refers to the author of this work as *stupidus auctor quidem anonymus (Helvetius creditur),* a certain stupid anonymous author, thought to be Helvetius.
51. Turrion, 1989, 307–8.
52. S.v. "cuarango," *Diccionario de la lengua española,* 19th ed.
53. Hospital real de Nuestra Señora de Esqueba hasta fin de este año de 1703, 1703–13.
54. Letters dated Braunschweig, 7 Aug. and 31 Oct. 1989. For any errors in the presentation or interpretation of these data I alone am responsible.
55. S.v. "Taxe," *Muret-Sanders enzyklopädisches . . . Wörterbuch,* 1944.
56. Great Britain, Inspector General of Imports and Exports, 1974. The records for 1705 and 1712 are missing. I thank Professor Clifford M. Foust of the University of Maryland for an introduction to this body of data, now made available at the Columbia University Library.

Chapter 13. Epilogue

1. Leincker, 1705. (Incidentally, note on p. 11: "Brasiliam, florentissimam Americae septentrionalis regionem." As Chaucer wrote, the best clerics are not the wisest men.) Engelen, 1967–68. S.v. "emetinum," Weisenberg, [1853] 1969, 347–49, 240–41.
2. In the case of ipecacuanha the credit probably belongs to a Jesuit lay brother, Irmão Manoel Tristão (b. 1544; died between 1621 and 1631), who served the college at Bahia, Brazil, as apothecary and nurse. His manuscript collection of medical recipes found its way to Samuel Purchas. See Purchas, [1625] 1905–7, 16:417, 478. See also Chapter 6. Further details are to be found in Leite, 1938–50, 8:133–34, 9:167.
3. This resemblance was noted by Engelen, 1967–68, 37.
4. Peregrino da Costa, 1948, summarized in Leite, 1953, 89, n. 1. I have not seen the original.
5. Pankhurst, 1979, 297–313. S.v. "Hagenia abyssinica," Schneider, 1968–75, 2:23, 5 (pt. 2): 152.
6. Torti, 1712, 10, 424–32.
7. Letter from E. Milano (director of Biblioteca Estense), Modena, 27 Sept. 1988.

Appendix A. The Intermittent Fevers as Understood in the Seventeenth and Early Eighteenth Centuries

1. The reader is reminded that some of the Galenic passages quoted are samples and are contradicted or modified by passages that occur elsewhere in the Galenic corpus. For a very brief conspectus of seventy-seven kinds of fever listed in the index of the Kühn edition of Galen see Jarcho, 1980a, 132–38 (esp. 132–33). Galen's opinions are discussed anew in Brain, 1986.

2. Like many other Galenic dicta, this statement is recorded also in Hippocrates, 1973–82, 7: 569 (sect. 45), 7:587.

3. See also the discussion in K9. 678–79 and Jarcho, 1987b.

4. Galen says (K14. 730) that older writers sometimes classed it as continuous and sometimes as intermittent. Sir John Falstaff died of it. See Shakespeare's *King Henry the Fifth*, Act 2, Scene 1. See also Jarcho, 1987a.

5. Galen discusses the differential diagnosis and treatment of the intermittent fevers somewhat concisely in *De medendi methodo ad Glauconem*, bk. 1, chaps. 5–13 (K11. 18–41) and much more elaborately in *De methodo medendi*, especially bks. 8–11 (K10. 531–809).

6. The development of this notion by Fernel—with important consequences—is discussed by I. M. Lonie in Bynum and Nutton, 1981, 30–35.

7. See Shortt, 1948, 607–17.

8. Baglivi, 1732, 290–91 (De febribus messentericis). In the *Opera omnia* of 1727, it is at p. 33 (*De praxi medica*, bk. 1, chap. 9).

9. This matter is considered again in the discussion of Spigelius (see below).

10. Galen: *Ad Glauconem de methodo medendi* 1.5 (K11.19), 1.6 (K11.21); *De causis pulsuum* 2.1 (K9. 57–61); *De methodo medendi* 9. 304 (K10. 607–10); *De febrium differentiis* 1.9 (K7. 306). Zacutus Lusitanus, 1667, 2:587, assembled these statements and a few more in his discussion of tertian fever and reconciled them, to his satisfaction if not ours.

11. A sample of Mercatus's writing on internal medicine, translated into English with critique, is in Jarcho, 1980b, 87–102.

12. Mercatus uses the term *tertianam extensam*, while Kühn says *tertianam productam*, to translate Galen's *ektetamenon tritaion*.

13. Some of his incidental comments should be rescued from oblivion, for example, *non raro tyrones medicos hallucinari* (it is not unusual for inexperienced doctors to go haywire, 532).

14. A long list of such physicians is in Werlhof, 1745, 6–9.

15. S.v. "Spiegel, Adrian Van den," in *Dictionary of Scientific Biography*, 1975, 12:577–78. See also Favaro, 1925—26. The treatise is reproduced, with minimal editorial change, in Spigelius, 1645, 2:1–64; page references are to this edition.

16. For the definition and characteristics see Kühn's Galen 7. 356, 7. 363–367, and 17(1). 944. The diagnosis is discussed in 9. 673. See also Hippocrates, [1839–61] 1973–82, 2. 606–10.

17. Garrison, 1929, 271, speaks of "Spieghel's extensive account of malarial fever (*De semitertiana*, 1624)"; Morton, 1991, 805, refers to it as the "first extensive account of malaria." In the spring of 1607 Spigelius witnessed an outbreak of malignant fever "with red spots resembling mosquito bites" (2:57).

18. Hippocrates, 1988, 5:30–34, 34–37.

19. Spigelius and his opinions are discussed *in extenso* in Jarcho, 1987b.

20. *In magna frusta divideretur* (2:9).

21. *A duplici tertiana longitudine paroxysmorum et typo quotidianae permixtae* (2:17).

22. This is known from Harvey, 1886, 80.

23. Isler, 1968; Davis, 1973; s.v. "Willis, Thomas," *Dictionary of Scientific Biography*, 1976, 14: 404–9; Frank, 1980; Dewhurst, 1980; Dewhurst, 1981; Dewhurst, 1983, esp. xix–xxiii, 262–78.

24. The same text appears, without noteworthy change, in Willis, 1681a, 1:63–140 (preceded by a four-page intercalated preface). *This edition forms the basis of the present discussion.* A convenient English translation (with misbound illustrations) is Willis, 1681b, 53–178; a facsimile edition prepared by W. Feindel was issued in two volumes by the McGill University Press in 1965.

25. Probably this word and its Latin original are to be interpreted as signifying *diversity*, rather than *inhomogeneity*.

26. Puschmann, 1902, 2:63.

27. Pages cited in parentheses in this discussion are in Willis, 1681a, and in the case of those preceded by "SP," in Willis, 1681b, the translation by Samuel Pordage.

28. It is possible but not certain that at this point Willis was thinking of pernicious tertian fever.

29. Emphasis added. The original clause reads *quae a visceribus cruoris massae inspirantur.*

30. Willis, 1670, 47–69 (also in 1681a, 1:660–72).

31. The entry for Willis in the *Dictionary of Scientific Biography*, 1976, ascribes this opinion to the influence of Lower (who served as Willis's research assistant).

32. Here Willis uses *heterogeneous* to mean *alien*, that is, of foreign origin. It does not necessarily signify diversity of composition.

33. *Quando repullulat haec materia* (77). Although Willis's use of *repullulat* might suggest that he is thinking of live entities, the word *materia* in the same clause suggests the contrary.

34. One of the few to contest Willis's assertions was Jean Riolan, 1649, 226, who says that the ventricles are frequently obstructed by fleshy and fatty bits, and are the veins also.

35. See especially K7. 334, 7. 182, 9. 657, and 17 (2). 642.

36. See Galen K18(2). 279 on change from quartan to continuous, and 7. 466 on change from tertian to semitertian.

37. Could these be cases of lymphoma?

38. See, for example, Galen's remarks on putridity in putrid fevers (K10. 773ff. and 10. 751).

39. Aristotle, 1955, 157–329 (esp. 269, 275); 1952, esp. 295; 1953, 529, 291. For valuable comment see Ross, 1945, 99–111; and Aristotle, 1962, 9.

40. In his excellent discussion of this aspect Dewhurst, 1981, 25, has used the term "farmhouse empiricism." The use of analogy by Jesuits is considered in Chapter 1.

41. According to Jacques-Charles Brunet, 1861, 2: col. 611, a corrected second edition was prepared by Clerselier and published in Paris in 1677 by Argot, with Descartes's *Traité de l'homme.*

42. S.v. "Montmor, Henri Louis Habert de," *Dictionary of Scientific Biography*, 1970–80, 9:497–99. Brown, 1934, 64–134, mentions (p. 85) a discourse that Samuel Sorbière (1610–70) presented on 11 Feb. 1659, *du Froid des Fièvres intermittentes.*

43. See 1:567–650, esp. 613–32 and the description of the heart and circulation, 619–32.

44. Adam and Milhaud, 1934–63, 6:215–18.

45. Ibid., 6:225.

46. Ibid., 7:58–62.

47. Willis, 1681a, 2:4.

48. The full name is Abraham Zacutus Lusitanus. This analysis is based on the *Operum* of 1667. Principal supplementary sources are: Lemos, 1881; Lemos, 1909; Friedenwald, 1944, 307–21; Friedenwald, 1946, 154–55; Hirsch, 1962, 5:1021–22; Ferreira de Mira, 1947; Barbosa Machado, 1741–59, 3:797–98.

49. For a beautiful commendation of Galen, such as is rare nowadays, see Zacutus Lusitanus, 1667, 1:708.

50. Zacutus wrote *lethalis sane affectus, prorsus dirus*. Doubtless he had in mind the Horatian *crescit indulgens sibi dirus hydrops* (*Carmina* 2.2.13).

51. The word *scirrhus* in this context signifies induration, which might be accompanied by enlargement.

52. Lemos, 1909, 22; Friedenwald, 1944, 1:297–304.

53. Friedenwald, 1944, 1:310 n.

54. The reader is warned that there are not a few errors in pagination in the *Opera;* the page references in the tables of contents are not invariably to be trusted.

55. This order is found in the Edwin Smith papyrus (see Breasted, 1930) and persisted at least as late as Morgagni's *De sedibus,* 1761. It is still used nowadays in the internist's physical examination.

56. For further discussion, see Jarcho, 1989a.

57. On at least a few occasions Zacutus's reports encountered disbelief and even overt hostility. Nor was he altogether free from credulity. See Reis, 1670, 935.

58. Professor Paul Potter of London, Ontario, suggests as the source section 38 of Galen's second commentary on the *Prognostikon* (K18/2. 165f.).

59. Zacutus gives the source as "6 epid[emics] sect 1, text 9"; repeated search in Hippocrates, [1839–61] 1973–82, did not confirm this reference. Stuart F. Kitchen (in Boyd, 1949, 1018) wrote as follows: "In our experience the onset of quartan attacks has been ordinarily gradual, thus differing from the situation in many of the *vivax* and *falciparum* infections."

60. Blancardus, [1683] 1973, defines this as a vein that goes to a finger from branches in the arm. Dorland's *Medical dictionary,* 27th ed., defines it as "a small vein of the little finger and dorsum of the hand."

61. Friedenwald, 1944, 319, item VII.

62. This appears under *De pulueribus expurgantibus.*

63. Zacutus erred. Ebenum was known to the Greeks and Arabs. S.v. "Lithospermum," in Schneider, 1968–75, 5/2:264–65.

64. Psalm 19:2.

65. For evidence of Zacutus's wide reading and his intense interest in newly discovered regions and their products, see *De Medicorum Principum Historia,* book 4, quaestio 47 (1:774–75). Not even the letters of Alvarado to Cortes escaped him.

66. *Passiflora quadrangularis L.* The common names *granadilho* and *maracuja açu* are recorded in Sánchez-Monge y Parellada, 1981, 214, item 2676. See also Balbach, 1972, 1009–11, no. 684; Hoppe, 1975, 1:803–4. I have found no modern observations, or even folklore, which credit this plant with febrifugal properties.

67. A full list of new drugs, botanical and mineral, advocated by Zacutus is in Lemos, 1909.

68. Garrison, 1924, 272. The same statement appears in Garrison, 1929, 271.

69. Petraeus, 1618, disputatio 5, no. 22, p. 99.

70. I have considered this phenomenon briefly in "Dr. Isac Lampronti of Ferrara," *Koroth* (Jerusalem) 8:203–6, 1985.

71. Yerushalmi, 1971.

72. For further bibliographic information see Barbosa Machado, 1741–59, 2:20–21. See also Menéndez Pelayo, 1967, 2:209–214.

73. I thank the Universidad Complutense de Madrid for the privilege of consulting this very rare book in microfilm.

74. For a slightly later Spanish mention of the same malady see Barrionuevo, 1968–69, 2:109, who reported, under date of 6 Feb. 1655, that the count of Oñate had *unas tercianas sincopales*.

75. Galen, K10. 821, 836, 839. Avicenna, [1507] book 4, fen 1, tract 2, chaps. 56, 57. Mercatus, 1619–20, 2:417–20.

76. *Aphorisms* 4.43 (Hippocrates, 1923–31, 4:146–47). For a perceptive account of malaria in ancient Greece, see Bruce-Chwatt and Zulueta, 1980, 17–21.

77. Jarcho, 1987b.

78. *Sensu et motu privatus.*

79. *Pulsus omnimodus defectus (asphygiam dicunt) decem, et undecim horis durans.*

80. Patin, 1707, 3:320 (letter no. 496, 28 Aug. 1669), 265 (letter no. 465, 11 Oct. 1667).

81. S.v. "Sydenham, Thomas," in *Dictionary of Scientific Biography,* 1970–81, 13:213–15.

82. Bayle and Thillaye, 1967, 1:488–89.

83. Barbeyrac, 1751, 232–51.

84. [Barbeyrac?], [1770?], item 1, fol. 6r, 7r, 3v, 9r.

85. The publisher, John Crook, sold Jesuits' bark at his shop in St. Paul's churchyard.

86. This work reappeared in many editions, including the *Opera omnia,* edited by Gulielmus Alexander Greenhill, London: Sydenham Society, 1844. I have usually used—despite its exasperating index—the English version (Sydenham, 1848–50). Page references cited here are to that edition. In addition to the biographical notice cited in note 81 above, another valuable guide is D. G. Bates, 1975, "Thomas Sydenham, the development of his thought," unpublished thesis, Baltimore, Johns Hopkins University.

87. Sydenham's concepts of constitution, at once intricate and obscure, are discussed in Bates, 1975, 61–78, 104, 111–13, 129–31; see note 86 above.

88. In this context the word *contagion* refers to a noxious object and not to the process of transmission.

89. Rush wrote: ". . . instead of which I believe a disease . . . to consist in the confused and irregular operations of disordered and debilitated nature" (Sydenham, 1809, iv–v).

90. The reader will find it instructive to consult Keele, 1974.

91. A somewhat similar opinion was expressed by Charles Goodall (1642–1712). See Davis, 1974.

92. Readers may countenance a curiosum at this point. Sydenham's discussions of acute diseases are arranged by series of years, for example, 1661–64, 1665–66, 1667–69. In his time the legal year began on Annunciation Day, 25 March; in England the change to 1 January did not occur until 1752. Therefore Sydenham's presentations presumably omitted any cases that occurred in the first 12 weeks of each series. It remains for some diligent scholar to ascertain whether or not this peculiarity proved significant.

93. According to the calendrical practice that prevailed in England in Sydenham's time, this refers to the period beginning on March 27 and not to the period beginning on 1 January. See note 92 above.

94. Botallo, 1660, 169–72.

95. For Ramazzini see, for example, 1690; a list of other writings in [1713] 1940, 527, includes translations published originally in the German *Miscellanea curiosa*. Baglivi, [1696] 1704, 143, mentions constitution, but it is hazardous to assume Sydenhamian origin. Jarcho, 1989b, 4, discusses a consultation attributed to Ippolito Francesco Albertini, University of Bologna MS 2089, 1:5, lines 7–8. Sydenham's influence on Morgagni is discussed in Jarcho, 1984a, lxx.

96. Additional details are given in Corradi, [1865–94] 1972–73, 4:763–67, 5:591.

97. Borelli, an Italian and a Roman Catholic, says (159) that Harvey is worthy of *eternal glory*.

98. I have used the 1685 edition; page references are to it.

99. The reader will observe that the meaning of the term *convulsive* has changed somewhat.

100. "Quae in paroxysmis quartanae febris contingunt, et quae in spinali medulla molestissimam passionem inducunt" (proposition 218, p. 321).

101. Additional comments on autopsy experience are in letters exchanged by Borelli and Malpighi in 1661. Malpighi, 1698, 27–34.

102. Cullen, 1778, 1 (sect. 46):38.

103. Unless otherwise indicated, page numbers in the discussion of Bellini refer to this edition.

104. The essay on fevers also appeared, as a separate work, in an anonymous English translation (Bellini, 1720).

105. In the periodic continued fever, according to Bellini, the cause produces a recurrence before the previous one has ended (*antequam prior plane desierit*); in the periodic intermittent the recurrence does not appear until some time after the preceding one has definitely ended (*non nisi aliquo spatio temporis, postquam prius desiit*).

106. "Febris maligna cacoethes, seu mali moris: et varias ejus species, nempe morbum Hungaricum, sudorem Anglicum, febrem malignam cum spasmo . . . vide apud rei medicae scriptores" (229).

107. This arrangement is used also in Bellini, 1695. It is an obvious indication of Bellini's mathematical tendencies and may be an indication of Borelli's influence.

108. *Lentor ille, qui in sanguine supponitur* (prop. 18). A convenient explanation is to be found in Bellini, 1720, xx ff.

109. See esp. sections 6 and 7, pp. 136–38.

110. Boerhaave's introduction appeared also in the fifth edition, 1730.

111. Boerhaave, 1757, 169–286. See esp. Aphorismi 574, 577, 581, 755 (pp. 209, 221).

112. Those who do not find their way to the original may want to see the beautifully written review in *Acta eruditorum*, 1684, 334–36.

113. Anasarca, ascites, and so forth are referred to as sicknesses rather than as secondary epiphenomena or complications derived from a sickness and clearly subordinate to it.

114. Other editions recorded, but not examined by me, are Leipzig, 1695; Geneva, 1696; Amsterdam, 1698.

115. *Famoso illo, et multiplici experientia comprobato.*

116. Sydenham, 1848–50, 2:57–118.

117. These works were issued in Amsterdam in 1696 in a three-volume set, of which the treatise on phthisis (originally issued in 1689) comprises the first volume. Many subsequent editions are recorded.

118. The word *hypothesis*, expressing frank avowal of speculation or uncertainty, recurs frequently in Morton's discussions, e.g., pp. 31 and 43 (*hypothesin nostram*).

119. This comparison, a standard item among fermentationists, is noticed above in the discussion of Willis.

120. So often in medical theorizing the theorist assumes that the head consists of nothing but the brain and the meninges.

121. This notion is deeply imbedded in our own contemporary folklore; a Sicilian barber who used to cut my hair ca. 1976 accepted it as obvious. The Galenic sources are discussed in Siegel, 1968, 97, 102. See also Galen K2. 204 and 11. 402. It should be noticed that in accepting such opinions, Morton was accepting part of the Galenic circulation. That he also accepted the Harveian is evident at many points in his writings.

122. A diagrammatic synopsis, titled "Schema Morborum Generale," appears between pp. 44 and 45 of Morton's text.

123. Cf. Galen, *De morborum causis*, chap. 1 (K7. 4).

124. On 20 Dec. 1692 Dr. Thomas Molyneux of Dublin wrote to John Locke "concerning Dr. Morton, and his late Exercitations on Fevers. As for his General Theory of them, I esteem it, as all others of this kind, a sort of mere waking Dream, that Men are strangely apt to fall into, when they think long of a Subject, beginning quite at the wrong End." The later (practical) parts of Morton's book, Molyneux wrote, "must certainly be of great Moment." Dewhurst, 1966, 178.

125. Galen: *Ad Glauconem de medendi methodo* 1.9 (not 1.8 as Zacutus says); K11.28–29. Zacutus Lusitanus, 1667, 1: 707–8.

126. Galen: *Hippocratis epidem. VI et Galeni in illum commentarius I*, K17/1. 873–85. Additional comment in K7. 539–41 and 9. 647–52. Avicenna [1507] 1964, also mentions palpatory signs in pure tertian; see bk. 4, fen 1, tract 2, chap. 38.

127. For example, Sydenham, 1848–50, 1:50.

128. An obscure article (not untinged with skepticism) by Johannes Muralt helps us understand why Galenic doctrine was satisfying to many physicians as an explanation of the symptoms of intermittent fever and as a guide to treatment. See Muraltus, 1689, 2–16.

129. See, for example, these case reports in *Miscellanea curiosa seu ephemerides:* (a) Pechlin, J. N.: De quartanae contumacia 9 (1678): 87–88. (b) Muraltus, J.: Febris duplex tertiana (Decuria 2) 7 (1688): 407–10. (c) Krugius, T.: De non mutato pulsu et urina in febre intermittente tertiana (Decuria 2) 10 (1691): 5–8. (d) Ledelius, S.: De quadriga quartaniorum (Decuria 3) 2 (1694): 59–60. (e) Lanzoni, J.: De febri quartana larga uvarum assumptione curata (Decuria 3) 4 (1696): 153. Among what we nowadays distinguish as physical signs, these reports usually ignored all but the condition of the pulse and bodily warmth or coldness. Instead, the authors concentrated on what we consider to be symptoms, and on treatment. However, within these limits they were by no means deficient in observation, and it is a serious error to regard them as such.

130. Mercatus, 1611, 526, 539. Piquer, 1751, 234–37.

131. "Despite theoretical divergences, however, physicians [in antiquity] continued as always to show eclectic tendencies in their practical activities." Cohen and Drabkin, 1948, 467. Medical eclecticism in the eighteenth century is discussed briefly in Jarcho, 1984a, lxvii–lxviii.

Bibliography

Abad, C. M. 1943. El magisterio del Cardenal de Lugo en España con algunos datos más salientes de su vida y siete cartas autógrafas ineditas. *Miscelaneo Comillas* [Universidad Pontificia Comillas] 1: 331–70.

Abreu, Alexo de. 1623. *Tratado de las siete enfermedades . . . de la terciana y febre maligna.* Lisbon: Craesbeeck.

Ackerknecht, E. 1967. *Medicine at the Paris hospital, 1794–1846.* Baltimore: Johns Hopkins Press.

Adam, C., and Milhaud, G. 1934–63. *Descartes: Correspondance.* 8 vols. Paris: Alcan (vols. 1–2). Paris: Presses universitaires de France (vols. 3–8).

Adelmann, H. 1966. *Marcello Malpighi and the rise of embryology.* Ithaca: Cornell University Press.

Aikawa, M., Suzuki, M., and Gutierrez, Y. 1980. Pathology of malaria. In *Malaria*, ed. J. P. Kreier. 2: 47–102. New York: Academic Press.

Albertini, I. F. 1731 [reprinted 1748]. Animadversiones super quibusdam difficilis respirationis vitiis a laesa cordis et praecordiorum structura pendentibus. *De Bononiensi Scientiarum et Artium Instituto atque Academia Commentarii* 1:382–404.

———. 1828. Hippolyti Francisci Albertini: Opuscula. Ed. M. Romberg. Berlin: Hirschwald.

Alibert, I. L. 1807. *A treatise on malignant intermittents*, 3d ed. Trans. Charles Caldwell. Philadelphia: Fry & Kammerer.

Allbutt, T. C. 1870. Medical thermometry. *British and Foreign Medico-Chirurgical Review* 45:429–41.

Antidotarium gandavense, nobilissimi amplissimique senatus iussu . . . editum. 1663. Ghent: Manilius.

Appleby, J. 1983. Ivan the Terrible to Peter the Great: British formative influence on Russia's medico-apothecary system. *Medical History* 27:289–304.

Archivo de Indias, Sevilla. 1980–86. *Catálogo de pasajeros a Indias durante los siglos XVI, XVII, y XVIII.* 7 vols. Madrid: Ministerio de Cultura, Dirección de Archivos.

Archivo General de Simancas. 1937. *Catalogo XV. Papeles sobre la introducción y distribución de la quina en España.* Valladolid: Vicente.

Arcos, G. 1933. *La medicina en el Ecuador.* Quito: Fernández.

Argelati, F. 1745. *Bibliotheca scriptorum mediolanensium.* Milan: in aedibus Palatinis.

Aristotle. 1952. *Meteorologica.* Ed. and trans. H. D. P. Lee. Loeb Classical Library. Cambridge: Harvard University Press.

———. 1953. *Generation of animals.* Ed. and trans. A. L. Peck. Loeb Classical Library. Cambridge: Harvard University Press.

———. 1955. *On coming-to-be and passing-away.* Ed. and trans. E. S. Forster. Loeb Classical Library. Cambridge: Harvard University Press.

———. 1962. *The Nicomachean ethics.* Ed. D. A. Rees. Oxford: Clarendon Press.

Arnobius of Sicca. 1949. *The case against the pagans.* Trans. and ed. G. E. McCracken. New York: Newman Press.

Astrain, A. 1916. *Historia de la Compañía de Jesús en la asistencia de España.* Madrid: Administración de Razón y Fe.

Astruc, J. 1767. *Mémoires pour servir à l'histoire de la Faculté de médecine de Montpellier.* Ed. M. Lorry. Paris: Cavelier.

Auda, D. 1740. *Practica de' speziali,* 2d ed. Ed. Giovanni Battista Capello. Venice: de' Paoli.

Avicenna. [1507] 1964. *Liber canonis* [Venice.] Facsimile. Hildesheim: Olms.

Bacon, F. 1624. *De dignitate et augmentis scientiarum.* Paris: Mettayer.

Badaro, R., Falcoff, E., Badaro, F., Carvalho, E., et al. 1990. Treatment of visceral leishmaniasis with pentavalent antimony and interferon gamma. *New England Journal of Medicine* 322:16–21.

[Badus, S.] 1656. *Saggio d'alcuni rimedij preservativj dalla peste dedicato all'illustriss[imi] signori protettori della spedale di Pammatone.* Genoa: Guasco [sic].

Badus, S. 1663. *Anastasis corticis Pervviae, seu chinae chinae defensio, Sebastiani Badi Genviensis, patrii vtriusque nosochomij olim medici, et publicae sanitatis in ciuitate consultoris. Contra ventilationes Iacobi Chifletii, gemitvsque Vopisci Fortvnati Plempii, illustrium medicorum.* Genoa: Calenzani.

———. See also Baldus, S.

Baglivi, G. 1704. *De praxi medica,* 4th ed. Leyden: Haring.

———. [1696] 1704. De usu, et abusu vesicantium. [Rome]. In *De praxi medica.* Leyden: Haring.

———. 1727. *Opera omnia medico-practica et anatomica.* Venice: Tomasinus.

———. 1732. *Opera omnia,* 17th ed. Bassani.

Bagrow, L. 1964. *History of cartography.* Rev. R. A. Skelton. Cambridge: Harvard University Press.

Bailly, C. 1987. *Théophraste Renaudot, un homme d'influence au temps de Louis XIII et de la Fronde.* Paris: Le Pré au Clercs.

Baker, G. 1785. Observations on the late intermittent fevers; to which is added a short history of the Peruvian bark. *Medical Transactions of the Royal College of Physicians of London* 3:141–216.

Balbach, A. 1972. *A flora nacional na medicina domestica.* São Paulo: Edificação do Lar.

Baldinger, E. 1778. Geschichte der Chinarinde. *Magazin vor Aertzte.* 2 vols. Leipzig: Jacobäer & Son.

Baldus, S. 1656. *Cortex Pervviae redivivvs, profligator febrium, assertus ab impugnationibus Melippi Protimi Medici Belgae.* Genoa: Guaschi.

Ballonius, G. 1640. *Epidemiorum et ephemeridum libri duo.* Paris: Quesnel.

Bantug, J. 1953. *A short history of medicine in the Philippines during the Spanish regime, 1565–1898.* Manila: Colegio Medico-Farmacéutico de Filipinas.

Barba, P. [1642?] *Vera praxis de curatione tertianae stabilitur: falsa impugnatur: liberantur hispanici medici a calumniis.* [Louvain?]

Barbette, P. 1675. *The practice of the most successful physitian Paul Barbette . . . with the notes and observations of Frederick Deckers.* London: Broome.

Barbeyrac, C. 1751. *Medicamentorum constitutio, seu formulae Caroli Barbeyrac . . . cura et studio doctoris medici Monspesulanae.* Lyons: de Tournes.

[Barbeyrac, C.?] [ca. 1770?] *Methodus formulae praescribendi.* [Montpellier?] Ms. in medical library, Yale University.

Barbosa Machado, D. 1741–59. *Bibliotheca lusitana.* Lisbon: Da Fonseca, Rodriguez, et al.

Barckhausen, J. 1696. *Pharmacopoeus synopticus,* 2d ed. Utrecht: Halma.

Bardus, H. 1634. *Medicus politico catholicus.* Genoa: Farroni.

Barrionuevo, J. 1968–69. *Avisos.* Ed. A. Paz y Melía. Madrid: Ediciones Atlas.

Bartholinus, T. 1654. *Historiarum anatomicarum rariorum, centuriae I et II.* Amsterdam: Henricus.

———. 1661. *Historiarum anatomicarum et medicarum rariorum centuria V et VI.* Copenhagen: Gödianus.

———. 1663. *Epistolarum medicinalium . . . centuria I et II.* Copenhagen: Godicchenius.

———. 1667. *Epistolarum medicinalium . . . centuria III et IV.* Copenhagen: Godicchenius.

Bastien, J. 1987. *Healers of the Andes.* Salt Lake City: University of Utah Press.

Bates, D. 1981. Thomas Willis and the fevers literature of the seventeenth century. In *Theories of fever from antiquity to the enlightenment,* ed. W. F. Bynum and V. Nutton. *Medical History* [London] suppl. 1.

Battisti, C., and Alessio, G. 1950–57. *Dizionario etimologico italiano.* 5 vols. Florence: Barbèra.

Bayle, A. L. J., and Thillaye, A. J. [1855] 1967. *Biographie médicale.* [Paris.] Facsimile. 2 vols. Amsterdam: Israël.

Bellini, L. 1683. *De urinis et pulsibus, de missione sanguinis, de febribus, de morbis capitis, et pectoris.* Bologna: Pisarrius.

———. 1695. *Opuscula aliquot ad Archibaldum Pitcarnium.* Pistoia [Pistorii]: Gatti.

———. 1717. *De urinis et pulsibus, de missione sanguinis, de febribus* . . . , 4th ed. Leyden: Kerckhem. Also 5th ed., 1730.

———. 1720. *A mechanical account of fevers.* [Trans. anonymously.] London: Bell.

Belon [also Bellon], P. 1681. *A new mystery in physick discovered, by curing of fevers and agues by quinquina or Jesuites powder.* Trans. and rev. Dr. Belon. London: William Crook[e].

Benedictus, J. 1649. *Epistolarum medicinalium libri decem.* Rome: Phaeus.

———. 1650. *Consultationum medicinalium.* Venice: Bertanos.

Beng, J. T. [1684] 1965. *Über indonesische Volksheilkunde an Hand der Pharmacopoeia Indica des Hermann Nikolaus Grim(m).* Frankfurt am Main: Govi Verlag.

Bergen, H. v. 1826. *Versuch einer Monographie der China.* Hamburg: Hartwig & Müller.

Berger, J. G., and Stieler, H. 1711. De china china ab iniquis judiciis vindicata. In Haller, 1757–60. 5:41–59.

Bernier, J. 1689. *Essais de médecine où il est traité de l'histoire de la médecine et des médecins . . . De l'utilité des remèdes, et de l'abus qu'on en peut faire.* Paris: Langronne.

———. 1691. *Supplémens . . . avec des corrections.* Paris: Langronne.

Beverovicius, J. 1641. *Epistolicae quaestiones.* Rotterdam: Leers.

Bigatti, G. 1926. Gli antichi ricettari della "Spezieria de Brera" in Milano. *Notiziario dell' antica farmacia de Brera* (Sept.–Oct.): 93–98.

Biss[el?], I. [1653?] *Responsio libelli pulveris febrifugi ventilati a Ioanne Iacobo Chifletio archiducali doctore medico.* MS in National Library of Medicine, Bethesda.

Blake, J. B. 1979. *A short title catalogue of eighteenth century printed books in the National Library of Medicine.* Bethesda: National Library of Medicine.

Blancardus, S. [1683] 1973. *Lexicon medicum.* [Jena.] Facsimile, Hildesheim: Olms.

Blanco Juste, F. J. 1935. Las actas de Chinchon. *10th International Congress of the History of Medicine,* 1 (fasc. 1): 241–57.

Blegny, N. de. 1680. *La découverte de l'admirable remède anglois, pour la guérison des fièvres.* Paris: Blageart & d'Hourry.

———. 1682. *Le remède anglois pour la guérison des fièvres.* Paris and Brussels: Frick. Paris: Padeloup.

———. 1685. Remedium anglicum pro curatione febrium; ex mandato Regiae Majestatis publici juris factum. Additis observationibus domini primarii regis medici. *Zodiacus Medico-Gallicus* 5:1–20. [Geneva: Chouet.]

———. 1687. Remedium anglicanum pro curatione febrium. In *Febris china chinae expugnata,* ed. F. Nigrisoli, 1–48. Ferrara: Pomatelli.

Boccabadati, A. 1833. Elogio di Francesco Torti. *Memorie della reale accademia di scienze, lettere e d'arte di Modena* 1 (p. 3): 125–47.

Boehmer, P. 1738. *De cortice cascarillae. Praeside Friderico Hoffmanno.* Halle: Grunert.

Boerhaave, H. 1757. *Opera omnia medica.* Venice: Basilius.

Bohn, J. 1710. *Disquisitio traditionis vulgaris de praematuriore intermittentium fuga suspecta.* In *Circulus anatomico-physiologicus seu economia corporis animalis . . . accesserunt dissertationes physiologicae.* Leipzig: Fritsch.

Boisseau, R. P. 1933. *Le renouveau de l'antimoine; thérapeutique tropicale.* Thesis. [Bordeaux.] Paris.

Borelli, G. 1649. *Delle cagioni delle febbri maligne di Sicilia negli anni 1647, 1648.* Cosenza: Rosso.

Borelli, J. A. 1685. *De motu animalium. Editio altera.* Leyden: Gaesbeeck et al.

Borghesi, G. 1705. *Lettera scritta de Pondisceri a' 10 di febbraio 1704.* Trans. from Latin by Mario di Crescimbeni. Rome: Zenobij.

Botallo, L. 1660. *Opera omnia medica et chirurgica.* Leyden: Gaasbeeck.

Bouley, G., Lataillade, F., Espargilière, M., and Guimond-Darbois, F. 1982. Jean-Adrien Helvetius et l'administration du quinquina. *Revue de l'histoire de Pharmacie* 29:272–74.

Bouvet, J. 1697. *Portrait historique de l'Empereur de la Chine.* Paris: Michallet.

Bouvet, M. 1934. *Histoire de la pharmacie de l'Hôtel-Dieu de Paris.* Paris: Pharmacie Française.

———. 1937. *Histoire de la pharmacie en France des origines à nos jours.* Paris: Editions Occitana.

Bovonier, F. 1656. *Questio medica an febribus intermittentibus inutilis Chinchinae pulvis.* (Praeses Daniel Arbinet.) Thesis. Paris.

Boxer, C. R. 1952. *Salvador de Sá and the struggle for Brazil and Angola, 1602–1686.* London: University of London.

———. 1957. *The Dutch in Brazil, 1624–1654.* Oxford: Clarendon Press.

———. 1965. *The Dutch seaborne empire 1600–1800.* London: Hutchinson.

Boyd, M. 1949. *Malariology.* 2 vols. Philadelphia: Saunders.

Brain, P. 1986. *Galen on bloodletting; a study of the origins, development and validity of his opinions, with a translation . . .* Cambridge: Cambridge University Press.

Braudel, F. 1982. *The wheels of commerce. Civilization and capitalism, 15th–18th century,* vol. 2. Trans. S. Reynolds. New York: Harper & Row.

Bravo de Sobremonte, G. 1654. *Resolutiones medicae in quatuor partes tributae.* Lyons: Borde et al.

———. 1671. *Disputatio apologetica pro dogmaticae medicinae praestantia . . . huic accesserunt tractatus duo.* Cologne: Friessem.

Breasted, J. H. 1930. *The Edwin Smith surgical papyrus.* 2 vols. Chicago: University of Chicago Press.

Brinkman, G. 1957. *The social thought of John de Lugo.* (Studies in Sociology, no. 41.) Washington, D.C.: Catholic University of America, School of Social Science.

Broeckx, C. 1855. Notice sur Roland Storms. *Annales de la société de médecine d'Anvers* 16:5–24.

Brown, H. 1934. *Scientific organizations in seventeenth-century France (1620–1680).* Baltimore: Williams & Wilkins.

Browne, S. 1698. Letter to James Petiver. Fort St. George, Sept. 20. British Library. Sloane MS 4062, fol. 288–291v.

Browne, Sir Thomas. 1946. *The letters of Sir Thomas Browne*. Ed. Geoffrey Keynes. London: Faber & Faber.

Bruce, J. 1810. *Annals of the honorable East-India Company, from their establishment by the charter of Queen Elizabeth, 1600, to the union of the London and English East-India Companies 1707–8*. 3 vols. London: Black, Parry & Kingsbury.

Bruce-Chwatt, L. J. 1982. Oliver Cromwell's medical history. *Transactions and Studies of the College of Physicians of Philadelphia*, 5th ser., 4:98–121.

———. 1985. *Essential malariology*, 2d ed. New York: Wiley.

———. 1988. Cinchona and its alkaloids: 350 years. *New York State Journal of Medicine* 88:318–22.

Bruce-Chwatt, L. J., and Zulueta, J. de. 1980. *The rise and fall of malaria in Europe; a historico-epidemiological study*. New York: Oxford University Press.

Brunacius, G. 1661. *De cina cina, seu pulvere ad febres, syntagma physiologicum*. Venice: Pezzana.

Brunet, J.-C. 1861. *Manuel du libraire*. Paris: Didot.

Brunner, C., and von Muralt W. 1969. *Aus den Briefen hervorragender schweizer Ärzte des 17 Jahrhunderts*. Basel: Schwabe.

Burger, R. L. 1989. Long before the Inca. *Natural History*, Feb., 66–73

[Burton, R.] [1651] 1838. *The anatomy of melancholy . . . by Democritus Junior. The sixteenth edition, printed from the authorized copy of 1651, with the author's last corrections, additions, &c. &c*. London: Blake.

Buxhoeveden, S. [Sof'ya Karlovna]. 1932. *A cavalier in Moscow*. London: Macmillan.

Bynum, W., and Nutton, V. ed. 1981. Theories of fever from antiquity to the enlightenment. *Medical History*, suppl. 1.

Cabanès, A. 1910. *Remèdes d'autrefois*, 2d ed. Paris: Maloine.

Cabriada, J. de. (A supplementary title page is dated 1686.) *Carta filosófica médica química en que se demuestra que de los tiempos y experiencias se han aprendido los mejores remedios contra las enfermedades de la nova antigua medicina*. Madrid: Bedmar y Baldivia.

Calancha, A. de. 1638. *Coronica moralizada del orden de S. Augustin en el Peru*. Barcelona: Lacavalleria.

Caldera de Heredia, G. 1663. . . . . *Tribunalis medici illustrationes et observationes practicae*. Antwerp: Meursius.

Canezza, A. 1925. *"Pulvis Jesuiticus." Note storiche sulla scoperta e diffusione della china*. Rome: Fide Romana.

———. 1932. Il terzo centenario della corteccia di china in Roma (1632–1932). *Capitolium* 8:591–98.

———. 1933. *Gli arcispedali di Roma*. Rome: Stianti.

Canguilhem, G. 1963. The role of analogies and models in biological discovery. In *Scientific change*, ed. A. C. Crombie, 507–20. London: Heinemann.

Cantù, M. C., and Righini Bonelli, M. L. [1981?]. *The Accademia del Cimento (1657–1667)*. [Florence]: Nardini.

Cardella, L. 1792–97. *Memorie storiche de' cardinali della santa Romana chiesa*. Rome.

Cardoso, Ferdinandus [Isaac]. 1639. *De febre syncopali, tractatio noviter discussa, utiliter disputata. Controversiis, observationibus, historijs referta.* Madrid: Didacus Diaz de la Carrera.

Carpaneto di Langasco, C. 1953. *Pammatone. Cinque secoli di vita ospedaliera.* Genoa: Ospedali Civili.

Carter, Henry R. 1914. *Quinine prophylaxis for malaria.* (Reprint from *Public Health Reports.*) Washington, D.C.: U.S. Public Health Service.

Castelli, P. 1654. *Responsio chimica . . . de effervescentia et mutatione colorum in mixtione liquorum chimicorum.* Messina: Pyreae.

Castiglioni, A. 1941. *A history of medicine.* Trans. and ed. E. Krumbhaar. New York: Knopf.

Castro, Andreas Antonius. 1636. *. . . De febrium curationie libri tres.* Villa Viçosa: Carvalho.

Castro Sarmento, Jacobo de. [1735] 1758. *Materia medica physico-historicomechanica.* [London] London: Strahan.

Celli, A. 1933. *The history of malaria in the Roman campagna.* Ed. Anna Celli-Fraentzel. London: Bale & Danielsson.

Celli-Fraentzel, A. 1928. Die Malaria in 17 Jahrhundert in Rom und in der Campagna in Lichte zeitgenossischer Anschauungen. *Archiv für Geschichte der Medizin* 20:101–19.

Charas, M. 1676. *Pharmacopée royale galenique et chymique.* Paris: the author.

———. 1704. *Pharmacopée royale galenique et chymique.* Lyon: Anisson & Posuel.

———. 1730. Nouvelle préparation de quinquina et la manière de s'en servir pour la guérison des fièvres. *Mémoires de l'Académie Royale des Sciences* 10.

Cheylud, E. 1897. *Histoire de la corporation des apothicaires de Bordeaux (1355–1802).* Bordeaux: Mollat. Paris: Picard.

Chifletius, J. J. 1653. *Pulvis febrifugus orbis Americani iussu serenissimi principis Leopoldi Guilielmi . . . proregis ventilatus.* [Louvain.]

Chinchón, Conde de [Luis Gerónimo Cabrera Bobadilla Cerda y Mendoza]. 1640. *Relación que dio el Sr Conde de chinchon del estado en que dexo el Gouierno de Peru.* Holograph MS, 52 fols. Archivo General de las Indias, Seville, legajo LIMA 52, no. 27-A.

[Chomel, J. B. L.]. 1762. *Essai historique sur la médecine en France.* Paris: Lottin.

Chomel, N. 1732. *Dictionnaire oeconomique,* 3d ed. Ed. J. Marret. Amsterdam: Covens & Martin, 1732.

Cirillo, N. 1738. *Consulti medici.* Naples: de Bonis.

Cobo, B. 1956. *Historia del nuevo mundo.* 2 vols. Madrid: Ediciones Atlas.

Cogrossi, C. 1711. *Della natura, effetti, ed' uso della corteccia del Perù, ò sia china china: considerazioni fiscio-mechaniche e mediche.* Crema: Carcheno.

———. 1716. *Giunta al trattato della china-china.* Crema: Carcheno.

———. 1718. *Nuova ginunta al trattato della china-china.* Crema: Carcheno.

Cohen, M. R., and Drabkin, I. E. 1948. *A source book in Greek science.* New York: McGraw-Hill.

Cole, W. 1693. *Novae hypotheseos, ad explicanda febrium intermittentium symptomata et typos excogitatae hypotyposis. Una cum aetiologia remediorum; speciatim vero de curatione per corticem peruvianum . . .* London: Browne & Smith.

Collegium Physicorum, Milan. 1668. *Prospectus pharmaceuticus, sub quo Antidotarium Mediolanense spectandum proponitur.* Milan: Ferrarius.

———. 1698. *Prospecti pharmaceutici editio secunda.* Milan: Quintus.

Collet, J. 1933. *The private letter books of Joseph Collet, sometime governor of Fort St. George, Madras.* Ed. H. Dodwell. London: Longmans, Green.

Colmenero, J. 1697. *Reprobacion del pernicioso abvso de los polvos de la corteza de el qvarango, o china china, ilustrada con muchas eficaces razones . . . que demuestran su mucha pernicie cierta.* Salamanca: Garcia.

Colonne, F.-J.-M. 1929. *Dominique Guglielmini.* Thesis. Paris: Jouve.

Condamine, [C. M.] de la. 1740. Sur l'arbre de quinquina. *Histoire de l'Académie Royale des Sciences. Année 1738,* 226–43. Paris: Imprimerie Royale.

Conygius, Antimus [pseudonym of Fabri, Honoratus]. 1655. *Pulvis peruvianus vindicatus de ventilatore eiusdemque suscepta defensio ab Antimo Conygio hortatu Germani Poleconii.* Rome: Corbelletti.

Cook, A. S. 1989. Alexander Dalrymple's appointment as East India Company hydrographer. *Abstracts, 13th International Conference on the History of Cartography, June 26 to July 1.*

Coquerelle, J. 1901. *Guy Patin.* Compiègne: Lefebvre.

Corradi, A. [1865–94] 1972–73. *Annali delle epidemie occorse in Italia.* [8 vols. Bologna: Gamberini & Parmeggiani.] Facsimile, 5 vols. Bologna: Forni.

Corte, B. [1718] 1972. *Notizie istoriche a' medici scrittori milanesi.* [Milan: Malatesta] Facsimile, Bologna: Forni.

Costa, H. de la. 1961. *The Jesuits in the Philippines, 1581–1768.* Cambridge: Harvard University Press.

Cramer, C. A. 1713. *De usu corticis chinae febrifugo cauto ac suspecto.* Halle: Salfeld.

Crawford, D. 1914. *A history of the Indian medical service, 1600–1913.* London: Thacker.

Crescimbeni, G. M., ed. 1720–21. *Notizie istoriche degli arcadi morti.* Rome: De Rossi.

Cullen, W. 1778. *First lines of the practice of physic.* Edinburgh: Creech.

Cullum, L. 1956. Georg Joseph Kamel: Philippine botanist. *Philippine Studies* 4:319–39.

da Orta. See Orta, Garcia da.

Daval, J. 1684. *Questio medica. Petro Perreau . . . praeside. An Anglica praescribendi corticis Peruviani methodus explodenda?* [Paris?] In the British Library.

Davis, A. 1971. The virtues of the cortex in 1680; a letter from Charles Goodall to Mr. H. *Medical History* 15:293–304.

———. 1973. *Circulation physiology and medical chemistry in England 1650–1680.* Lawrence, Kans.: Coronado Press.

Deák, G. 1989. *Picturing America.* 2 vols. Princeton: Princeton University Press.

de Backer, A. 1890–1932. *Bibliothèque de la Compagnie de Jésus.* Ed. C. Sommervogel. Brussels: Schepens. Paris: Picard.

Debus, A. 1977. *The chemical philosophy.* 2 vols. New York: Science History Publications.

Dedouvres, L. 1932. *Le père Joseph de Paris, capucin d'éminence grise.* Paris: Beauchesne.

De Jonge, J. K. J. 1862–1909. *De opkomst van het Nederlandsch gezag in Oost-Indie.* 16 vols. in 13. 's-Gravenhage: Nijhoff.

Dekkers, F. 1673. *Exercitationes medicae practicae circa medendi methodum.* Leyden and Amsterdam: Gaesbeek.

De Launay, L. 1564. *De la faculté et vertu de l'antimoine.* La Rochelle: Berton.

———. 1566. *Responce av discours de maistre Jacques Grevin . . . touchant la faculté de l'antimoine.* La Rochelle: Berton.

Delaunay, P. 1906. *Vieux médecins Sarthois.* Paris: Champion.

De Leon, A. [1627]. *Libro de papeles curiosos impressos de las Indias.* In Biblioteca Nacional, Madrid.

de Lugo, J. 1751. *Opera omnia.* Venice: Pezzana.

de Meeüs, A. 1962. *History of the Belgians.* Trans. G. Gordon. London: Thames & Hudson.

De Renzi, S. [1845–49] 1966. *Storia della medicina italiana.* [Naples: Tipografia del Filiatre Sebezio] Facsimile, Bologna: Forni.

Descartes, R. [1637] 1963. *Discours de la methode pour bien conduire la raison, et chercher la vérité dans les sciences* [Leyden: Maire]. In *Oeuvres philosophiques,* ed. F. Alquié, 1: 567–650. Paris: Garnier.

———. 1664. *Le monde de Mr Descartes, ou le traité de la lumière, et des autres principaux objets des sens. Avec un discours du mouvement local, et un autre des fiévres* [sic], *composez selon les principes du méme* [sic] *auteur.* Paris: Girad [Giraud].

———. 1934–63. *Correspondance.* Ed. C. Adam and G. Milhaud. Paris: Alcan. (Vols. 3–8, Paris: Presses Universitaires de France.)

———. See also Hall.

De Tipaldo, E. 1834–45. *Biografia degli Italiani illustri . . . del secolo XVIII, e de contemporanei.* 10 vols. Venice: Alvisopoli.

Dewhurst, K. 1962. Some letters of Dr. Charles Goodall (1642–1712) to Locke, Sloane, and Sir Thomas Millington. *Journal of the History of Medicine* 17: 487–508.

———. 1963. *John Locke (1632–1704) . . . a medical biography, with an edition of the medical notes in his journals.* London: Wellcome Historical Medical Library.

———. 1966. *Dr. Thomas Sydenham (1624–1689). His life and original writings.* Berkeley: University of California Press.

———, ed. and trans. 1980. *Thomas Willis's Oxford lectures.* Oxford: Sandford.

———, ed. 1981. *Willis' Oxford casebook (1650–52).* Oxford: Sandford.

————, ed. 1983. *Richard Lower's* Vindicatio, *a defence of the experimental method*. Oxford: Sandford.

Dictionnaire des sciences médicales. 1812–22. 60 vols. Paris: Crapart & Pancoucke.

[Dieuxyvoie, B.: *An febri quartanae peruvianus cortex?* Thesis. Paris, 1658. Cited in Raynaud, 1862, 218.]

Di Pietro, P. 1949. La corteccia di china ai tempi di Francesco Torti (1658–1741). *Mese sanitario* 1 (10): 3–8.

————. 1952. Il maestro di F. Torti, Antonio Frassoni. *Minerva Medica* 43 (Varia): 688–92.

————. 1957. Contributo alla storia degli studi anatomici in Modena. *Atti e memorie, deputazione storia patria per le antiche prov. Modenesi*, 8th ser., 9: 81–87.

————. 1958. Vita ed opere di Francesco Torti, medico modenese (1658–1741). *Bolletino della Società Medico-Chirurgica di Modena* 58:460–78.

————. 1981. Le fonti bibliografiche nella "de morbis artificum" di Bernardino Ramazzini. *History and Philosophy of the Life Sciences* 3:95–114.

Dircks, H. 1865. *The life, times, and scientific labours of the second marquis of Worcester*. London: Quaritch.

Documentación indiana. See Spain.

Dolfi, P. 1670. *Cronologia di famigli nobili di Bologna*. Bologna: Ferroni.

Dominian, H. 1958. *Apostle of Brazil. The biography of Padre José de Anchieta, S. J. (1534–1597)*. New York: Exposition Press.

Dousset, J. C. 1985. *Histoire des médicaments des origines à nos jours*. Paris: Payot.

Duhr, B. 1907–28. *Geschichte der Jesuiten in den Ländern deutscher Zunge*. 4 vols. in 6. Freiburg: Herder (vols. 1–2). Munich-Regensburg: Manz (vols. 3–4).

Dulieu, L. 1975. *La médecine à Montpellier*. Vol. 3. *L'Époque classique*. Avignon: Presses Universelles.

————. [n.d.] *Les thèses de l'université de médecine de Montpellier*. Photocopy of typescript, 32 and 113 pp. In National Library of Medicine, Bethesda.

Dumas, G. 1936. *Histoire du Journal de Trévoux depuis 1701 jusqu'en 1762*. Paris: Boivin.

Duran-Reynals, M. L. 1946. *The fever bark tree; the pageant of quinine*. Garden City: Doubleday.

Durling, R., comp. 1967. *A catalogue of sixteenth century books in the National Library of Medicine*. Bethesda: National Library of Medicine.

El Archipiélago filipino. Colección de datos geográficos, cronológicos y científicos . . . por algunos padres de la mision de la Compañia de Jesús en estas islas. 1900. Washington, D.C.: Imprenta del Gobierno.

Elgood, C. 1951. *A medical history of Persia and the eastern caliphate*. Cambridge: Cambridge University Press.

Eloy, N. 1778. *Dictionnaire historique de la médecine ancienne et moderne*. 4 vols. Mons: Hoyois.

Emery, M. 1888. *Renaudot et l'introduction de la medication chimique. Étude historique d'après des documents originaux.* Montpellier: Imprimerie Centrale du Midi.

An encyclopedia of world history. 1968. Ed. W. L. Langer. Boston: Houghton Mifflin.

Engelen, S. 1967–68. Die Einführung der Radix ipecacuanha in Europa. Dissertation. Düsseldorf.

The English remedy; or, Talbor's wonderful secret, for cureing of agues and feavers . . . Now tr. into English. 1682. London: Wallis. 1682.

Estes, J. W. 1989. *The medical skills of ancient Egypt.* Canton, Mass.: Science Publications.

Esteyneffer, J. de (Johannes Steinhöffer). [1712] 1978. *Florilegio medicinal de todas las enfermedades,* ed. Carmen Anzures y Balanos. [Guillena Carrascosa] Academia Nacional de México.

Fabri, H. See Conygius, A.

Falloppius, G. 1600–1606. *Opera omnia.* Frankfurt: Wechel.

———. 1606. *Tractatus de ulceribus.* Frankfurt: Wechel.

Fantuzzi, G. 1781–94. *Notizie degli scrittori bolognesi.* Bologna: d'Aquino.

Favaro G. 1925–26. Contributi alla biografia di A. Spigelio. *Atti del Reale Istituto Veneto di Scienze, Lettere ed Arti* 85 (pt. 2): 213–54.

Fernández, T. 1698. *Defensa de la china china y verdadera respuesta a las falsas razones que para su reprobación trae el Doct[or] Don Joseph Colmenero.* Madrid: Martinez Abad.

Fernel, J. 1554. *Pathologia.* In *Medicina.* Paris: Wechelius.

Ferreira de Mira, M. B. 1947. *História de medicina Portuguesa.* Lisbon: Empresa nacional de publicidade.

Filiatro (pseudonym of Christoval Tixedas). 1688. *Verdad triunfante, respuesta apologetica, escrita por Filiatro, en defensa de la carta filosofica medicochymica del Doctor Ivan de Cabriada. Manifiestase lo irracional de la medicine dogmatica, y racional del aduanista enmascarado.* (Madrid, 1687). Barcelona: Ferrer.

Fischer, H. 1988. *Metaphysische, experimentelle und utilitaristische Traditionen in der Antimonliteratur . . .* (1520–1820). (Braunschweiger Veröffentlichungen zu Geschichte der Pharmazie und der Naturwissenschaften.) Brunswick.

Fletcher, J. 1969. Medical men and medicine in the correspondence of Athanasius Kircher (1602–80). *Janus* 56:259–77.

Flores, Salvador Leonardo de. [1698.] *Desempeño a el metodo racional en la curacion de la calenturas tercianas, que llaman notas.* Seville: de Blas.

Flückiger, F., and Hanbury, D. 1874. *Pharmacographia.* London: Macmillan. Second edition, 1879.

Fonseca, G. 1623. *Medici oeconomia, in qua omnia quae ad perfecti medici munus attinent brevibus explanantur.* Rome: Phaeus.

Fonseca Henriquez, F. 1714. *Medicina lusitana.* Lisbon: Deslandesiana.

Fonssagrives, J.-B. 1859. Étude médico-litteraire sur le poème du quinquina de La Fontaine. *Bulletin Général de Thérapeutique Médicale et Chirurgicale* 56:298–301, 395–99.

Fouquet, [Marie]. 1676. *Recueil des receptes.* Lyon: Certe.

———. 1703. *Recueil des receptes.* Toulouse: Boude.

Frank, R. G., Jr. 1980. *Harvey and the Oxford physiologists.* Berkeley: University of California Press.

Fraser, D. 1987. Epidemiology as a liberal art. *New England Journal of Medicine* 316:309–14.

Freyer, J. 1698. *A new account of East India and Persia in eight letters, begun 1672 and finished 1681.* London: Chiswell.

Friedenwald, H. 1944. *The Jews and medicine; essays.* Baltimore: Johns Hopkins Press.

———. 1946. *Jewish luminaries in medical history; and a catalogue.* Baltimore: Johns Hopkins Press.

Gaddi, P. 1868. Carteggio di Marcello Malpighi. *Memorie della Regia Accademia di Scienze, Lettere, ed Arte in Modena* 9:3–48.

Galen. [1822–33] 1964–65. *Opera omnia.* Greek text and Latin translation, ed. C. G. Kühn. [Leipzig: Cnobloch, 20 vols. in 22.] Facsimile, Hildesheim: Olms.

Gams, P. B. 1957. *Series episcoporum ecclesiae catholicae.* Graz: Akademische Druck- und Verlagsanstalt.

Garcia da Orta. See Orta.

Garrison, F. H. 1917. *An introduction to the history of medicine,* 2d ed. Philadelphia: Saunders. Also 4th ed., 1929; 3d ed., 1924; 1st ed., 1913.

Gathercoal, E., and Wirth, E. 1947. *Pharmacognosy,* 2d ed. Philadelphia: Lea & Febiger.

Gicklhorn, J., and Gicklhorn, R. 1954. *Georg Kamel, S. J., 1661–1706; Apotheker, Botaniker, Arzt und Naturforscher.* Eutin, Holstein: Internationale Gesellschaft für Geschichte der Pharmazie.

Gigli, G. 1958. *Diario romano (1608–1670).* Ed. Giuseppe Ricciotti. Rome: Tuminelli.

Goodman, A. G., et al. 1985. *Goodman and Gilman's pharmacological basis of therapeutics,* 7th ed. New York: Macmillan.

Gordon, R. 1859. *Passages from the diary of General Patrick Gordon of Auchleuchries.* Aberdeen: Spalding Club.

Gramann, M. 1666. *Dissertationem inauguralem de quartana intermittente . . . praeside . . . Guernero Rolfincio . . . proponit . . . Michael Gramann . . . Magni Moscoviae imperatoris designatus archiater.* Jena: Krebs. Foliation added manually, 327r–354v. Examined in microfilm obtained from British Library and deposited at the New York Academy of Medicine.

Granado, V. M. [1975?] *Loja. Plan regulador.* Guayaquil: Senefelder.

Granel, F. 1964. *Pages medico-historiques montpelliéraines.* Montpellier: Causse & Castelnau.

Granjel, L. 1978. *La medicina española del siglo XVII.* Salamanca: Ediciones Universidad de Salamanca.

———. 1983. *Historia de la medicina vasca.* Salamanca: Instituto de la Medicina Española.

Gray, J. 1737. An account of the Peruvian or Jesuits bark . . . extracted from some papers given him by Mr. William Arrot. *Philosophical Transactions of the Royal Society of London* (no. 446), 81–86.

Gray Herbarium Index, Harvard University. 1968. Boston: Hall.

Great Britain, Inspector General of Imports and Exports. 1974. *Customs 3.* 1696–1780. 82 vols. With introduction by W. E. Minchinton and C. J. French. In Public Record Office, London. Microfilm, East Ardsley, England, E. P. Microform Ltd.

Grmek, M. 1989. *Diseases in the ancient Greek world* [1983]. Trans. M. and L. Muellner. Baltimore: Johns Hopkins University Press.

Guarini, B. 1613. *La idropica*[.] *Commedia.* Venice: Crotti. (The original is in the Library of Congress.)

———. 1950. *Opere.* Ed. Luigi Fassò. Turin: Unione Tipografico-Editrice Torinese.

Guerra, F. 1977a. El descubrimento de la quina. *Medicina e Historia* [Barcelona] (no. 69), 7–26.

———. 1977b. The introduction of cinchona in the treatment of malaria. *Journal of Tropical Medicine and Hygiene* 80:112–18, 135–40.

———. 1982. *Historia de la medicina*, vol. 1. Madrid: Ediciones Norma.

Guglielminus, D. 1701. *De sanguinis natura et constitutione.* Venice: Poletus.

———. 1719. *Opera omnia mathematica, hydraulica, medica et physica.* 2 vols. Geneva: Cramer, Perachon & socii.

Guiart, J. 1947. *Histoire de la médecine française.* Paris: Nagel.

Guitton, G. 1953. *Les Jesuites à Lyon sous Louis XIV et Louis XV.* Lyon: Procure.

Güldenklee. See Timaeus.

Haas, P. J. 1845. Notice sur la vie et les ouvrages de Vopiscus Fortunatus Plempius. *Annuarie de l'université Catholique de Louvain* 9:209–32.

Haggis, A. W. 1941. Fundamental errors in the early history of cinchona. *Bulletin of the History of Medicine* 10:417–59, 568–92.

Hall, T. S. 1986. *A biomedical index to the correspondence of René Descartes.* 15 pp. Bethesda: National Library of Medicine.

Haller, A. v. [1774–77] 1969. *Bibliotheca anatomica* [Zürich]. Facsimile, Hildesheim: Olms.

———. 1776–78. *Bibliotheca medicinae practicae.* 4 vols. Basel: Schweighauser. Bern: E. Haller.

———. 1757–60. *Disputationes ad morborum historiam et curationem facientes.* 7 vols. Lausanne: Bousquet.

Haring, C. 1918. *Trade and navigation between Spain and the Indies in the time of the Hapsburgs.* Cambridge: Harvard University Press.

Harris, S. J. 1988. Jesuit ideology and Jesuit science: religious values and scientific activity in the Society of Jesus, 1540–1773. Thesis. Madison: University of Wisconsin.

Harris, W. 1683. *Pharmacologia anti-empirica; or a rational discourse of remedies both chymical and galenical.* London: Chiswell.

Harvey, G. 1678. *Casus medico-chirurgicus; or, a most memorable case of a noble-man deceased.* London: Rooks.

———. 1683. *The conclave of physicians. The first part detecting their intrigues, frauds, and plots . . . also a peculiar discourse of the Jesuits bark.* London: Partridge.

————. 1689. *The art of curing diseases by expectation.* London: Partridge.

Harvey, W. 1886. *Praelectiones anatomiae.* London: Churchill.

Hatin, L. 1853. *Histoire du journal en France,* 2d ed. Paris: Jannet.

Hazon, J.-A. 1778. *Notice des hommes les plus célèbres de la faculté de médecine en l'Université de Paris.* Paris: Morin.

Hedges, W. 1887–89. *The diary of William Hedges . . . during his agency in Bengal; as well as on his voyage out and return overland (1681–1687).* 3 vols. London: Hakluyt Society.

Heilbron, J. L. 1979. *Electricity in the 17th and 18th centuries: A study of early modern physics.* Berkeley and Los Angeles: University of California Press.

Held, G. 1715. Cortex peruvianus, vulgo china chinae dictus, polychrestum remedium. *Academiae Caesareo-Leopoldinae Carolinae Naturae Curiosorum Ephemerides,* Centuriae 3 and 4, Observ. 170, pp. 383–86.

[Helvetius, J. A.?] 1694a. *La kinakina, e le di lei stupende qualità . . . Il tutto portato dal francese in Italiano.* Trans. C. Ricani. Parma: dall'Oglio and Rosati.

Helvetius, J. A. 1694b. *Méthode pour guérir toute sorte de fièvre sans rien faire prender par la bouche.* Paris: Oudot.

Henke, F., and Lubarsch, O. 1926–70. *Handbuch der speziellen pathologischen Anatomie und Histologie.* Berlin: Springer.

Henriquez, F. 1714. *Medicina lusitana.* Lisbon: Deslandesiana.

Henriquez de Villacorta, F. 1670. *Opera medica.* 2 vols. in 1. Lyons: Anisson.

Heredia, Petrus Michaelis de. 1689–88 [*sic*]. *Operum medicinalium.* Rev. D. Petrus Barea [Barca] de Astorga. (1st ed. 1665.) Lyons: Borde & Arnaud.

Héritier, J. 1987. *La sève de l'homme; de l'age d'or de la saignée aux débuts de l'hématologie.* Paris: Denoël.

Hernández Morejon, A. 1842–52. *Historia bibliográfica de la medicina española.* 7 vols. Madrid: Jordan.

Hernándo y Ortega, T. 1982. *Dos estudios históricos (vieja y nueva medicina).* Madrid: Espasa-Calpe.

Higby, G. J. 1986. Heroin and medical reasoning: The power of analogy. *New York State Journal of Medicine* 86:137–142.

Hippocrates. 1923–31. Loeb Classical Library edition, trans. W. H. S. Jones and E. T. Withington. 4 vols. Cambridge: Harvard University Press.

————. [1839–61] 1973–82. *Oeuvres complètes d'Hippocrate.* Ed. and trans. Émile Littré. 10 vols. [Paris: Baillière.] Facsimile, Amsterdam: Hakkert.

————. 1988. Loeb Classical Library edition, trans. Paul Potter, vols. 5, 6. Cambridge: Harvard University Press.

Hirsch, A. 1883–86. *Handbook of geographical and historical pathology.* Trans. C. Creighton. 3 vols. London: New Sydenham Society.

Hirsch, A. 1962. *Biographisches Lexikon der hervorragenden Ärzte,* 3d ed. 6 vols. Munich and Berlin: Urban & Schwarzenberg.

Hoefer, W. 1657. *Hercules medicus sive locorum communium liber.* Vienna: Kürner.

Hoffmann, F. 1687. Thesaurus pharmaceuticus. In *Pharmacopoea Schrödero-Hoffmanniana*, ed. I. I. Mangetus. Geneva: De Tournes.

———. 1695. *Fundamenta medicinae.* Halle: Hübner.

———. 1729–34. *Medicina rationalis systematica,* 2d ed. Halle: Ranger.

Hoppe, H. A. 1975. *Drogenkunde,* 8th ed. Berlin: De Gruyter.

Hospital real de Nuestra Señora de Esqueba hasta fin de este año de 1703. 1703–13. MS. Ayuntamiento de Valladolid. Legajo 19–38 (1703), 19–37 (1704), 19–36 (1712), 19–35 (1713).

Houghton, J. 1727–28. *Husbandry and trade improv'd.* London: Woodman & Lyon.

Humboldt, A. von. 1807. Über die Chinawälder in Sudamerika. *Gesellschaft naturforschenden Freunde zu Berlin. Magazin* 1.

Huxham, J. 1756. *Medical and chemical observations upon antimony.* London: Hinton.

———. 1765. *Johannis Huxham . . . liber De Febribus.* Ed. G. C. Reichel. Venice: Basilius.

———. [1757] 1988. *An essay on fevers,* 3d ed. [London: Hinton.] Reissued, with intro. by S. Jarcho. Canton, Mass.: Science History Publications.

Index-Catalogue of the library of the Surgeon-General's Office, United States Army. 1880–1961. 61 vols. in 5 series. Washington, D.C.: Government Printing Office.

Inventari dei manoscritti delle biblioteche d'Italia. 1890–. Florence: Olschki.

Isler, H. 1968. *Thomas Willis, 1621–1675, doctor and scientist.* New York: Hafner.

Ives, E. 1773. *A voyage from England to India, in the year 1754 . . . with an appendix containing an account of the diseases prevalent in Admiral Watson's squadron.* London: Dilly.

Jaramillo Arango, J. 1949a. Estudio crítico acerca de los hechos básicos de la historia de la quina. *Anales de la sociedad peruana de historia de la medicina* 10: 31–88.

———. 1949b. A critical review of the basic facts in the history of cinchona. *Journal of the Linnean Society of London* 53:272–309.

Jarcho, S. 1956. Workmen's compensation among pirates and buccaneers. *Academy Bookman* [New York Academy of Medicine] 9:5–8.

———. 1970. A cartographic and literary study of the word *malaria. Journal of the History of Medicine* 25:31–39.

———. 1972. Seventeenth-century medical journalism as exemplified by the *Ephemerides Naturae Curiosorum. Journal of the American Medical Association* 220:64–68.

———. 1980a. Some ancient and medieval statements about fever. In *Times, places and persons; aspects of the history of epidemiology,* ed. A. M. Lilienfeld, 132–38. Baltimore: Johns Hopkins University Press.

——— 1980b. *The concept of heart failure from Avicenna to Albertini.* Cambridge: Harvard University Press.

———. 1982. A note on the autopsy of Oliver Cromwell. *Transactions and Studies of the College of Physicians of Philadelphia,* 5th ser., 4:228–31.

————. 1984b. Laveran's discovery in the retrospect of a century. *Bulletin of the History of Medicine* 58:215–24.

————. 1986. *Italian broadsides concerning public health.* Mt. Kisco, N.Y.: Futura.

————. 1987a. Falstaff, Kittredge, and Galen. *Perspectives in Biology and Medicine* 30:197–200.

————. 1987b. A history of semitertian fever. *Bulletin of the History of Medicine* 61: 411–30.

————. 1989a. The style of Zacutus Lusitanus and its origins. *Journal of the History of Medicine* 44:291–95.

————. 1989b. *Clinical consultations and letters by Ippolito Francesco Albertini, Francesco Torti, and other physicians.* University of Bologna ms 2089–1. Boston: Francis A. Countway Library.

————, ed. and trans. 1984a. *The clinical consultations of Giambattista Morgagni.* Boston: Francis A. Countway Library of Medicine. Charlottesville: University Press of Virginia.

Jefferys, T. 1762. *A description of the Spanish islands and settlements on the coast of the West Indies.* London: T. Jefferys.

Jiang, J. B., Jacobs, G., Liang, D.-S., and Aikawa, M. 1985. Qinghaosu-induced changes in the morphology of *Plasmodium inui. American Journal of Tropical Medicine and Hygiene* 34:424–28.

Johnson, S. 1739. The life of Boerhaave. *Gentleman's Magazine.*

Johnston-Saint, P. 1929. An outline of the history of medicine in India. *Journal of the Royal Society of Arts* 77: 844–69.

Jones, David. 1979. *Paraguay. A bibliography.* New York: Garland.

Jones, J. 1683. *Novarum dissertationum de morbis abstrusioribus tractatus primus. De febribus intermittentibus . . .* London: Kettilby.

Joncquet, D. 1659. *Hortus, sive index onomasticus plantarum, quas excolebat Parisiis annis 1658 & 1659.* Paris: Clouzier.

Jorge, R. 1937. "Receituário brasilico." *Petrus Nonius* 1:13–18.

Juanini, J.-B.: 1685. *Dissertation physique ou l'on montre les mouvemens de la fermentation . . . et les causes qui alterent la pureté de l'air de Madrid.* Trans. J. J. Courtial. Toulouse: Desclassan.

Jüngken, J. 1732. *Corpus pharmaceutico-medicum universale.* Frankfurt: Knoch.

Jussieu, J. de. 1849. *Histoire des arbres à quinquina de Loxa, 1738.* In *Histoire naturelle des quinquinas, ou monographie du genre Cinchona,* ed. H. A. Weddell. Paris: Masson.

Katterbach, B. 1931. *Referendarii utriusque signaturae.* Vatican City: Bybliotheca Apostolica Vaticana.

Kay, M. 1989. The *Florilegio Medicinal:* source of southwest ethnomedicine. *Pharmacy in History* 31:27–31.

Keatinge, R., ed. 1988. *Peruvian prehistory, an overview of the pre-Inca and Inca society.* Cambridge: Cambridge University Press.

Keele, K. D. 1974. The Sydenham-Boyle theory of morbific particles. *Medical History* 18:240–48.

Keevil, J. 1957–63. *Medicine and the navy, 1200–1900.* 4 vols. Edinburgh and London: Livingstone.

Kettering, S. 1986. *Patrons, brokers, and clients in seventeenth-century France.* New York: Oxford University Press.

King, Lester S., ed. and trans. 1971. *Fundamenta medicinae. Friedrich Hoffmann.* London: Macdonald.

Klayman, D. 1985. Qinghaosu (Artemisinin): An antimalarial drug from China. *Science* 228:1049–55.

Klerk de Reus, G. 1894. Geschichtlicher Ueberblick der administrator, rechtlichen und finanziellen Entwicklung der Niederländisch-Ostindischen Compagnie. *Bataviaasch Genootschap van Kunsten en Vetenschappen. Verhandelingen.* Batavia: Albrecht & Rusche.

Krivatsy, P. 1989. *A catalogue of seventeenth century printed books in the National Library of Medicine.* Bethesda: U.S. Department of Health and Human Services, National Library of Medicine.

Kronick, D. 1976. *A history of scientific and technical periodicals,* 2d ed. Metuchen, N.J.: Scarecrow Press.

Krugius, T. 1691. De non mutato pulsu et urina in febre intermittente tertiana. *Miscellanea curiosa seu ephemerides.* Decuria 2, 10: 5–8.

Lacuna, A. 1553. *Epitome omnium Galeni Pergameni operum.* Lyons: Rouillius.

La Fontaine, J. de. 1682. *Poème du quinquina et autres ouvrages en vers.* Paris: Thierry & Barbin.

———. 1883–92. *Oeuvres.* Ed. Henri Regnier. Paris: Hachette.

Lancisi, J. M. 1717. *De noxiis paludum effluviis eorumque remediis.* Rome: Salvioni.

Langasco. See Carpaneto.

Lange, Christian J. 1704. *Opera omnia medica.* Leipzig: Gleditsch.

Langius, C. 1704. *Opera omnia medica theoretico-practica.* Leipzig: Gleditsch.

Larrieu, F. 1889. *Gui Patin.* Paris: Picard.

La Wall, C. H. 1932. The history of cinchona. *American Journal of Pharmacy* 104:23–43.

Ledelius, S. 1694. De quadriga quartaniorum. *Miscellanea medico-physica sive ephemerides.* Decuria 3, 2: 59–60.

Leincker, J. H. 1705. *Dissertatio medica inauguralis de ipecacuanha americana, et germanica.* Praeses, G. W. Wedel. Jena.

Leite, S. 1938–50. *Historía da Companhia de Jesus no Brasil.* Rio de Janeiro: Civilização Brasileira, Instituto Nacional do Livro.

———. 1953. *Artes e ofícios dos jesuitas no Brasil, 1549–1760.* Lisbon: Broteria. Rio de Janeiro: Livros de Portugal.

———. 1965. *Suma histórica da Companhia de Jesus no Brasil (assitência de Portugal), 1549–1760.* Lisbon: Junta de Investigações do Ultramar.

Lémery, N. 1683. *Cours de chymie,* 5th ed. Paris: Michallet.

———. 1707. *Traité de l'antimoine.* Paris: Boudot.

———. 1716. *Dictionaire ou traité universel des drogues simples,* 3d ed. Amsterdam: Aux depens de la compagnie.

———. 1717. *Trattato dell' antimonio.* Trans. Salvaggio Canturani. Venice: Ertz [Hertz].

Le Moine d'Espine, [J.] 1710. *Le negoce d'Amsterdam,* 2d ed. Amsterdam: Brunel.

Lemos, Maximiano Junior. 1881. *A medicina em Portugal até aos fins do seculo XVIII.* Inaugural dissertation. Porto: Impresa Commercial.

Lemos, Maximiano. 1909. *Zacuto Lusitano: A sua vida e a sua obra.* Porto: Tavares Martins.

Le Roi, J. A., ed. 1862. *Journal de la santé du roi Louis XIV de l'année 1647 à l'année 1711 écrit par [Antoine] Vallot, [Antoine] d'Aquin et [Guy-Crescent] Fagon.* Paris: Durand.

Le admirables qualitez du kinkina, confirmées par plusieurs expériences, et la manière de s'en servir dans toutes les fièvres . . . 1689. Paris: Jouvenet.

Lettres édifiantes et curieuses, écrites des missions étrangères, new ed. 1819. Lyons: Vernarel & Cabin.

Lévy-Valensi, J. 1933. *La médecine et les médecins Français au XVII siècle.* Paris: Baillière.

Lilienfeld, A. M., ed. 1980. *Times, places and persons; aspects of the history of epidemiology.* Baltimore: Johns Hopkins University Press.

Lind, J. 1762. *An essay on the most effectual means of preserving the health of seamen in the royal navy.* London: Wilson.

———. 1768. *An essay on diseases incidental to Europeans in hot climates . . . to which is added an appendix concerning intermittent fevers.* London: Becket & de Hondt.

Lindeboom, G. A. 1968. *Herman Boerhaave; the man and his work.* London: Methuen.

Linnaeus, C. 1742. *Genera plantarum,* 2d rev. ed. Leyden: Wishoff & Wishoff. Also 2d ed., Paris: David, 1743; 4th ed., Halle: Kümmel, 1752.

Lister, M. 1684. *De fontibus medicatis Angliae,* rev. ed. London: Kettilby.

———. 1697. *Octo exercitationes medicinales,* 2d ed. London: Smith & Walford.

Litta, P. 1819. *Famiglie celebri italiane,* vol. 4. Milano: Ferrario.

Lloyd, G. E. R. 1973–74. Analogy in early Greek thought. In *Dictionary of the history of ideas,* ed. P. P. Wiener. New York: Scribner's.

Loomis, A. L., and Thompson, W. G. 1897. *A system of practical medicine,* vol. 1. New York and Philadelphia: Lea.

Lutteroth, H. 1858. *Russia and the Jesuits, from 1772 to 1820.* London: Seeley, Jackson, & Halliday.

Maclagan, E. 1932. *The Jesuits and the great mogul.* London: Burns Oates & Washbourne.

Madras Government. 1908–11. *Selections from the records of the Madras Government. Dutch records.* 15 vols. Madras: Government Press.

Madras Record office (presidency). 1919. *Records of Fort St. George. Public despatches to England 1694–96.* Ed. H. Dodwell. Madras: Government Press.

Malcorps, F. J. 1853. Notice sur Herman van der Heyden. *Annales de la Société de Médicin d'Anvers,* 449–61.

Malpighi, M. 1698. *Opera posthuma.* Amsterdam: Gallet.

Malvezin, T. 1892. *Histoire du commerce de Bordeaux depuis les origines jusqu'à nos jours.* 4 vols. Bordeaux: Bellier.

Mandosio, P. 1696. *Theatron in quo . . . pontificum archiatros . . . spectandos exhibet.* Rome: De Lazaris.

Mangetus, I. I., ed. 1687. *Pharmacopoea Schrödero-Hoffmanniana.* Geneva: De Tournes. Appendix . . . continens Frederici Hoffmanni thesaurum pharmaceuticum.

Mangetus, J. 1703. *Bibliotheca pharmaceutica-medica.* Geneva: Chouët et al.

———. 1731. *Bibliotheca scriptorum medicorum.* Geneva: Perachon & Cramer.

Manno, A. 1898. *Bibliografia di Genova.* Genoa: R. Istituto Sordo-Muti.

Marini, G. 1784. *Degli archiatri pontificj.* Rome: Pagliarini.

Markham, C. 1874. *A memoir of the lady Ana de Osorio, countess of Chinchon.* London: Trübner.

———. 1880. *Peruvian bark, a popular account of the introduction of chinchona* [sic] *cultivation into British India.* London: Murray.

Master, S. 1911. *The diaries of Streynsham Master, 1675–1680, and other contemporary papers relating thereto.* London: Murray.

Mazzuchelli, G. 1753–63. *Gli scrittori d'Italia.* Brescia: Bossini.

Meade, R. 1751. *Monita et praecepta medica.* London: Brindley.

Melippus. See Protimus.

Mémoires pour l'histoire des sciences et des beaux-arts. 1701–67. Printed at Trévoux. 265 vols. in 290. Paris: Geneaux.

Menéndez Pelayo, M. 1967. *Historia de los heterodoxos españoles,* 2d ed. Ed. Rafael García y García de Castro. Vol. 2. Madrid: Biblioteca de autores cristianos.

Menéndez-Pidal, G. 1944. *Imagen del mundo hacia 1570.* Madrid: Gráficas Ultra.

Mercatus, L. 1611. *Praxis medica.* Venice: Iunta [Giunta] et al.

———. 1619–20. *Operum,* vol. 2. Frankfurt: Palthenius.

Mercurius Politicus. 1650–59. London.

Mettam, R. 1988. *Power and faction in Louis XIV's France.* Oxford: Blackwell.

Migne, J. P. 1844. *Patrologiae cursus completus,* 1st ser. [Latin], vol. 5. Paris: Sirou.

———. 1857. *Troisième et dernière encyclopédie théologique.* Vol. 31, *Dictionnaire des cardinaux.* Paris: Migne.

Minot, J. 1691. *De la nature et des causes de la fiévre* [sic], *du legitime usage de la saignée et des purgatifs. Avec des experiences sur le quinquina, et des reflexions sur les effets de ce remede,* 2d ed. Paris: d'Houry.

Miscellanea curiosa seu ephemeridum medico-physicarum academiae caesareo leopoldinae naturae curiosorum decuriae, ann. VII et VIII. 1702. Frankfurt and Leipzig.

Moens, A. 1911. *Memorandum on the administration of the coast of Malabar . . . April 1, 1781.* Trans. P. Groot and A. Galletti. In *Selections from the records of the Madras government. Dutch records no. 13.* Madras: Government Press.

Monardes, N. [1565] 1568. *Dos libros.* [Seville: Trugillo.] Seville: Diaz.

Monginot, F. de [pseudonym of François de La Salle]. 1680. *De la guérison des fièvres par le quinquina*. Paris: Guignard.

Morão, Simão Pinheiro. [ca. 1677] 1965. *Queixas repetidas em ecos dos Arrecifes de Pernambuco contra os abusos médicos que nas suas capitanias se observam*. [Pernambuco.] Ed. Jaime Walter. Lisbon: Junta de Investigações do Ultramar.

Moreau, R., ed. and com. 1625. *Schola salernitana, hoc est de valetudine tuenda . . . Adiectae sunt animadversiones nouae et copiosae Renati Moreau*. Paris: Blasius.

———. 1647a. *Tabulae methodi generalis curandorum morborum*. Paris: Boisset.

———. 1647b. *Tabulae methodi universalis curandorum morborum in aula cameracensi regia*. Paris: Variquet.

Morejon. See Hernández Morejon, A.

Morgagni, J. B. 1761. *De sedibus, et causis morborum per anatomen indagatis*. Venice: Remondini.

———. 1769. *The seats and causes of diseases*. Translated by B. Alexander. London: Millar & Cadell. Facsimile, New York: Hafner, 1960; reissued New York: Futura, 1980.

Morton, L. 1991. *A medical bibliography*, 5th ed. Ed. J. M. Norman. Aldershot: Scolar Press.

Morton, R. 1689. *Phthisiologia*. London: Smith.

———. 1692. *Pyretologia, seu exercitationes de morbis universalibus acutis*. London: Smith.

———. 1694. *Pyretologia. Pars altera: sive exercitatio de febribus inflammatoriis universalibus*. London: Smith & Walford.

Muraltus, J. 1689. Febres fugatae per corticem peruvianum. *Miscellanea curiosa sive ephemerides*. Decuria 2, 8: 2–16.

Nardi, J. 1656. *Noctes geniales, annus primus*. Bologna: Ferronii.

New Cambridge modern history. 1970. Vol. 4. Cambridge: University Press.

Newton, A. P. 1933. *The European nations in the West Indies, 1493–1688*. London: Black.

Nieremberg, J. E. 1890. *Varones ilustres de la Compañía de Jesús*, 2d ed. Bilbao: Administración de "El mensajero del Corazon de Jesús."

[Nigrisoli, F., ed.] 1687, 1700. *Febris china chinae expugnata, seu illustrium aliquot virorum opuscula, quae verum tradunt methodum, febres china chinae curandi*. Ferrara: Pomatelli. (2d ed. augmented, Ferrara: Lilius.)

Nolhac, P. de. 1911. *Histoire du chateau de Versailles*. Paris: Marty.

Notiziario dell' antica farmacia di Brera. [Milan:] 1924–26. 3 vols. (In annex of Biblioteca comunale, Milan.)

Novombergskiy, N. 1905. *Materialy po istorii meditsiny v Rossii*. St. Petersburg: Stasyulevich. Microfilm no. 486, New York Academy of Medicine.

Nutton, V. 1983. The seeds of disease: An explanation of contagion and infection from the Greeks to the Renaissance. *Medical History* 27:1–34.

Nutton, V. 1990. The reception of Fracastoro's theory of contagion. *Osiris*, 2d ser., 6:196–234.

Ogg, D. 1960. *Europe in the seventeenth century*, 8th ed. London: Adam & Charles Black.

Oliver, W. 1704. A letter . . . to Mr. James Petiver, F. R. S. concerning the Jesuits bark. *Philosophical Transactions* 24 (no. 290): 1596.

O'Malley, C. 1964. *Andreas Vesalius of Brussels*. Berkeley: University of California Press.

Orta, Garcia da [1563] 1911. *Colloquies on the simples and drugs of India*. [Goa.] Ed. of Lisbon [1891]-1895, ed. Conde de Ficalho. Trans. Sir Clements Markham. London: Sotheran.

Ortelius, A. 1570. *Theatrum orbis terrarum*. Antwerp. 2d ed., 1579. 3d ed. 1584.

Osler, W. 1969. *Bibliotheca Osleriana*. Montreal: McGill-Queens University Press.

Oviedo y Valdes, G. F. de. [1535–57] 1944–45. *Historia general y natural de las Indias*, vols. 13, 14. Asunción: Editorial Guarania.

Packard, F. 1925. *Guy Patin*. New York: Hoeber.

Padberg, J. W. 1974. The general congregations of the Society of Jesus; a brief survey of their history. *Studies in the Spirituality of Jesuits* 6:22–27.

Pallegoix, J. 1854. *Description du royaume Thai ou Siam, comprenant la topographie, histoire naturelle . . . et précis historique de la mission*. 2 vols. Paris.

Pankhurst, R. 1979. Europe's discovery of the Ethiopian taenicide—*Kosso*. *Medical History* 23:297–313.

Pardal, R. 1937. *Medicina aborígen americana*. Buenos Aires: Anesi.

Paredes Borja, V. 1947. *La contribución del Ecuador a la materia médica: la quina*. Quito: Casa de la Cultura Ecuatoriana.

———. 1963. *Historia de la medicina en el Ecuador*. Quito: Casa de la Cultura Ecuatoriana.

Pastor, L. von. [1938] 1955. *The history of the popes*. Trans. Ernest Graf. London: Routledge & Kegan Paul, reprint.

Patin, G. 1707. *Lettres choisies de feu Mr. Guy Patin*. The Hague: van Bulderen.

———. 1718. *Nouvelles lettres de feu Mr. Guy Patin*. 2 vols. The Hague: Gosse.

———. 1907. *Lettres de Guy Patin 1630–1672*, new ed. Ed. P. Triaire. Paris: Champion.

Pelletier, P., and Caventou, J. 1820. *Recherches chimiques sur les quinquinas*. *Annales de Chimie et de Physique* (Paris) 15:289–318, 337–65.

Peregrino da Costa, P. J. 1948. Medicina portuguesa no extremo-oriente— Sião, Molucas, Japão, Cochinchina, Pequim e Macau (século XVI a XX). *Boletim do Instituto Vasco da Gama* (nos. 63, 64): 1–236. Bastora, India Portuguesa: Tipografia Rangel.

Perez Arbelaez, E. 1959. Alejandro de Humboldt y las quinas del nuevo reino de Granada. *Bolivar* (Bogotà) 12: 123–34.

Per la storia della malaria nell' agro Romano. 1926. *La Civiltà Cattolica*, Anno 77, 2: 246–54, 525–34.

Perreau, J. 1655. *Rabbat-ioye de l'antimoine triumphant; ou examen de l'antimoine*. Paris: Meturas.

Pescetto, G. B. 1846. *Biografia medica ligure*. Genoa: R. Istituto Sordo-Muti.

Peters, W., ZeLin, L., Robinson, B., and Warhurst, D. 1986. The chemotherapy of rodent malaria, XL. The action of artemisinin and related sesquiterpenes. *Annals of Tropical Medicine and Parasitology* 80:483–89.

Peter the Great. 1887–1912. *Pis'ma i bumagi imperatora Petra Velikogo*. [Letters and papers of the emperor Peter the Great.] 6 vols. St. Petersburg: Imperial Printing Shop.

Petraeus, H. 1618. *Agonismata medica*. Marpurgi Cattorum [Marburg]: Egenolphus.

Peyer, J. C. 1686. De febrium tertianarum et quartanarum intermittentium remedio. *Ephemerides Naturae Curiosorum*, Decade 2, year 4 (obs. 102): 201–2. Nuremberg.

Pharmacopoea Amstelredamensis. 1636, 1660. Amsterdam: Blaeu.

———. 1639. Amsterdam: Wetstenius.

Pharmacopoea Belgica. 1659. London: Farnham.

Pharmacopoea Hagiensis. 1659. Hague: Tongerloo.

Pharmacopoea Harlemensis. 1693. Haarlem: van Kessel. Amsterdam: ten Hoorn.

Pharmacopoea Ultrajectina. 1656. Utrecht: Zyll & Ackersdyck.

Pharmacopoeia Augustana. 1613. Ed. R. Minderer. Augsburg: Mangus.

Pharmacopoeia Collegii Regalis Londini. 1677. London: Newcomb et al.

Pharmacopoeia Londinensis. Or, the new London dispensatory. 1678. Trans. William Salmon. London: Dawks.

Piquer, A. 1751. *Tratado de las calenturas segun la observacion, y el mecanismo*. Valencia: Garcia.

Piso, C. 1648. *Historia naturalis Brasiliae, auspicio et beneficio Illustris[simi] I. Mauritii Com[itis] Nassau*. Leyden: Hackius. Amsterdam: Elzevirius.

———. 1658. *De Indiae utriusque re naturali et medica*. Amsterdam: L. & D. Elzevirius.

Pitcairne, A. 1701. *Dissertationes medicae*. Rotterdam: Leers.

Plempius, V. F. 1642. . . . *Animadversio in veram praxim curandae tertianae propositam a Doctore Petro Barba regiae majestatis, et serenissimi Hispaniarum Infantis Ferdinandi . . . cubiculario medico*. Louvain: Zeger.

Plomer, H. R. 1907. *A dictionary of the booksellers and printers who were at work in England, Scotland and Ireland from 1641 to 1667*. London: Blades, East, & Blades.

Pluchon, P., ed. 1985. *Histoire des médecins et pharmaciens de marine et des colonies*. Toulouse: Privat.

Posthumus, N. W. 1943. *Nederlandsche Prijsgeschiedenis*. Leiden: Brill.

———. 1946–64. *Inquiry into the history of prices in Holland*. 2 vols. Leiden: Brill.

Pringle, J. 1752. *Observations on diseases of the army*. London: Millar & Wilson.

Protimus, Melippus [pseudonym of Vopiscus Fortunatus Plempius]. 1655. *Antimus Conygius* [pseudonym of Honoratus Fabri] *peruviani pulveris defensor repulsus a Melippo Protimo Belga, exequias peruviano pulveri febrifugo* . . . [Louvain.] Unpaginated MS in National Library of Medicine, bound with Antimus Conygius: *Pulvis peruvianus vindicatus*, Rome: Corbelleti.

Public Record Office, London. 1960. *Descriptive list of exchequer, Queen's remembrancer, port books.* Part 1, 1565–1700. London: Public Record Office.

Publick Intelligencer. 1658–59. London.

Puccinotti, F. 1842. *Storia delle febbri intermittenti perniciose di Roma negli anni* MDCCCXIX MDCCCXX MDCCCXXI [1819–21]. Ed. G. Nicolucci. Naples: Jovene.

Purchas, S. [1625] 1905–7. *Hakluytus posthumus, or Purchas his pilgrimes.* Glasgow: MacLehose.

Puschmann, T. 1902. *Handbuch der Geschichte der Medizin,* vol. 2. Ed. Max Neuburger and Julius Pagel. Jena: Fischer.

Raius, Johannes [John Ray]. 1686–1704. *Historia plantarum.* 3 vols. London: Faithorne, vols. 1, 2; Smith & Walford, vol. 3.

Ramazzini, B. 1690. *De constitutione anni 1690.* Modena: Cassiani.

———. [1713] 1940. *De morbis artificum Bernardini Ramazzini diatriba.* Ed. and trans. W. C. Wright as *Diseases of Workers.* The work originally appeared in 1700. Chicago: University of Chicago Press.

———. 1714. De abusu chinae chinae. In *Constitutionum epidemicarum mutinensium annorum quinque,* 2d ed. Padua: Conzatti.

———. 1716a. De principum valetudine tuenda. In *Opera omnia, medica, et physica.* Geneva: Cramer & Perachon.

———. 1716b. *Opera omnia, medica, et physica.* Geneva: Cramer & Perachon.

———. 1717. *Opera omnia, medica et physiologica.* Geneva: Cramer & Percahon. Also 3d ed., London: Paul & Isaac Vaillant, 1718.

———. 1940. *Diseases of workers.* Trans. and rev. W. C. Wright. Chicago: University of Chicago Press.

———. 1964. *Epistolario; pubblicato . . . a cura di Pericle di Pietro.* Modena: Toschi.

Ratio atque institutio studiorum Societatis Iesu. Auctoritate septimae congregationis generalis aucta. 1635. Antwerp: Meursius.

Ray. See Raius.

Raynal, G. T. F. 1780. *Histoire philosophique et politique des établissements et du commerce des Européens dans les deux Indes.* Geneva: Pellet.

Raynaud, M. 1862. *Les médecins au temps de Molière.* Paris: Didier.

Reddy, D. V. S. 1947. *The beginnings of modern medicine in Madras.* Calcutta: Thacker & Spink.

Redi, F. 1712–30. *Opere di Francesco Redi.* Venice: Ertz [Hertz].

Reis, Gaspar Franco dos. 1670. *Elysius jucundarum campus, omnium literarum amoenissima varietate refertus.* Frankfurt am Main: Haered. Beyeri.

Relaciones históricas y geográficas de America Central. 1908. Madrid: Suárez.

[Renaudot, T.] 1664. *A general collection of discourses of the virtuosi of France . . . by the most ingenious persons of that nation.* Trans. G. Havers. London: Dring & Starkey.

Renaudot, T. 1665. *Another collection of philosophical conferences of the French virtuosi. . . .* Trans. G. Havers and J. Davies. London: Dring & Starkey.

(Translation of *Receuil général des questions traités dans les conférences du Bureau d'adresse.*)

Renouard, P.-V. [1846] 1856. *Histoire de la médecine.* [Paris.] Eng. trans. C. G. Comegys. Cincinnati: Moore, Wilstach, Keys.

Restaurand, R. 1681. *Hippocrate de l'usage du chinachina, pour la guérison des fièvres.* Lyon: Esprit Vitalis.

Ricani, C., trans. 1694. [Helvetius, A.?] *La kinakina, e le di lei stupende qualità.* Parma: dall' Oglio & Rosati.

Richter, W. 1813–17. *Geschichte der Medizin in Russland.* Moscow: Wsewolojsky.

Riddle, J. M. 1985. *Dioscorides on pharmacy and medicine.* Austin: University of Texas Press.

Riding, A. 1988. Brazil now a vital crossroad of Latin cocaine traffickers. *New York Times,* 28 Aug. 1988 (sect. 1): 1, 18 (with map).

Riolan, J. 1649. *Encheiridium anatomicum et pathologicum.* Leyden: Wyngaerden.

———. 1651. *Curievses recherches svr les escholes en medecine, de Paris, et de Montpellier.* Paris: Meturas.

———. 1661. *Manuel anatomique et pathologique.* Paris: Meturas.

Riverius, L. 1656. *Observationum centuria quarta,* ed. Simon Jacoz. The Hague: Jacoz.

———. 1690. *Opera medica universa.* Lyon: Huguetan.

Rolfincius, G. 1658. *Ordo et methodus cognoscendi et curandi febres generalis.* Jena: Krebs.

Romano, Gaetano M. 1843. *Dizionario di erudizione storico-ecclesiastica.* Venice: Tipografia emiliana.

Rompel, J. 1905. Kritische Studien zur ältesten Geschichte der Chinarinde. *XIV Jahresbericht des öffentlichen Privat Gymnasium an der Stella Matutina zu Feldkirch.* Feldkirch.

———. [1929] 1932. Der Arzt Baldo und die Chinarinde. [*Stimmen der Zeit* (Freiburg im Breisgau) 117: 124–36.] Reprinted in *Pharmaceutisch Weekblad,* 382–98.

———. 1931. Kardinal de Lugo als Mäzen der Chinarinde. I. Aus dem Leben der Kardinal. *75 Jahre Stella Matutina.* Festschrift, Band I, 416–52. Feldkirch: Selbstverlag Stella Matutina.

Ross, D. 1945. *Aristotle.* London: Methuen.

Rothmann, C. 1663. *Alpha et omega. Anti-quartii peruviani historia . . . sub praesidio . . . Pauli Ammann.* Leipzig: Wittigau.

Rowell, M. 1978. Russian medical botany before the time of Peter the Great. *Sudhoffs Archiv* 62:339–58.

Royal Society, London. 1700–74. *A list of the Royal Society, 1717, from Lists of Fellows.* Photocopy.

———. 1660–1800. *Journal books of scientific meetings.* Microfilm.

Royle, F. 1839. *Illustrations of the botany and other branches of natural history of the Himalayan mountains.* London: Allen.

Ruiz López, H. 1792. *Quinologia, o, tratado del arbol de la quina o cascarilla.* Madrid: Marin.

Russell, P. 1952. Italy in the history of malaria. *Rivista di parassitologia* 13:93–104.

Salado Garces, D. 1678. *Apologetico discurso, con que se prueba que los polvos de quarango se deben vsar por febrifugio de tercianas nothas, y de quartanas.* Seville: Lopez de Haro.

Salado Garzes [*sic*], D. 1679. *Estaciones medicas, en las quales para mayor confirmacion del Apologetico Discurso, con que se prueba que los polvos de quarango se deben usar por febri-fugio de tercianas, y quartanas, se desatan unas agudas notas de vn docto Sevillano medico* . . . Seville: Lopez de Haro.

Salle, François de la. See Monginot.

Salmon, W. 1671. *Synopsis medicinae.* London: Godbid. Also 2d ed., London: Dawks, 1680.

Sánchez-Monge y Parellada, E. 1981. *Diccionario de plantas agricolas.* Madrid: Ministerio de Agricultura, Servicio de Publicaciones Agrarias.

Santos Filho, L. 1977. *História geral da medicina brasiliera,* vol. 1. São Paulo: Editora da Universidade de São Paulo.

Satinoff, E. 1977. Quinine-induced hypothermia in cold-exposed rats. *Pharmacology, Biochemistry and Behavior* 6:539–43.

Saunders, W. 1782. *Observations on the superior efficacy of the red Peruvian bark, in the cure of agues and other fevers.* London: Johnson & Murray.

Scarborough, J. 1985. Galen's dissection of the elephant. *Koroth* 8 (11–12):123–34.

Schelenz, H. [1904] 1965. *Geschichte der Pharmazie* [Berlin.] Facsimile, Hildesheim: Olms.

Schelhammer, G. C. 1693. *De genuina febres curandi methodo dissertatio.* Jena: Bielckius.

Schneider, W. 1968–75. *Lexikon zur Arzneimittelgeschichte.* 7 vols. in 9. Frankfurt: Govi Verlag.

Schondorff, J. 1694. *Disputatio inauguralis medica de chinae chinae, usu et abusu* . . . *praeside Dr. Frederico Hoffmanno.* Halle: Salfeld.

Schouten, W. [1676] 1725. *Oost-indische voyagiën.* [Amsterdam.] French trans.: *Voyage du Gautier Schouten aux Indes Orientales, commencé l'an 1658 et fini l'an 1665.* 2 vols. Rouen: Le Boucher.

Schreiber, W., and Mathus, F. 1987. *Infectio. Infectious diseases in the history of medicine,* 2d ed. Basel: Hoffmann-La Roche.

Schröder, I. 1649–50. *Pharmacopoeia medico-chymica.* 2 vols. Ulm: Gerlinus.

Sebastiani, G. 1672. *Seconda speditione all' Indie Orientali.* Rome: Mancini.

Sebes, J. 1961. *The Jesuits and the Sino-Russian treaty of Nerchinsk (1689). The diary of Thomas Pereira, S. J.* Rome: Institutum Historicum S. I.

Senac, J. B. 1749. *Traité de la structure du coeur.* Paris: Briasson.

———. [1759] 1805. *De reconditum febrium intermittentium, tum remittentium natura, et de earum curatione.* [Amsterdam.] Trans. C. Caldwell: *A treatise on the nature, and the treatment of intermitting and remitting fevers.* Philadelphia: Kimber & Conrad.

Service, M. W. 1989. *Demography and vector-borne diseases.* Boca Raton: CRC Press.

Sévigné, Mme. Marie de. 1972–78. *Correspondence*. Paris: Gallimard.

Seyfarth, C. 1926. Die Malaria. In F. Henke and O. Lubarsch. *Handbuch der speziellen pathologischen Anatomie und Histologie*, ed. 1 (pt. 1): 178–248. Berlin: Springer.

Sheridan, J. J. 1922. Quinine. *Fordham Monthly* 29: 310–14.

Shortt, H. E. 1948. The pre-erythrocytic cycle of *Plasmodium cynomolgi*. *Proceedings of the Fourth International Congresses on Tropical Medicine and Malaria*, 607–17. Washington, D.C.: U.S. Government Printing Office.

Siegel, R. 1968. *Galen's system of physiology and medicine*. Basel: Karger.

Siegel, R., and Poynter, F. N. L., 1962. Robert Talbor, Charles II, and cinchona; a contemporary document. *Medical History* 6:82–85.

Snapper, I. 1946. On the influence of stilbamidine upon multiple myeloma. *Journal of Mount Sinai Hospital* 13: 119–27.

Società Italiana per l'Esercizio Telefonico. 1985–96. *Genova e Provincia*.

Soers, M. 1641. *Repetitio de tertiana praeside Clariss. Viro Dom. D. Vopisco Fortunato Plempio . . . repetet Martinus Soers Breensis*, Louvain, 26 Nov.

———. 1642. *Stricturae in ceritum quemdam Eburonem inconditum blateronem. Controversiae de curanda tertiana inter D. D. Petrum Barbam et V. F. Plempium agitatae*. Louvain: Zeger, 14 pp.

Sollmann, T. 1948. *A manual of pharmacology*, 7th ed. Philadelphia: Saunders.

Sommervogel, C. 1864–65. *Table méthodique des Mémoires de Trévoux*. Paris: Durand.

———. 1884. *Dictionnaire des ouvrages anonymes et pseudonymes publiés par des religieux de la compagnie de Jésus*. Paris: Librairie de la société bibliographique.

Soproni, R. 1667. *Li scrittori della Liguria*. Genoa: Calenzani.

Spain, Ministerio de Cultura. 1990. *Documentación indiana en Simancas*. Valladolid: Iglesia de las Francescas.

Spate, O. 1983. *Monopolists and freebooters*. London: Croom & Helm.

Spigelius, A. 1624. *De semitertiana libri quatuor*. Frankfurt: de Bry.

———. 1633. *Isagoges in rem herbariam libri duo*. Leyden: Elzeviriana.

———. 1645. *Opera quae extant omnia*. Ed. J. A. van den Linden. 2 vols. in 1. Amsterdam: Blaeu.

Spon, J. 1682. *Observations on fevers and febrifuges*. Trans. J. Berrie. London: Pardoe.

Sprengel, K. 1821–38. *Versuch einer pragmatischen Geschichte der Arzneykunde*, 3d ed. Halle: Gebauer.

Stahl, G. 1726. *Untersuchung der übel curirten und verderbten Kranckheiten*. Leipzig: Eyssel.

Stakelberg, N. 1940–41. *Bibliografiya malyarii, 1771–1935*. Ed. E. N. Pavlovsky. Moscow: Academy of Sciences USSR.

Steele, A. R. 1964. *Flowers for the king. The expedition of Ruiz and Pavon and the flora of Peru*. Durham: Duke University Press.

Stepan, N. 1981. *Beginnings of Brazilian science*. New York: Science History Publications.

Stieb, E. W. 1958. Drug adulteration and its detection in the writings of Theo-

phrastus, Dioscorides and Pliny. *Journal Mondial de Pharmacie* 2:117–
34.

Stisser, J. 1687. *Febrium intermittentium consideratio nova. Iatricae hodiernae placitis accommodata.* Brunswick: Gruber.

Storia di Milano. 1953–66. [Milano:] Fondazione Treccani degli Alfieri.

Streit, R. 1916–71. *Bibliotheca missionum.* 28 vols. in 29. Münster: Aschendorf.

Stübler, E. 1926. *Geschichte der medizinischen Facultät der Universität Heidelberg, 1386–1925.* Heidelberg: Winter.

Sturmius, R. 1659. *Febrifugi Peruviani vindiciarum.* Delft: Oosterhout.

Suardo, J. A. 1935. *Diario de Lima.* Ed. Ruben Vargas Ugarte. Lima: Vasquez.

Suárez de Ribera, F. 1724. *Medicina ilustrada chymica observada ó teatro farmacologo médico-práctico chymico Galénico.* Madrid: del Hierro.

———. 1726. *Medicina invencible legal, o theatro de fiebres intermitentes complicadas.* Madrid: del Hierro.

Suppan, L. 1931. Three centuries of cinchona. In *Celebration of the three hundredth anniversary of the first recognized use of cinchona.* St. Louis: Missouri Botanical Garden.

Sur le chacril. 1723. *Histoire de l'Académie Royale des Sciences, Année MDCCXIX* [1719]. Amsterdam: De Coup.

Sydenham, T. 1666. *Methodus curandi febres propriis observationibus superstructa.* London: Crook.

———. 1809. *The Works of Thomas Sydenham.* Trans. and ed. B. Rush. Philadelphia: Kitt.

———. 1848–50. *The works of Thomas Sydenham.* Trans. and ed. R. G. Latham from the Latin edition of Dr. [William Alexander] Greenhill. 2 vols. London: Sydenham Society.

Sylvius, F. de le Böe. 1679. *Opera medica.* Amsterdam: Elzevirius & Wolfgang.

Talbor, R. 1672. *Pyretologia, a rational account of the cause and cure of agues.* London: Robinson.

———. 1682. *The English remedy: or, Talbor's wonderful secret, for cureing of agues and feavers. . . . now translated into English for publick good.* London: Wallis for Hindmarsh.

Thieme, U. 1916. *Allgemeines Lexikon der bildenden Künstler,* vol. 12. *Leipzig: Seemann.*

Thwaites, R., ed. 1896–1901. *The Jesuit relations and allied documents.* 73 vols. Cleveland: Burrows.

Timaeus von Güldenklee, B. 1667. *Casus medicinales praxi triginta sex annorum observati. Accessere et medicamentorum singularium quae in casibus proponuntur descriptiones.* 9 parts in 1 vol. Leipzig: Kirchner.

Tiraboschi, G. 1781–86. *Biblioteca modenese.* 6 vols. Modena: Società tipografica.

Torres Saldamando, E. 1882. *Los antiguos Jesuitas del Perú.* Lima: Imprenta Liberal.

Torti, F. [1695] 1743. Dissertatio epistolaris prima circa mercurii motiones in barometro. [Modena: Soliani.] In *Therapeutice specialis,* 4th ed. Venice: Basilius.

————. 1708. Synopsis libri cui titulus Therapeutice Specialis. *La Galleria di Minerva overo notizie universali, di quanto e stato scritto da letterati di Europa* 6: 316–17. [The dating here is nominal and not to be regarded as exact. See Chapter 8.]

————. 1709. *Synopsis libri cui titulus, Therapeutice specialis ad febres quasdam perniciosas, inopinatò, ac repente lethales.* Modena: Soliani.

————. 1712. *Therapeutice specialis ad febres quasdam perniciosas, inopinato, ac repentè lethales, una verò China China, peculiari methodo ministrata, sanabiles, aucta curationum historiis, quaestionibus, ac animadversionibus practicis, aliisque plurimis, variam hujusmodi febrium habitudinem, intermittentium quoque omnium, quin et continuarum naturam, et Chinae Chinae praestantiam, actionemque, respicientibus, nec non usum, et abusum illius in singulis febrium, aliorumque plurium morborum, praesertim recurrentium, speciebus.* 736 pp. Modena: Soliani. Also 2d ed., Modena: Soliani, 1730; 3d ed., Venice: Basilius, 1732; 4th ed. (with biography by L. A. Muratori), Venice: Basilius, 1743.

————. 1715. *Ad criticam dissertationem de abusu chinae chinae Mutinensibus medicis perperam objecto a clarissimo quondam viro Bernardino Ramazzino in Patavina Universitate practicae medicinae professore primario responsiones jatro-apologeticae Francisci Torti medici Mutinensis.* Modena: Soliani.

————. 1720. Letter to J. Mangetus. MS. Modena, 25 Feb. Biblioteca Estense, Modena, Codice miscellanei.

————. [1695] 1743. *Dissertatio epistolaris prima circa mercurii motiones in barometro.* [Modena.] In *Therapeutice specialis,* 4th ed.

————. [1698] 1743. *Dissertatio altera triceps circa mercurii motiones in barometro.* [Modena.] In *Therapeutice specialis,* 4th ed.

————. 1821. *Therapeutice specialis.* 2 vols. Ed. C. C. J. Tombeur and O. Brexhe. Liège: Bassompierre.

Tozzi, L. 1693. In *Hippocratis aphorismos commentaria.* 2 vols. Naples: Parrinus & Mutius.

Trousseau, A. 1865. *Clinique médicale de l'Hôtel-Dieu de Paris,* 2d ed. 3 vols. Paris: Baillière & Fils.

————. 1868–72. *Lectures on clinical medicine.* Trans. Sir John R. Cormack and others. 5 vols. London: New Sydenham Society.

Trousseau, A., and Pidoux, H. 1855. *Traité de thérapeutique et de matière médicale,* 5th ed. Paris: Béchet jeune. Also 6th ed., 1858.

Tschirch, A. 1907–25. *Handbuch der Pharmacognosie,* 3 vols. in 6. Leipzig: Tauchnitz.

Turrión, M. L. de A. 1989. Quina del nuevo mundo para la corona española. *Asclepio* 41:305–24.

Underwood, E. A. 1946. Obituary of Alec W. Haggis. *Proceedings of the Linnean Society of London,* 157th session, 1944–45, pt. 3.

Valdizan, H. 1915. La corteza Peruana. *La Crónica Médica* [Lima] 32: 73–82, 102–12, 129–36, 189–97.

Valdizan, H., and Maldonado, A. 1922. *La medicina popular peruana (documentos ilustrativos).* Lima: Torres Aguirre.

Valega, J. 1939. *El virreinato del Perú.* Lima: Editorial Cultura Ecléctica.

Valentini, B. 1696. Discursus academicus de china chinae. *Miscellanea medico-physica sive ephemerides Germanicae* [Ephemerides naturae curiosorum] decuria 3, annus 3, appendix, 41–60. Nuremberg.

Valles Covarrubias, F. 1589. *In aphorismos Hippocratis commentarii VII praeterea ejusdem commentarii omnes.* Cologne: Ciotti.

Vallisneri, A. 1733. *Opere fisico-mediche.* Venice: Coleti.

van der Heyden, H. 1643. *Discours et advis sur les flux de ventre douloureux . . . Sur le trousse-galant; dict cholera morbus . . . les fièvres tierces et quatres . . .* Ghent: Manilius. Supplement, 1645.

Vargas Ugarte, R. 1928. Una fecha olvidada. El tercer centenario de descubrimento de la quina. 1631–1931. *Revista histórica* [Lima] 9:291–301.

———. 1963–65. *Historia de la Compañía de Jesús en el Perú.* 4 vols. Burgos.

Vernadsky, G. 1959, 1969. *A history of Russia,* vols. 4, 5. New Haven: Yale University Press.

Vogel, R. 1764. *Historia materiae medicae ad novissima tempora producta,* new ed. Frankfurt and Leipzig: Goebhard.

Wafer, L. [1699] 1903. *A new voyage and description of the isthmus of America.* [London.] Ed. G. P. Winship. Cleveland: Burrows.

Waring, E. 1878–79. *Bibliotheca therapeutica.* 2 vols. London: Sydenham Society.

Warren, M. 1729. *Ad amicum epistola, in qua curandi methodus et ratio in febribus nuper grassantibus; corticis peruviani periculum, incertitudo, et insalubritas breviter explicatur.* Cambridge: Typis academicis.

Waskin, H., Harpaz, R., and Navin, T. R. 1987. *Leishmaniasis in the United States, 1976–1985.* American Society of Tropical Medicine and Hygiene, 36th annual meeting, Los Angeles. Presentation no. 372.

Watkin, E. 1957. *Roman Catholicism in England, from the Reformation to 1950.* New York: Oxford University Press.

Weddell, H. A. 1849. *Histoire naturelle des quinquinas, ou monographie du genre Cinchona.* Paris: Masson.

Weisenberg, A. [1853] 1969. *Handwörterbuch der gesammtem Arzneimittel.* [Jena.] Facsimile, Hildesheim: Olms.

Weiss, C. 1844. *L'espagne depuis le règne de Philippe II jusqu'à des Bourbons.* Paris: Hachette.

Welch, W. H. [1897] 1920. Definition, synonyms, history and parasitology [of malaria]. In *A system of practical medicine,* ed. A. L. Loomis and W. G. Thompson. New York and Philadelphia: Lea. Reprinted in *Papers and addresses by William Henry Welch,* ed. W. C. Burket, 2:463–531. Baltimore: Johns Hopkins Press.

Werlhof, P. 1732, 1745. *Observationes de febribus praecipue intermittentibus.* Hannover: Foersteriani.

———. 1759. De limitanda febris laude et censura corticis Peruviani. In *Tractatus varii.* Venice: Basilius.

———. 1775–76. *Opera medica.* 3 vols. Hannover: Helwing.

Whittemore, N. 1713. *An almanack for the year of our Lord 1713.* Boston.

Wilkins, E. 1974. *A history of Italian literature*, rev. ed. Cambridge: Harvard University Press.

Willis, T. 1659. De febribus. In *Diatribae duae . . . prior agit de fermentatione . . . altera de febribus.* London: Roycroft.

———. 1660. *Diatribae duae*, 2d ed. London: Roycroft. Also 3d ed., The Hague: Vlacq, 1662.

———. 1670. De sanguinis incalescentia sive accensione. In *Affectionum, quae dicuntur hystericae et hypochondriacae.* London: Allestry. (Also in *Opera omnia*, vol. 1, see below.)

———. 1681a. *Opera omnia.* 2 vols. Lyons: Huguetan.

———. 1681b. *The remaining medical works.* Trans. S[amuel] P[ordage]. London: Dring.

Wolfart, P. 1695. *Discursus academicus de china chinae . . . sub praesidio Michaelis Bernhardi Valentini.* Giessen: Müller.

Wolff, J. 1907. *Die Lehre von der Krebskrankheit*, vol. 1. Jena: Fischer. (English trans. 1989 Barbara Ayoub, *The science of cancerous disease.* Canton, Mass.: Science History Publications.)

Wooton, A. C. [1910] 1971. *Chronicles of pharmacy.* [London: Macmillan.] Republished Boston: Milford House.

Wunderlich, C. 1857. Die Thermometrie bei Kranken. *Archiv für physiologische Heilkunde* 1:5–16.

———. 1868. *Das Verhalten der Eigenwärme in Krankheiten.* Leipzig: Wigand.

Wunderlich, C., and Seguin, E. 1871. *Medical thermometry and human temperature.* New York: Wood.

Yerushalmi, Y. 1971. *From Spanish court to Italian ghetto. Isaac Cardoso: A study in seventeenth-century marranism and Jewish apologetics.* New York: Columbia University Press.

Zacutus Lusitanus. 1667. *Operum.* 2 vols. Lyons: Huguetan & Barbier.

Zegarra, F. C. 1879. Doña Francisca Henriquez de Rivera. *Revista peruana* 1:383–84, 445–61.

Zendrini, B. 1715. *Trattato della chinachina, con una prefazione intorno à pregiudicj ch s' hanno per l'arte medicinale, e al modo più sicuro d'apprenderla.* Venice: Ertz [Hertz].

———. 1741. *Leggi e fenomeni, regolazioni ed usi delle acque correnti.* Venice: Pasquali.

Index